VULNERABLE OLDER ADULTS

Health Care Needs and Interventions

Patricia M. Burbank, DNSc, RN, is a professor in the College of Nursing at the University of Rhode Island and faculty member in the Rhode Island Geriatric Education Center. Currently, she directs the Gerontological Clinical Nurse Specialist concentration and is the project director of the Gerontological Nurse Practitioner program. Her clinical background has been in community health nursing and gerontology. She has authored three books related to older adults; one has been recently translated into Japanese. Research and publications have been in the areas of meaning in life among older adults, including collaborative cross-cultural research in Korea, and health behavior change in older adults. She is a consultant to Senior Action in a Gay Environment–Rhode Island (SAGE-RI), participating in assessment of needs and program planning with older lesbians, gay men, bisexuals, and transgenders in Rhode Island.

VULNERABLE OLDER ADULTS

ADULTS

Health Care Needs and Interventions

Patricia M. Burbank, DNSc, RN
Editor

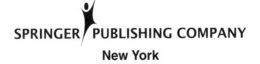

SPRINGER PUBLISHING COMPANY

New York

Springer Publishing Company, Inc.
11 West 42nd Street
New York, NY 10036

Acquisitions Editor: Sheri W. Sussman
Managing Editor: Mary Ann McLaughlin
Production Editor: Print Matters, Inc.
Cover design by Joanne E. Honigman
Typeset by Compset

06 07 08 09 10/ 5 4 3 2 1

Library of Congress Cataloging-in-Publication Data

Vulnerable older adults: health care needs and interventions / [edited by] Patricia M. Burbank.
    p.; cm.
  Includes bibliographical references and index.
  ISBN 0-8261-0208-5 (hc)
    1. Older people—Medical care. 2. Older people—Health and hygiene. 3. Aging. 4. Geriatric nursing. I. Burbank, Patricia M.
  [DNLM: 1. Health Services for the Aged. 2. Aged. 3. Geriatric Nursing—methods. 4. Vulnerable Populations. WT 31 V991 2006]
  RA564.8.V85 2006
  613'.0438—dc22

                                                                          2006042390

Printed in the United States of America by Bang Printing.

*Dedicated to Joanne,
Ben, Amanda, and Rick*

Contents

Part II: Aging Prisoners

Part IV: Lesbian, Gay, Bisexual, and Transgender Older Adults

Contributors

G. Burkholder, PhD
Assistant Dean for Student Success
School of Psychology
Walden University
Tucson, AZ

C. A. Emlet, PhD, ACSW
Associate Professor of Social Work
University of Washington, Tacoma
Tacoma, WA

P. Fournier, MA
LNHA Executive Director
Village at Waterman Lake
Greenville, RI

M. Gragert, PhD, RN
Associate Professor
University of North Dakota
   College of Nursing
Grand Forks, ND

C. Holtzer, MD
Director of Geriatric Education
Roger Williams Medical Center
Assistant Professor
Boston University School of
   Medicine
Clinical Assistant Professor
Boston University School of
   Medicine
Providence, RI

D. C. Martins, PhD, RN
Assistant Professor
Department of Community
   Nursing
College of Nursing
University of Massachusetts,
   Dartmouth
North Dartmouth, MA

**K. M. Nokes, PhD, RN, CS,
   FAAN**
Hunter-Bellevue School of
   Nursing
Hunter College
New York, NY

J. Ritzau, MD
Geriatrician
Roger Williams Medical Center
Clinical Assistant Professor
Boston University School of
   Medicine
Providence, RI

T. Smyer, DNSc, RN
Associate Professor
South Dakota State University
College of Nursing
Brookings, SD

J. Stoukides, MD, RPh
Director of Geriatric Service
Roger Williams Medical Center
Clinical Assistant Professor
Boston University School of
  Medicine
Providence, RI

M. A. Sullivan, MS, RN
Geropsychiatric Clinical Nurse
  Specialist
Elmhurst Extended Care
Providence, RI

Preface

As the population of older adults grows, high-risk groups within this population also become larger. The health care system, already struggling to meet the demands of the aging population in general, is often unable to meet the special needs of these vulnerable, high-risk groups. This book explores the concept of vulnerability and addresses five groups of vulnerable older adults: those who are frail; those incarcerated in prisons; homeless older adults; gay, lesbian, bisexual, and transgender elders; and those who are HIV positive or have AIDS. Each of these populations is described and their health care needs are discussed along with specific strategies to meet these needs. For each vulnerable population group, the current research and theoretical approaches are summarized to give health professionals a concise picture of health care needs and strategies for care of these older adults. Themes of an interdisciplinary team approach to care, cultural considerations, and neglect and abuse are integrated throughout. Lastly, strategies and resources to assist health professionals to care for each group of vulnerable older adults are included.

These categories of vulnerability may overlap, as it is possible that an older person may be in up to four of these five categories at the same time. An older prisoner may also be frail; have AIDS; and be gay, lesbian, bisexual, or transgender, for example. The broad scope of populations addressed in this book makes it applicable to all health professionals and organizations providing services to, and caring for, older adults. Regardless of setting, health care professionals and staff care for members of the lesbian, gay, bisexual, and transgender (LGBT) elder community, often without being aware that these orientations exist. Although most health professionals do not interact with elders who are in prisons or who have HIV/AIDS, these are growing populations who require further attention. Frail older adults are prominent in many health care settings and have complex care needs. In addition to use by health care professionals, administrators, and staff in facilities that care for older adults in each of these groups, students in a variety of disciplines, including medicine, nursing, social work, gerontology, community planning, health care administration, correctional health, and criminal justice, will find this book useful.

Many older adults in these five populations have been forgotten or "given-up on" by society. Their situations seem hopeless at times. This book provides recent research on the nature and complexity of their problems and offers strategies to rekindle hope for improvement in their conditions. Resources are described to assist in decreasing and sometimes even reversing their vulnerable status. Older prisoners can receive cost-effective quality health care; older adults who are homeless can find comfort in age-appropriate services; older LGBT adults can receive affirming quality health care; older people with HIV/AIDS can be diagnosed and treated earlier with improved quality of life; and the frail need not always be consigned to a downward spiral toward death.

P. Burbank

Foreword

Vulnerability is not a term that we hear often in discussions of health care for American older adults. Typically, the debate on geriatric care focuses on "disease management," geriatric syndromes (e.g., falls, incontinence), or on the locus of care, be it hospital care, home care, or care in nursing homes. Neither our educational system, which prepares health care practitioners, nor current streams for reimbursement for health care take into consideration classification of patients by their "susceptibility to harm." In this unique book, Patricia Burbank and her colleagues make a strong case for the need to focus, one might even say to refocus, our objectives on a subset of older adults whom they identify as vulnerable, specifically those older adults in prisons; those who are homeless; gay, lesbian, bisexual, or transgender; those who are HIV positive or have AIDS; and those who are frail. The authors make a compelling argument about the commonalities of needs for health care among these groups of older adults, who they identify by their increased risk for adverse health outcomes.

Nurses and physicians involved in education, and health care practitioners delivering care to groups of vulnerable older adults will find *Vulnerable Older Adults: Health Care Needs and Interventions* an invaluable resource. The authors begin the text with a focus on general strategies to care for what they identify as frail and complex patient groups. Clearly the care for vulnerable older adults cries out for an interprofessional approach to care, and the text places a strong emphasis on interdisciplinary practice. Equally important, the authors' approach is to emphasize both the weaknesses and the strengths inherent in vulnerable populations, helping educators and practitioners identify and build on strengths as they teach novice practitioners, and attempt to create systems of care responsive to the needs of the vulnerable older adults.

It has been said that one measure of a society is the care it provides to its most vulnerable members. By taking on this challenge, Burbank and her colleagues have opened the door to addressing the needs of the most vulnerable among our older population.

Mathy Mezey, RN, EdD, FAAN

Introduction

People in the United States are living longer, and older adults are healthier than ever before in history. The current population of Americans over the age of 65 years is 36 million (12% of the population). It is predicted that the population will grow to 71.5 million by the year 2030 (20% of the U.S. population). Women who survive to the age of 85 years can expect to live for 7 more years (92 years of age) and males 6 more years (91 years of age) (Federal Interagency Forum on Aging-Related Statistics, 2004). Unfortunately, this improvement in health status and longevity is not enjoyed by all members of the older population. Some subgroups of older adults age more quickly, have higher mortality rates, and more health problems than other groups. These are our most vulnerable older adults, many of whom are forgotten or rejected by society. These vulnerable elders are those who are marginalized, have few financial resources, have reduced access to quality health care, or have few physiological and psychosocial reserves. Five groups of especially vulnerable older adults are addressed in this book: those who are frail; incarcerated; homeless; lesbian, gay, bisexual, or transgender (LGBT); and those who are HIV positive or have AIDS.

THE CONCEPT OF VULNERABILITY

The concept of vulnerability in the health literature has been applied in different ways to describe a variety of populations. The most common use of the word is in referring to those who are "susceptible to harm" (Leffers et al., 2004). For this book, vulnerability is defined as an increased risk of adverse physical, psychological, or social health outcomes, similar to Aday's (2001) definition.

The concept of vulnerability can be thought of as having two aspects: an individual focus and an aggregate focus (deChesnay, 2005). As a state of increased risk, vulnerability is fluid and may change rapidly at the individual level, although it is more stable at the population level. Individuals can move in and out of a state of vulnerability although at the aggregate level populations are designated as vulnerable based on characteristics that are often inherent in the nature of the population. "To be a member of a vulnerable population does not necessarily mean that one is vulnerable" (deChesnay, 2005, p. 3). Some members of vulnerable population groups may be at high risk in some contexts or settings and not in others. Vulnerable populations, then, are those groups of people at greater-than-average risk of developing adverse health outcomes because of their marginalized sociopolitical status; their limited access to resources, especially economic; and/or their demographic characteristics such as age and gender (Aday, 2001; deChesnay, 2005; Sebastian, 1996).

The health disparities that exist among different groups of people contribute to increased vulnerability. *Healthy People 2010* (U.S. Department of Health and Healing Services, 2000), the primary document that outlines the principle areas of focus for the decade, has a goal of eliminating health disparities. They identify disparities of focus as gender, race and ethnicity, income and education, disability, geographic location, and sexual orientation. These disparities are discussed throughout each of the chapters. The objectives in the volume are organized into 28 focus areas. Five of these focus areas: access to quality health services, HIV, injury and violence prevention, physical activity and fitness, and substance abuse are also addressed directly in chapters throughout this book. Nine other focus areas include chronic illnesses or conditions common among older adults. By addressing these priorities, the vulnerability of older adults in these five population groups can be reduced.

The five vulnerable populations addressed in this book are not mutually exclusive. Several of them may overlap, as individuals may be members of more than one vulnerable group. This situation increases and complicates the person's risk for adverse health outcomes.

ISSUES OF VULNERABLE POPULATIONS

Oppression and marginalization are known to be issues for all but one of the groups of elders (frail elders) addressed here. Older adults in prisons are stigmatized, taken advantage of, and are sometimes victims of violence because of their weakness. Homeless people of all ages are marginalized and viewed as undesirable figures in society at large as well as in the health care system. Discrimination against lesbian, gay, bisexual, and transgender people (LGBT) is well documented. People with HIV/AIDS are also stigmatized and sometimes shunned despite sound knowledge about communicability of the virus. Lastly, the prejudice of ageism itself is alive and well in American society and applies to all groups discussed in this book. Status and power are generally lost as one travels through the older adult years. Frail older adults are not generally thought of as being oppressed; however, they have the double status of being old and ill. Thus they have lost status and power, and are further limited by their condition.

Race and ethnicity are important considerations in each of these vulnerable populations, with the prison population having the greatest percentage of minority elders. Adding membership in a minority racial or ethnic group to any of these five populations of older adults increases their risk and vulnerability to adverse health outcomes. Minority populations of older adults in the United States are expected to increase dramatically over the next 50 years with percentages of Blacks increasing by 50%, the Asian population doubling, and percentage of Hispanics tripling. Currently, the non-Hispanic White population accounts for 83% of the population aged 65 and over, Blacks 8%, Asians 3%, and Hispanics 6%. By 2050 the rates are projected to be 61% non-Hispanic White, 12% Black, 8% Asian, and 18% Hispanic (Federal Interagency Forum on Aging-Related Statistics, 2004). Cultural issues are addressed in each chapter as they pertain to each group of vulnerable elders.

GENERAL STRATEGIES

Because of the complex issues in care of older adults and the focused scope of practice of health professionals, an interdisciplinary approach to care has been recognized as the most effective way of meeting these challenges (Burbank et al., 2002). Calls for increased interdisciplinary collaboration are being made with growing frequency by a number of national organizations (Clark, 2002). The health care needs of these five groups of vulnerable older adults are especially complex and often involve multiple systems of health care, making interdisciplinary collaboration even more essential. An interdisciplinary team approach to care is discussed in the chapters addressing strategies for each population group.

Although the focus in the chapters describing health issues is on identifying problems and needs of older adults in these population groups, it is recognized that all individuals in each of these groups have strengths as well as needs. Some might argue that "vulnerable population" is just another label used to promote a system of health care that the consumers of care may consider "patronizing" (deChesnay, 2005). A strengths-based approach to care, while acknowledging vulnerability and needs, also assesses strengths and builds on these to create more effective strategies. For example, among frail older adults, the expectation and acceptance of frailty and weakness is a hindrance to beginning exercise. Focusing on identifying strengths is essential if the decline of frailty is to be slowed or halted. The strengths of older adults in each of these populations are assets that can be mobilized to improve their health and quality of care.

CHAPTER OVERVIEW

The subgroups of older adults addressed in this book (frail, prisoners, homeless, LGBT elders, and those with HIV/AIDS) are not parallel. Frailty is a condition that can affect anyone along with other disease processes. HIV/AIDs is an infectious disease afflicting older people. Older adults in prisons and those who are homeless are similar in that they both are characterized by environments or settings. Lastly, LGBT older adults are linked by characteristics that define their nature as human beings and set them apart as a marginalized group within society. What all of these groups do have in common is their vulnerable status and their need for strategies to improve their health outcomes.

There are two chapters for each of the five population groups; the first reviews issues and needs of the elders in the group, and the second describes strategies designed to meet these needs. Although all of the chapters are based on reviews of the research literature, research is sorely lacking for most of the groups of older adults. This should be taken as a call for research into these important areas.

The first chapter is on issues and problems of frail older adults, authored by John Stoukides, Cynthia Holzer, Jennifer Ritzau, and Patricia Burbank. The first three authors are all geriatricians with clinical practices, academic appointments, and extensive backgrounds with frail older adults. They discuss definitions of frailty and review new theories related to its causes and antecedent conditions. The major features of frailty and concomitant clinical problems are also described. Consequences or outcomes of frailty are discussed, presenting a clinical picture of the syndrome.

The same authors, along with Patricia Burbank, a gerontological clinical nurse specialist, educator, and researcher, write the second chapter on strategies for care of frail older adults. The chapter begins with an overview of comprehensive geriatric assessment, including an interdisciplinary team approach. Frailty assessment tools are also discussed. Then two types of interventions are reviewed: those that address issues common to frailty such as falls, polypharmacy, depression, delirium, dementia, and caregiver issues; and those that are associated with health in general such as exercise and nutrition. Although frailty is generally viewed as a downward spiral, research is presented here to indicate that it is possible to forestall the decline of frailty and may, in some cases, be possible to reverse the downward trajectory.

The third chapter is on health care issues and needs of older adults who are prisoners, authored by Tish Smyer and Marcia Gragert, nurse educators with clinical and research experience with the prison population. Because of the harsh lifestyle and physiological changes associated with people who are incarcerated, they are considered to be "older adults" at age 50. This chapter presents demographics and background information of this growing population, including information on the disproportionate numbers of minorities in the prison system. Subcultures within the prison are described and the physical and mental health needs of aging prisoners are discussed.

Chapter 4, also by Tish Smyer, Marcia Gragert, and Diane C. Martins, a nurse educator with clinical experience working with prison populations, describes the accompanying strategies and resources for older adults who are prisoners. Health care of prisoners is mandated by law, making correctional health care a balancing act between ethical delivery of care and limited financial resources. This chapter describes the general health care within correctional facilities along with issues of primary prevention, specialty units, long-term care, and hospice programs. Current programs, such as early release to meet the special needs of older prisoners, are also discussed along with suggestions for improvement of care.

Issues of older adults who are homeless are addressed in chapter 5 by Diane C. Martins, whose research and clinical experience focus on homeless people and Mary A. Sullivan, a geropsychiatric clinical nurse specialist with extensive experience with homeless elders. For this group as well, age 50 is considered "elderly." The numbers of seniors among the homeless population are small but growing with the decline of availability of affordable housing and increasing poverty among certain segments of older adults. These authors define homelessness and discuss its prevalence and risk factors. Common physical and mental health issues are described with a call for more attention to the needs of this very vulnerable population.

In the accompanying chapter, chapter 6, also by Diane C. Martins and Mary A. Sullivan, interventions and resources for homeless older adults are explored. Using a critical perspective, they report that there is a lack of services that address the needs of this client group and a general reluctance on the part of health care professionals to care for older homeless people. Stategies at three levels are described to meet the immediate health needs of the individual homeless person, to empower the homeless to use their resourcefulness, and to provide interventions to eradicate homelessness. An interdisciplinary approach is discussed as essential.

Chapter 7 is on health care issues and needs of lesbian, gay, bisexual, and transgender (LGBT) older adults written by Patricia Burbank, who has consultation and research experience with this population, and Gary Burkholder, an experimental psychologist and educator with teaching and research expertise with this group. The dearth of literature on this topic limits the level of description; however, the authors provide definitions of key terms and describe demographics of this population. Physical, psychosocial, and spiritual health issues are addressed for gay men, lesbians, bisexuals, and transgender older adults. Stigma and bias against the LGBT population are also discussed, as they are at the core of reduced access and quality of health care to this group of elders.

Specific strategies for improving the health of the LGBT older population are covered in chapter 8, by the same authors with Peter Fournier, a social worker, rehabilitation counselor, and administrator of a life care community and nursing home. Communication techniques, assessment guidelines, and standards for practice with the LGBT population are discussed. Education about LGBT issues and self-awareness of attitudes are also included to assist health care providers to become culturally competent in caring for this population group. Organizational changes for improving care along with policy and legal issues are suggested. Lastly, this chapter outlines current activities to ensure access to LGBT-affirming health care.

Chapter 9, by Charles A. Emlet, a social worker and researcher on HIV/AIDS in older adults, and Kathy Nokes, a nurse educator with extensive clinical and research experience in care of people with HIV/AIDS, addresses health issues of older adults with HIV or AIDS. A discussion of the various aspects of diversity among this population, including the disproportionate number of cases of AIDS and HIV among persons of color, is also included. Health–related issues, such as age-related changes, transmission risks, diagnostic issues, symptom management, and psychosocial factors, are also described.

The last chapter, chapter 10, also by Kathy Nokes and Charles A. Emlet, addresses strategies and interventions for those older adults with HIV/AIDS. This chapter includes strategies targeting both the individual level and the larger system level. Specific interventions for caring for the needs of older adults with HIV/AIDS are discussed, as well as strategies for prevention and education. Five different sectors offering care to this population are also described with a call for increased interdisciplinary, coordinated care across sectors.

Through the perspectives of these authors, insights can be gained into the needs of these five different vulnerable populations of older adults. Armed with knowledge about their needs, readers are encouraged to apply the strategies suggested here or to design their own to improve quality of health care and ultimately the health of these important groups of elders.

P. Burbank

REFERENCES

Aday, L. (2001). *At risk in America*. San Francisco: Jossey-Bass.

Burbank, P. M., Owens, N. J., Stoukides, J., Evans, E. B., Leinhaas, M. M., & Evans, J. M. (2002). Developing an interdisciplinary geriatric curriculum: The perils and payoffs of collaboration. *Educational Gerontology, 28*, 451–472.

Clark, P. (2002). Introduction to the special issue of educational gerontology: Interdisciplinary geriatric education in the health care professions. *Educational Gerontology, 28*, 427–432.

deChesnay, M. (2005). Vulnerable populations: Vulnerable people. In M. deChesnay, *Caring for the vulnerable*. Boston: Jones and Bartlett.

Federal Interagency Forum on Aging-Related Statistics. (2004). *Older Americans 2000: Key indicators of well-being*. Federal Interagency Forum on Aging-Related Statistics. Washington, DC: U.S. Government Printing Office.

Leffers, J. M., Martins, D. C., McGrath, M. M., Brown, D. G., Mercer, J., Sullivan, M. C., et al. (2004). Development of a theoretical construct for risk and vulnerability from six empirical studies. *Research and Theory for Nursing Practice: An International Journal, 18*(1), 15–34.

Sebastian, J. (1996). Vulnerability and vulnerable populations. In M. Stanhope & J. Lancaster (Eds.). *Community health nursing: Promoting Health of individuals, aggregates, and communities* (4th ed.), St. Louis: Mosby.

U.S. Department of Health and Human Services (2000). *Healthy People 2010: Understanding and Improving Health* (2nd ed). Washington, D.C.: U.S. Government Printing Office.

PART I

Frail Older Adults

CHAPTER ONE

Health Issues of Frail Older Adults

J. Stoukides, C. Holzer, J. Ritzau, and P. Burbank

Frailty decreases quality of life for older adults, impacts families and caregivers, and stretches the capabilities of health care systems and financing. In general, the condition of frailty among older adults is associated with increased vulnerability to adverse outcomes, including being at high risk for dependency, institutionalization, falls, injuries, acute illness, hospitalization, slow recovery from illness, and mortality (Fried, Ferrucci, Darer, Williamson, & Anderson, 2004). Although limitations in defining frailty make it difficult to determine its prevalence, it is clear that the incidence of frailty increases with advancing age. One study using stringent exclusion criteria reported the prevalence of frailty to be 7% of the population over age 65 and 20% of those over age 80 (Fried et al., 2001). A study of Medicare claims data found that 47% of older adults were frail prior to their deaths (Lunney, Lynn, & Hogan, 2002). In another study, a cohort analysis of data from the Epidemiological Studies of the Elderly study showed that 20% of those who had died had a frail trajectory before their deaths (Lunney, Lynn, Foley, Lipson, & Guralnik, 2003).

Frail older adults, although a minority within their own age group, disproportionately represent the majority of consumers within the health care system. They visit primary care providers more often, consume 50% of all hospital care, receive over 80% of home care services, and occupy 90% of all nursing home beds in the United States (Mezey &

Fulmer, 1998). Recognizing the magnitude of the problems associated with frailty, the National Institute of Aging (NIA) identified the reduction of frailty as a top priority for research in 2003 (NIA, 2003).

Currently there are more than 4.2 million older adults (1.5% of the total population) aged 85 or older, the age group at highest risk for frailty. It is estimated that by the year 2050, over 19.3 million adults will be 85 or older, comprising 5% of the total population and 20% of those aged 65 and older (U.S. Census Bureau, 2004). If 20% of this population becomes frail, an already overburdened health care system will need to provide care for 3.9 million frail older adults.

This chapter begins with a description of the syndrome of frailty including its theoretical and operational definitions, a discussion of the etiology and antecedents of frailty, and the major features and concomitant clinical problems associated with the syndrome. In addition, consequences or outcomes are also presented resulting in a clinical picture of common issues and problems associated with frailty and increased vulnerability for this group of older adults. The following chapter will present strategies for health care providers geared at preventing frailty and treating frail older adults. The ultimate goals in understanding frailty are to provide information to health care providers to assist them in improving the quality of life for those who are frail and their caregivers, to slow the progression of frailty, and to prevent the onset of frailty in at-risk older adults.

DEFINING FRAILTY

The concept of frailty among older adults has had an interesting development over the past 35 years. The idea of frailty first emerged in the 1970s and gained popularity because it was a useful term to describe a condition that clinicians easily recognized, however, it was difficult to define (Hogan, MacKnight, Bergman, & Steering Committee, Canadian Initiative on Frailty and Aging, 2003). Through the years, the concept of frailty has continued to lack clarity of definition and has been characterized in a variety of ways. Recently, efforts were made to more carefully define the concept theoretically and to operationalize it through measures that would be useful for clinical assessments and/or research studies. Currently, efforts have been directed at conceptualizing frailty as having biological and physiological bases and searching for antecedents and biological markers that may be early indicators of the syndrome (National Institute on Aging, 2003; Wilson, 2004). The ultimate aim of research efforts is to identify older adults at risk of becoming frail and develop therapeutic measures to prevent frailty or to forestall functional decline as long as possible.

In their review of definitions of frailty, Hogan et al. (2003) described definitions as focusing on dependency, vulnerability, or disease states. Different definitions of frailty have emphasized a variety of characteristics. When the main features of these definitions are considered together, they depict a more comprehensive picture of the syndrome of frailty. These main features from several definitions are:

- Increased vulnerability for adverse outcomes, such as disease, disability, and death; highest risk of functional decline (Buchner & Wagner, 1992; Ferrucci et al., 2003; Fried et al., 2004; Rockwood, Hogan, & MacKnight, 2000)
- Instability, "unstable disability" (Rockwood et al., 2000; Schuurmans, Steverink, Lindenberg, Frieswijk, & Slaets, 2004)
- Involves multisystem dysfunction (Buchner & Wagner, 1992; Fried et al., 2001, 2004)
- Heterogeneity (Rockwood et al., 2000)
- Associated with chronological aging (Rockwood et al., 2000)
- Decline in reserves; loss of adaptive capacity; decline in ability to maintain homeostasis; decreased resistance to stressors; increased vulnerability to challenges from environment (Campbell & Buchner, 1997; Carlson et al., 1998; Ferrucci et al., 2002, 2003; Fretwell, 1990; Fried et al., 2001, 2004; Hamerman, 1999)
- Atypical disease presentation (Jarrett, Rockwood, Carver, Stolee, & Cosway, 1995)
- Dependence on others for daily activities (ADLs), often institutionalized (Tennstedt & McKinley, 1994; Woodhouse & O'Mahoney, 1997)

Although these features are not drawn from an inclusive list of definitions, they cover the range of characteristics of frailty included in the various definitions and present a picture of the syndrome of frailty.

A hallmark of frailty is loss of adaptive capacity resulting in functional decline (Wilson, 2004) and increased vulnerability to adverse outcomes. According to Fried et al. (2004), there is currently general agreement that frailty is a physiological state of increased vulnerability to stressors that results from decreased reserves and dysregulation in multiple physiological systems. This causes difficulty in maintaining homeostasis when confronted with stressors. Interindividual variation among older patients prevents us from using any single marker, such as age, diagnosis, or functional disability to predict frailty (Costa & McCrae, 1985). Maintaining and regaining homeostasis is essential for warding off the vicious cycle of frailty (Wilson, 2004).

Recent research has focused on uncovering the biology of frailty to determine underlying factors that contribute to the onset of frailty. Frailty has been linked to chronic inflammatory states marked by elevations in serum interleukin-6 levels and reduced hemoglobin and hematocrit (Leng, Chaves, Koenig, & Walston, 2002). Research has also found associations between frailty and lower levels of hormones, such as insulin-like growth hormone I (IGF-I) and dehydroepiandrosterone (DHEA-S), both of which have also been linked to immune function (Leng et al., 2004). Although these studies have shown relationships between these immune markers, hormones, and frailty, no causal relationships have yet been established (Walston, 2004). On a cellular level, hypothetical causes of frailty include increases in free radical production and resulting DNA damage, telomere shortening, changes in gene expression, and cellular senescence (Wilson, 2004).

In another approach, research on the dynamics of physiological systems and using complexity theory has suggested that the aging process as well as disease processes result in a loss of complexity in fractal-like anatomical structures and physiological processes (Lipsitz, 2004; Lipsitz & Goldberger, 1992). A physiological reserve enables healthy individuals to compensate for age-related changes and losses from diseases; however, with a loss of complexity, adaptive capacity declines. When functional levels fall below a "frailty threshold," the older person can no longer adapt to stressors and becomes frail (Lipsitz, 2004).

It has been estimated that across most organ systems, 30% of normal function represents a threshold for adequate function. A 70% loss can occur before there is evidence of system failure. This has been translated to functional decline, indicating that 30% of baseline may be the frailty threshold (Bortz, 2002) as shown in Figure 1.1.

Wilson (2004) points out that physicians know frailty when they see it; however, efforts have been made to operationalize frailty and measure it for both clinical and research purposes. Fried et al.'s (2001) work on describing the frailty phenotype has resulted in an operational definition that incorporates the clinical indicators and outcomes of many of the features in the definitions of frailty. This definition seems to have gained empirical support and is becoming more widely accepted and utilized (NIA program announcement, 2003).

Frailty has been conceptualized as a cycle by Fried and Walston (1999) and Walston (2004). Walston's (2004) frailty cycle is an effort to identify key components of frailty that comprise the syndrome, predisposing or risk factors contributing to it, and functional outcomes (see Figure 1.2). Fried et al.'s (2001) five attributes of frailty (weight loss, muscle weakness, slow walking speed, exhaustion, and low physical activity) are incorporated into the model. This model emphasizes the

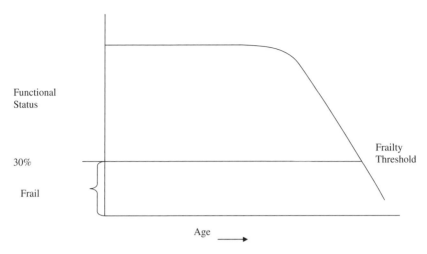

FIGURE 1.1   Frailty threshold.
Adapted from Fried and Walston (1999).

cyclical nature of frailty and shows how declines in a particular area or more than one area can initiate or perpetuate the cycle of general functional decline.

Sarcopenia, or the loss of muscle mass and function associated with aging, is believed to be a major contributor to frailty (Morley, Baumgartner, Roubenoff, Mayer, & Nair, 2001). Although the mechanisms causing sarcopenia are not yet clearly understood, the most important causal factors may be loss of motor neurons in the central nervous system (Roubenoff, 2003). Studies have shown that up to half of motor neuron units are lost in healthy adults in their 60s (Doherty, Vandervoort, & Brown, 1993). Other causes of sarcopenia are thought to include decreases in growth hormone, and estrogen/androgen secretion, decline in physical activity, increase in fat mass, increase in Interleukin-6 and decreased protein intake (Roubenoff, 2003). Sarcopenia occurs with normal aging, however, if allowed to progress unchecked it can lead to weakness, falls, disability, dependence, and frailty (Roubenoff & Hughes, 2000). Because of this, sarcopenia is a significant problem for older adults as well as the health care system, representing an estimated 1.5% of total health care expenditures (or $18.5 billion) for the year 2000 (Janssen, Shepard, Katzmarzyk, & Roubenoff, 2004).

Trigger events, such as acute illness, injury, or an adverse life event, can occur anywhere in the frailty cycle and cause further progression toward frailty. Chronic or acute stress, depression, low activity levels,

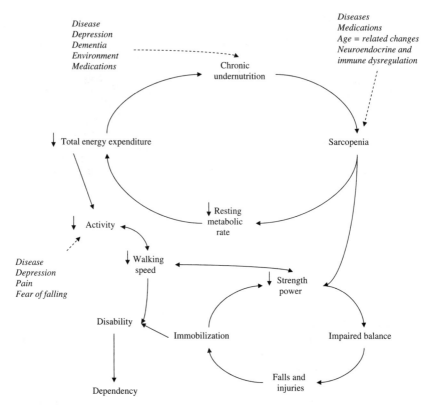

FIGURE 1.2 The cycle of frailty. The major components of the model are in text type, whereas factors that could precipitate or exacerbate these components are italicized and connected with dotted lines. Adapted from Fried et al. (2001).

or decreased protein and micronutrient intake can also act as triggers and accelerate frailty (Fried & Walston, 1999). Additional predictors of frailty include heavy drinking, prevalence of chronic conditions, fair–poor self-rated health, smoking, and social isolation (Strawbridge, Shema, Balfour, Higby, & Kaplan, 1998). It is easy to see how these factors may also initiate or perpetuate the cycle of frailty.

Frail older adults are generally the most in need of health care, including acute care, formal and informal support services, and long-term care. Consequences of frailty are increased morbidity and mortality, including a higher incidence of falls, depression, dementia, delirium, incontinence, functional impairment, and disability. Polypharmacy, or taking multiple medications, is also often problematic for frail elders with less adaptive capacity in organ systems and smaller therapeutic windows for medications. Frail older adults require a high level of care from either family caregivers or health care resources. Quality of caregiving becomes paramount and issues of abuse and neglect may surface. In the remaining part of the chapter, these health issues that frequently accompany frailty will be reviewed. Strategies for intervening with these problems as well as with frailty as a syndrome will be discussed in the following chapter.

COMORBIDITIES OF FRAILTY

Aging is a continuous process that begins in early adulthood. This process gradually leads to noticeable changes in many body systems. As early as the age of 40, the most visible signs of aging begin as changes in the skin and hair. By the decades of the 60s, 70s, and 80s, aging becomes a complex process involving physical, psychological, and social losses. The complexity of the biopsychosocial factors involved in the aging process makes it difficult to predict which older adults will age "normally" versus those who will become frail (Sloane, 2002). In addition, people become more unique as they age, so each individual situation must be carefully assessed (Ham, 2002).

The medical system is built around assumptions that are often incorrect for older patients. It is incorrectly assumed that patients have to present themselves to a physician to declare that they have a symptom or that something is wrong rather than taking a proactive, preventive approach to care. Many individuals, however, have denial, ignorance, fear, and negativity about aging. This can lead some older persons to tolerate problems they would not have tolerated when they were younger and avoid reporting these changes to their physicians (Ham, 2002). Because of this, an older person may have significant issues predisposing them to frailty before reporting any problems to their health care providers.

Once ill, some frail older patients may experience a "cascade," a word describing a process of functional decline. Often, despite effective treatment of an acute medical illness, frail older adults may decline in functional abilities, developing problems associated with confusion, immobility, incontinence, and malnutrition (Fretwell, 1990). For example, if a frail patient is hospitalized, the medical treatment and hospitalization itself will affect their outcome. Medications can interact with the patient's anxiety at having been relocated to a strange, new environment and can set off a complex series of events leading to an acute loss of mental and physical function (Fretwell, 1990). Moreover, additional medical and nursing interventions such as Foley catheters,

physical restraints, feeding tubes, broad-spectrum antibiotics, antico-
agulants, and antipsychotic drugs add to the number of medications
and to the potential for clinical and functional iatrogenesis. In this
situation, an older person, perhaps with a mild cognitive deficit, can
become confused, immobile, and incontinent within a few days of admission. As this process continues, it becomes increasingly difficult to
determine cause and effect and to intervene properly (Fretwell, 1990).
Frail older adults living independently in the community also experience a fragile health and social situation. Simple health problems, in
otherwise stable situations, can send the older adult and their families
into a spiraling downward slope, where existing structures fall apart
and new support systems must be instituted (Guttman, 1999). In this
section, specific problem areas associated with frailty will be discussed,
understanding that these may sometimes be either consequences or
antecedents of frailty as it progresses cyclically.

FALLS

Falls and fall-related injuries are common in the geriatric population
and can be associated with significant morbidity and mortality. Falls
have been defined as an unintentional change in position that would not
occur in an otherwise fit individual (Schneider & Mader, 2002). The incidence of falls increases steadily after middle age and is highest among
those who are 80 years of age or older (Rubenstein & Josephson, 2002).
Longitudinal studies have found that 30–60% of community-dwelling
older adults fall each year with approximately half of them experiencing
multiple falls (Hayes, 1994).

The incidence of falls among institutionalized older adults is approximately three times higher than among community-dwelling older
populations (Buckwalter, Katz, & Martin, 2004a). Among nursing home
populations, it is estimated that between 16 and 75% (overall mean = 43%)
of residents fall each year (Rubenstein & Josephson, 2002). Falls are
the leading cause of injury-related deaths among individuals older than
65 years. Approximately 1,800 residents of nursing facilities die each year
as a result of a fall (Hayes, 1994) and more than 20% of falls in nursing
home residents who are more than 85 years of age are fatal (Baker &
Harvey, 1985).

Hip fractures are the most common serious injury resulting from a
fall with a disproportionately higher incidence of hip fractures among
nursing home residents compared to community-dwelling elderly. Other
serious injuries associated with falling include lacerations, head trauma,
and soft tissue injuries. A fall can also lead to diminished quality of life,

including functional decline, reduced activity, social isolation, depression, and a feeling of helplessness (Buckwalter et al., 2004a).

A previous fall is the best predictor of future falls. Common risk factors associated with falls include acute medical illness or infection, advanced age, delirium, dizziness or feelings of faintness, fear of falling, female gender, functional dependence, history of previous falls, impaired mental status, impaired mobility, impaired musculoskeletal function, incontinence, polypharmacy, recent change in medications, and sensory loss (Buckwalter et al., 2004a; Tideiksaar, 1997). All of these risk factors are more prevalent among older adults who are frail.

Environmental factors may also contribute to an increased risk of falling. Some environmental factors that have been implicated are low or elevated bed heights, bed rails, low toilet seats, poorly illuminated areas, upended carpet or rug edges, uneven sidewalks or curb edges, highly polished or wet floors, icy walkways, use of ambulatory assistive devices, and mechanical restraints (Schneider & Mader, 2002).

Illnesses or diseases that increase the risk of falling are those that cause muscle weakness, pain, gait abnormalities, balance disturbances, foot problems, mental confusion, visual disturbances, dizziness, or postural hypotension. Any medical condition, acute or chronic, that causes general fatigue, malaise, and weakness increases a person's risk of falling. Studies have consistently found that polypharmacy increases a patient's risk of falling. Several classes of drugs have been implicated in connection with falls, including diuretics, narcotics, sedative hypnotics, antidepressants, antipsychotics, antihypertensive agents, cardiac medications, anticholinergic drugs, hypoglycemic agents, antiparkinsonian medications, and topical eye medications (Buckwalter, Katz, & Martin, 2004b).

Once an older person experiences a fall the syndrome of "fear of falling" may ensue. This syndrome threatens the physical and mental well-being of older persons. Fear of falling is associated with functional impairments and perhaps depression. Moreover, fear may lead to self-imposed restriction of daily activities and thereby cause excessive immobilization or reduction of social contacts. This inactivity may lead to a decline in physical capabilities and reduce overall fitness and trigger the onset of frailty (Bloem, Steijns, & Sits-Engelsman, 2003).

ADVERSE EFFECTS OF POLYPHARMACY

The effect of multiple medications on the frail older adult is frequently a topic of debate. There is little evidence to support the occurrence of adverse effects based solely on the number of medications prescribed for an older individual (Hanlon et al., 2004). Specific agents, however, may be associated with a marked decline in various functional domains in the older person. There are three domains of function in the older adult commonly affected by pharmacotherapy. They are: cognitive ability, depression and mood disorders, and changes or decline in physical function. It is clear that certain classes of drugs, most notably the sedative hypnotics, other psychoactive drugs, and drugs with anticholinergic side effects, have a detrimental effect on a patient's cognitive ability. All drug classes, however, should be taken into consideration when cognitive function has changed from a patient's baseline status. This need is accentuated in the frail older adults who often lack the cognitive reserve to handle the deleterious effects of medications, especially those commonly accepted as free of side effects in the less frail older person (Higashi et al., 2004).

The second area, depression and mood disorders, is also commonly thought to be linked to a patient's medication regimen. A small number of drugs have been reported in the literature as being associated with causing depressive syndromes; however, none have been identified as a primary cause of major depressive syndrome. As with cognitive effects of medication, virtually any medication can potentially be linked to the onset of depression, anxiety, or thought disorder. Drug classes most commonly linked to depression include antihypertensive, sedative hypnotic, and corticosteroids (Patten & Barbury, 2004).

Physical functional decline is the third domain of geriatric function commonly affected by pharmacotherapy. The potential for detrimental effects are more varied and difficult to assess, as physical function is dependent on a combination of organ systems being compromised. For example, frail older adults at baseline are prone to falls. A wide range of pharmacologic agents can impact a frail elder's ability to ambulate by affecting their muscle strength, cognitive ability, cardiovascular stability, or their sensory capacity. It is easy to see how the addition of a seemingly innocuous medication, such as an antihypertensive or a sleep aid can have wide-ranging effects on a frail elder's ambulation, which at baseline is already reduced.

Another key issue in the pharmacotherapy of frail older adults is compliance with a prescribed medication regimen. The issues relating to compliance are wide ranging and involve both under- and overutilization of the prescribed medications. Underutilization is the most commonly recognized area of noncompliance in elderly populations. It is crucial to understand the factors leading to failure to take medications as prescribed in order to establish a safe and effective treatment program. Reasons for underutilization can include the obvious issues of side effects, or overly complex dosing schedules. The less obvious reasons are also important to consider and involve the cost of therapy, ability of the patient to open the prescription vial, the person's ability to appropriately administer the dosage, and the patient's ability to remember that it is time for a given medication.

Overutilization of a prescribed medication is also an important area of noncompliance that must be considered. Excessive dosing can be attributed to a variety of causes, including perceived ineffectiveness of a medication, lack of understanding of the action of a particular medication, or confusion over which medication is used for which problem. Health care providers who fail to consider the general need for lower dosages in older adults may also contribute to excessive dosing through inappropriate prescribing. Cognitive issues also play a major role in both under- and overutilization. Multiple or missed doses may be due to a patient's desire to be compliant with their medication regimen; however, changes in cognitive function prevents them from remembering that the drug was recently taken.

DEPRESSION

Major depression and related disorders affect between 5 and 20% of persons over age 65, living in the community (Lammers, 2002). True clinical depression is not a part of the normal aging process but is associated with functional decline and increased mortality. Depression is even more common in acutely ill, hospitalized elderly patients with a prevalence of 36–46% (Raj, 2004). Nursing home residents also have a very high prevalence of 25–40% (Parmelee, Katz, & Lawton, 1992). The most serious consequence of depression is suicide. In 2000, persons aged 65 years and older composed 13% of the US population but accounted for 18% of all suicides (National Center for Injury Prevention and Control, 2004). White men aged 85 and older had the highest rates of all age groups with 59 deaths per 100,000 people, more than five times the national rate of 10.6 per 100,000 (Office of Statistics and Programming, NCIPC, CDC, 2004). Suicide risk factors among older adults include male sex, White race, medical comorbidity, substance abuse, and lack of support systems.

Major depression and other less specific depressive symptoms are associated with many medical illnesses, including stroke, thyroid disorders, Parkinson's disease, heart disease, and dementia. Approximately 60% of stroke patients and 45% of patients who have had a myocardial infarction suffer with either major or minor depression (Raj, 2004). Additionally, certain medications used to treat medical illnesses including cardiac medications; antihypertensives, psychotropic agents, analgesics, steroids, and alcohol are associated with causing depressive symptoms.

DEMENTIA

A major contributing factor to frailty is the presence of an underlying cognitive impairment. Dementia is defined as an impairment of memory with loss of other cognitive abilities or change in personality sufficiently severe to interfere with previously achieved levels of daily function (American Psychiatric Association, 2000). It is important to note, however, that the term dementia, commonly used as a diagnosis by medical professionals and by the lay public, is only descriptive, referring to the clinical state of the patient. More specific terminology must be utilized in order to accurately describe the cause of the underlying illness. It is equally important to avoid older obsolete terminology that has continued to linger in the description of an individual's clinical state (Dugu, Neugroschl, Sewell, & Marin, 2003). Terms such as senility, hardening of the arteries or cerebral arteriosclerosis, and organic brain syndrome do little to help determine the optimal treatment or give an accurate description for the underlying disease process. Some of the reason for the use of poorly descriptive terms to describe cognitive impairments in older adults comes from the lack of ability to give a definitive diagnosis of the more common causative diseases.

Alzheimer's disease is the most common cause of dementia and is currently believed to be the primary etiology in approximately two thirds of all demented patients. Alzheimer's is primarily a disease of aging with an incidence of about 0.7 to 3.5 per 1,000 of population at the age of 65 and doubling every 5 years. Currently it is believed that 50% of the population over the age of 85 is suffering from Alzheimer's (Kalaria, 2003). It is important to note, that with advances in medical technology, patients with Alzheimer's disease are living much longer today than they were in the 1900s. As patients survive longer with Alzheimer's disease, the effects of advancing cognitive frailty begin to take a considerable toll on the patient's physical status. Also, as individuals live longer with other diseases, the chances of developing Alzheimer's as a new comorbid condition also greatly increase with advancing age. Both of these clinical situations are common among the frail older adult population.

Other illnesses resulting in dementia include vascular dementia, which not only accounts for approximately 5% of all dementias as a sole causative entity but also is seen as a comorbidity with Alzheimer's disease in another 10% of the patients. The other degenerative disorders that result in dementia include diffuse Lewy body dementia, which accounts for an additional 15–20% of all dementias. The remaining 5% of patients include such syndromes as progressive supranuclear palsy, combined systems degeneration, Pick's disease and Creutzfeldt-Jakob disease.

The exact etiology from a clinical standpoint is less important than the understanding that patients with an underlying cognitive impairment may look well physically, but have a heightened level of cognitive vulnerability. This vulnerability will become increasingly apparent when the patient is stressed from physical, medical, and/or environmental challenges. In the event of an acute change in the patient's status consideration of the patient's baseline is essential in estimating recovery from an event. Interdisciplinary comprehensive functional assessment remains the standard for establishing baseline status.

DELIRIUM

Delirium is a word that is often used casually in our society to mean "acting crazy" or to denote someone who is somewhat confused. The clinical definition of delirium, however, is much more rigorous, it is defined as a disturbance of normal consciousness characterized by an abrupt onset, an inability to attend to stimuli, and a reduced awareness of the environment. Delirious patients are often disoriented, and their level of activity may be either increased (agitated) or decreased (apathetic or hypoactive) from their baseline. Delirium tends to fluctuate over the course of the day, and different observers at different times may see a totally different patient. Delirium does not just happen, and its presence should alert health care providers to search for the culprit problem. Delirium is often the first sign of serious illness in older people, and the final common pathway for many different conditions.

Delirium is very common in frail older patients because of their reduced reserves and reduced capacity to maintain homeostasis. Gustafson, Brannstrom, Norberg, Bucht, and Windbladh (1991) found very high rates of prevalence in elderly hip fracture patients in Sweden, yet despite this, physician's detection of delirium was only about 9% of delirious patients. Nurses, while better at detection than physicians, detected delirium at a rate of about 30% of those affected, clearly showing that most health care professionals under-recognize delirium (Gustafson et al., 1991).

Health care providers often think of the "three M's" when seeking causative agents for delirium: medications, metabolic disturbance, and medical illness. Because older patients are usually on multiple medications, setting apart which of the medications is causing the delirium is sometimes a challenge. One can easily conclude drugs that affect the central nervous system like hypnotics, antidepressants, neuroleptics, anticonvulsants and anti-Parkinsonian agents commonly cause delirium. In addition, however, many other drugs used to treat high blood pressure, irregular heart rhythms, asthma, excess stomach acid, and even some prescription eye drops can cause delirium. Many patients believe that over-the-counter drugs tend to be safer than prescription drugs, but several cold remedies, antihistamines, appetite stimulants, and antinausea drugs available without a prescription may precipitate delirium. Eliciting a patient's use of nonprescription as well as prescription drug use is an essential part of the history-taking (Lefkoff, Besdine, & Weltine, 1989).

Another major category of causative agents for delirium is infections. In the elderly, many medical illnesses do not present with the classic signs of illness, such as painful urination with a bladder infection or a productive cough or even fevers with pneumonia, but instead have a change in mental status as the presenting symptom of illness. Dehydration, thyroid abnormalities, kidney, and liver failure can also cause the same clinical picture. Other disturbances of various minerals in the body, such as high or low sodium and potassium will cause delirium. Central nervous system events, such as strokes, meningitis, head trauma, and intracranial bleeding are also sometimes causative agents.

Some patients are predisposed to developing delirium, and documented factors that increase a person's risk include preexisting dementia, concomitant medical illness, alcohol use, dependency in activities of daily living, hearing and visual impairment, and depression. Elie, Cole, Primeau, and Bellavance (1998) described these in a meta-analysis of patients who developed in-hospital delirium. Both dementia and delirium, and sometimes depression cause an alteration in cognition, and in several other ways, these three clinical syndromes overlap, causing confusion to clinicians. Several key features separate the three. Delirium is characterized by an abrupt onset, a duration of hours to weeks, has a fluctuating clinical course, an abnormal level of consciousness, and poor attention span. Dementia has an insidious onset, duration of months to years, very little fluctuation in the clinical course, and normal level of consciousness and a normal attention span (Sullivan & Korman, 1993). Depression has been called pseudodementia or pseudodelirium because it can mimic either. Confusion caused by depression usually has an abrupt onset, either of episodic or persistent duration, and appear clinically like either dementia or delirium (Cacchinon, 2000). Before a diagnosis of dementia can be made, delirium and depression must be ruled out.

Several studies have confirmed that delirious patients have a much higher morbidity and mortality than nondelirious patients, have worse functional status at discharge, and higher rates of nursing home placement at discharge (Francis & Kapoor, 1992; Inouye, Rushing, Foreman, Palmer, & Pompei, 1998; O'Keefe & Lavan, 1997). In the hospital, these patients often become malnourished, develop pressure ulcers, fall and fracture bones, and become deconditioned from lying in bed. Delirium can also be a trigger for frailty ushering in a host of problems such as those in previously functional older adults. A multidisciplinary team approach is essential to prevent these complications and minimize functional decline.

In summary, delirium in older patients is common and under-recognized. Early recognition and intervention using an interdisciplinary team approach is necessary to prevent disability and adverse outcomes, both in hospital and at discharge. Health care providers must remember that delirium is caused by some underlying abnormality, and aggressively seek to correct the underlying disorders so that the delirium can be resolved.

CAREGIVER ISSUES

Anyone familiar with geriatric clinical practice knows quite well how many of his/her patients would be unable to survive outside of institutions were it not for the involvement of caregivers. There are 8.5 million Americans who have some impairment in their ADLs or instrumental activities of daily living (IADLs), and the number is expected to rise to 21 million by 2030, meaning that two out of every five adults over 70 years will require some assistance (Shirey & Summer, 2000).

Who are these caregivers? The AHEAD study surveyed caregivers across the country and found that 72% of caregivers were family members, with 42% of those being adult children and 25% spouses. Most caregivers assist with care on a daily basis, and 21% assist with care several times a week. Most caregivers, approximately 80%, provide care for patients 5 hours a day, but up to 7% provide care 24 hours a day (Shirey & Summer, 2000). In addition, a survey of caregivers for frail older patients found that 72% were female, and over a third were more than 65 years of age (Stone, Cafferata, & Sangl, 1987). In many cases, caregivers are in poor health themselves, or have limited financial means to provide for care of an elderly person (Stone et al., 1987). Caregiving is timeconsuming, stressful, labor intensive, and often lonely. It is no wonder that caregivers have higher rates of depression than noncaregivers in the population (Gallagher, Rose, Rivera, Lovett, & Thompson, 1989), along with a higher burden of physical illness and increased mortality when compared to noncaregivers in the population. In addition, Shulz and Beach showed that caregiving is an independent risk factor for mortality and that study participants who reported experiencing caregiver strain had mortality risks 63% higher than those in noncaregiving controls (Shulz & Beach, 1999).

What is included in the job of being a caregiver? For patients who are just physically frail, this care may be limited to assisting with the

IADLs such as shopping, cooking, and cleaning. As patients become more impaired, however, caregiving must take on the ADLs of dressing, feeding, bathing, and toileting. The National Caregivers Survey found that only 2.8% of caregivers assisted only with IADLs, and the majority (42.2%) assisted with more than five ADLs (Stone et al., 1987). Such care, especially when the caregiver is older or frail himself/herself, is very physically intensive. In patients with cognitive impairment, caregiving may take on additional dimensions of managing estates, coordinating medical care and overseeing professional caregiving services, if they are in place.

Finding the right health care provider who can be an ally to the caregiver and help with the burden of managing care is essential. Geriatricians, physicians who have received additional education in the medical management of elderly patients, can be especially helpful in minimizing the impact of chronic diseases and maximizing patient functioning to decrease the level of care a patient may require. Provider awareness of caregiver stress is very important, as providing supportive services in the home reduces burnout and delays nursing home placement (Mittleman, Ferris, Shulman, Steinberg, & Levin, 1996). Professional caregivers coming into the home in the form of certified nursing assistants to help with showering and dressing may ease some of the burden of the caregiver. If rigorous personal care is not required, homemakers, nonmedical personnel who can provide housekeeping services, shop, and cook meals, and drive shut-ins to doctors' appointments can also be helpful. Respite-stays in nursing facilities can enable caregivers to take a much-needed break from their duties or meet other family obligations, and have also been shown to delay nursing home placement. At some point, a higher level of care than a caregiver can provide may mandate placing a patient in a long-term care facility. Providers' active involvement in these decisions can ease some of the guilt that many caregivers feel in having the loved ones placed in facilities.

ABUSE AND NEGLECT

Although it is assumed that most caregivers are kind, well-meaning, and take good care of the dependent older adults, there is a dearth of information about the care that is actually delivered at home by informal caregivers (Barer & Johnson, 1990). There is no doubt that abuse and neglect do happen in some cases. Frailty in the older adult population places the aged individual in an increasingly dependent relationship with their caregivers. This dependency, which results from their complex physical and cognitive needs, greatly increases the burden of care leading to increased caregiver stress and burnout. As stress levels rise, elder abuse and neglect may ensue. It is estimated that approximately 1.2 million elders are abused or neglected annually with the majority of these cases occurring in the frail population (Paris, 2003).

There are multiple risk factors common to frail older adults that have been shown to increase the likelihood of abuse. Physical frailty is a significant risk factor due to the elders' reduced ability to defend themselves or seek help. Also there is frequently an associated lack of self-care, which results in increased caregiver stress. Cognitive frailty is considered to be one of the more significant risk factors that results from the caregivers' lack of understanding of the cognitive dysfunction and the need for both physical and behavioral support in a person who may look perfectly well. Substance abuse on the part of the caregiver is frequently cited as the primary reason for abuse and neglect. Financial dependency on the part of the caregiver is another significant risk factor. This can result in attempts to maintain an unsafe living situation rather than pursuing an alternative placement due to concern over lost financial support. Finally increased social isolation can result in the lack of recognition of mistreatment (Carney, Kahan, & Paris 2003).

Clear instances of abuse and neglect are easy to identify based on obvious traumatic injury or poor physical care and are the less common occurrences. The more common and difficult-to-identify cases involve subtler issues (Mendonca, Velamoor, & Sauve, 1996). The occurrence of an exacerbation of an underlying chronic disease may not seem to be an obvious case of abuse to the treating physician. This type of presentation may represent an intentional omission of care in an attempt to harm the individual or it may be a manifestation of caregiver burnout. Constant vigilance for all members of the care team is essential in identification of this sort of issue (Fulmer, 2003).

SUMMARY

It is distressing to consider that 20–47% of older adults spend the last months or years of their lives as dependent and frail. The alternative of healthy, successful aging, as Rowe and Kahn (1998) describe, is much more desirable. In order to do this, a better understanding of the syndrome of frailty is necessary along with education to older adults, their families, and health care providers that frailty is not an inevitable age change. It may be possible for frailty to be prevented, for the progression of frailty to be slowed, and there is even evidence that it may be reversed once the frailty cycle has begun.

The syndrome of frailty has been generally accepted as a physiological state of increased vulnerability to stressors that results from decreased reserves and dysregulation in multiple physiological systems. This causes difficulty in maintaining homeostasis when confronted with stressors (Fried et al., 2004). Maintaining and regaining homeostasis is essential for preventing the vicious cycle of frailty (Ferrucci, cited in Wilson, 2004). Falls, comorbidities, issues with polypharmacy, depression, dementia, and delirium all impact the cycle of frailty, either as antecedents or as consequences, and perpetuate the cycle.

Caring for frail older adults is often done by other older adults and can be very challenging. While many family members take excellent care of their loved ones, frail older adults are at highest risk of abuse and neglect. For health care providers, astute assessments and vigilant care of frail elders, as well as addressing all of the issues that frequently accompany frailty, are essential. Providing education and support for the caregivers is also important in ensuring quality care for the frail elder. Future research will bring a more complete understanding of the mechanisms of frailty and guide health care interventions.

REFERENCES

American Psychiatric Association. (2000). *Diagnostic and statistical manual of mental disorders* (4th ed., text rev.). Washington, DC: American Psychiatric Press.

Baker, S. P., & Harvey, A. H. (1985). Falls injuries in the elderly. *Clinics in Geriatric Medicine, 1*, 501–527.

Barer, B. M., & Johnson, C. L. (1990). A critique of the caregiving literature. *Gerontologist, 30*, 26–29.

Bloem, B. R., Steijns, J. A., & Sits-Engelsman, B. C. (2003). An update on falls. *Current Opinions in Neurology, 16*, 15–26.

Bortz, W. M. (2002). A conceptual framework of frailty. *Journals of Gerontology: A Biological and Medical Sciences, 57*, M283–M288.

Buchner, D. M., & Wagner, E. H. (1992). Preventing frail health. *Clinical Geriatric Medicine, 8*, 1–17.

Buckwalter, K., Katz, I., & Martin, H. (2004a, Winter). Guide to the prevention and management of falls in the elderly: part I. *CNS/LTC, CNS News*, pp. 7–11.

Buckwalter, K., Katz, I., & Martin, H. (2004b, Spring). Guide to the prevention and management of falls in the elderly: part II. *CNS/LTC, CNS News*, 31–36.

Cacchinone, P. A. (2000). Cognitive and neurologic function. In A. G. Lueckenotte (Ed.), *Gerontologic nursing* (2nd ed.). St. Louis: Mosby.

Campbell, A. J., & Buchner, D. M. (1997). Unstable disability and the fluctuations of frailty. *Age and Ageing, 26*, 315–318.

Carlson, J. E., Zocchi, K. A., Bettencourt, D. M., Gambrel, M. L., Freeman, J. L., Zhang, D., & Goodwin, J. S. (1998). Measuring frailty in the hospitalized elderly: Concept of functional homeostasis. *American Journal of Physical Medicine and Rehabilitation, 77,* 252–257.

Carney, M. T., Kahan, F. S., & Paris, B. E. (2003). Elder abuse: Is every bruise a sign of abuse? *Mount Sinai Journal of Medicine, 70*(2), 69–74.

Costa, P. T., & McCrae, R. R. (1985). Concepts of functional or biological age: A critical review. In R. Andres, E. L. Bierman, & W. R. Hazzard (Eds.), *Principles of geriatric medicine* (pp. 30–37). New York: McGraw-Hill.

Doherty, T. J., Vandervoort, A. A., & Brown, W. F. (1993). Effects of aging on the motor unit: A brief review. *Canadian Journal of Applied Physiology, 18,* 331–358.

Dugu, M., Neugroschl, J., Sewell, M., & Marin, D. (2003). Review of dementia. *Mount Sinai Journal of Medicine, 70*(1), 45–53.

Elie, M., Cole, M. G., Primeau, F. J., & Bellavance, F. (1998). Delirium risk factors in elderly hospitalized patients. *Journal of General Internal Medicine, 13,* 204–212.

Ferrucci, L., Cavazzini, C., Corsi, A., Bartali, B., Russo, C. R., Lauretani, F., Bandinelli, S., Bandinelli, S., & Guralnik, J. M. (2002). Biomarkers of frailty in older persons. *Journal of Endocrinological Investigation, 25*(Suppl. 10), 10–15.

Ferrucci, L., Guralnik, J. M., Cavazzini, C., Bandinelli, S., Lauretani, F., Bartali, B., et al. (2003). The frailty syndrome: A critical issue in geriatric oncology. *Critical Review of Oncology and Hematology, 46,* 127–137.

Francis, J., & Kapoor, W. N. (1992). Prognosis after hospital discharge of older medical patients with delirium. *Journal of the American Geriatrics Society, 40,* 601–606.

Fretwell, M. D. (1990). Acute hospital care for frail older patients. In W. R. Hazzard, R. Andres, E. L. Bierman, & J. P. Blass (Eds.), *Principles of geriatric medicine and gerontology* (pp. 247–253). New York: McGraw-Hill.

Fried, L. P., Ferrucci, L., Darer, J., Williamson, J. D., & Anderson, G. (2004). Untangling the concepts of disability, frailty, and comorbidity: Implications for improved targeting and care. *Journals of Gerontology. Series A, Biological Sciences and Medical Sciences, 59*(3), 255–263.

Fried, L. P., Tangen, C. M., Walston, J., Newman, A.B., Hirsch, C., Gottdiener, J., Seeman, T., Tracy, R., Kop, W. J., Burke, G., & McBurnie, M. A. for the Cardiovascular Health Study Collaborative Research Group. (2001). Frailty in older adults: Evidence for a phenotype. *Journals of Gerontology A: Biological and Medical Science, 56,* M146–M157.

Fried, L. P., & Walston, J. (1999). Frailty and failure to thrive. In W. R. Hazzard, J. P. Blass, W. H. Ettinger, Jr., J. B. Halter, & J. G. Ouslander (Eds.), *Principles of geriatric medicine and gerontology* (4th ed., pp. 1387–1402). New York: McGraw-Hill.

Fulmer, T. (2003). Elder abuse and neglect assessment. *Journal of Gerontological Nursing, 29*(6), 4–5.

Gallagher, D., Rose, J., Rivera, P., Lovett, S., & Thompson, L. W. (1989). Prevalence of depression in family caregivers. *Gerontologist, 29,* 449–456.

Gustafson, Y., Brannstrom, B., Norberg, A., Bucht, G., & Windbladh, B. (1991). Underdiagnosis and poor documentiation of acute confusional states in elderly hip fracutre patients. *Journal of the American Geriatrics Society, 39,* 760–765.

Guttman, R. (1999). Case management of the frail elderly in the community. *Clinical Nurse Specialist, 13,* 174–178.

Ham, R. J. (2002). Illness and aging. In R. J. Ham, P. D. Sloane, & G. A. Warshaw (Eds.), *Primary care geriatrics: A case-based approach* (4th ed., pp. 29–50). St. Louis: Mosby.

Hamerman, D. (1999). Toward an understanding of frailty. *Annals of Internal Medicine 130,* 945–950.

Hanlon, J. T., Artz, M. B., Pieper, C. F., Lindblad, C. I., Sloane, R. J., Ruby, C. M., & Schmader, K. E. (2004). Inappropriate medication use among frail elderly inpatients. *Annals of Pharmacotherapy, 38*(1), 9–14.

Hayes, W. C. (1994). Biomechanics of falls and hip fractures in the elderly. In D. F. Apple & W. C. Hayes (Eds.), *Prevention of falls and hip fractures in the elderly* (pp. 41–65). Chicago: American Academy of Orthopaedic Surgeons.

Higashi, T., Shekelle, P. G., Solomon, D. H., Knight, E. L., Roth, C., Chang, J. T., et al. (2004). The quality of pharmacologic care for vulnerable older patients. *Annals of Internal Medicine, 140*(9), 152.

Hogan, D. B., MacKnight, C., Bergman, H., & Steering Committee, Canadian Initiative on Frailty and Aging. (2003). Models, definitions, and criteria of frailty. *Aging Clinical and Experimental Research, 15*(Suppl. 3), 3–29.

Inouye, S. K., Rushing, J. T., Foreman, M. D., Palmer, R. M., & Pompei, P. (1998). Does delirium contribute to poor hospital outcomes? A three-site epidemiologic study. *Journal of General Internal Medicine, 13,* 234–242.

Janssen, I., Shepard, D. S., Katzmarzyk, P. T., & Roubenoff, R. (2004). The healthcare costs of sarcopenia in the United States, *Journal of the American Geriatrics Society, 52*(1), 80–85.

Jarrett, P. G., Rockwood, K., Carver, D., Stolee, P., & Cosway, S. (1995). Illness presentation in elderly patients. *Archives of Internal Medicine, 155,* 1060–1064.

Kalaria, R. N. (2003). Comparison between Alzheimer's disease and vascular dementia: Implications for treatment. *Neurological Research, 6,* 661–664.

Lammers, J. E. (2002). Depression. In R. J. Ham, P. D. Sloane, & G. A. Warshaw (Eds.), *Primary care geriatrics: A case-based approach* (4th ed., pp. 309–322). St. Louis: Mosby.

Lefkoff, S., Besdine, R., & Wetle, T. (1989). Acute confusional states in the hospitalized elderly. *Annual Review of Gerontology and Geriatrics, 6,* 1–26.

Leng, S., Cappola, A. R., Anderson, R., Blackman, R., Koenig, K., Blair, M., & Walston, J. (2004). Serum levels of insulin-like growth factor-I (IGF-I) and dehydroepiandrosterone sulfate (DHEA-S), and their relationships with serum interleukin-6, in the geriatric syndrome of frailty. *Aging Clinical and Experimental Research, 16,* 153–157.

Leng, S., Chaves, P., Koenig, K., & Walston, J. (2002). Serum interleukin-6 and hemoglobin as physiological correlates in the geriatric syndrome of frailty: A pilot study. *Journal of the American Geriatrics Society, 50,* 1268–1271.

Lipsitz, L. A. (2004). Physiological complexity, aging, and the path to frailty. *Science of Aging Knowledge Environment, 16*, pe16, 21.

Lipsitz, L. A., & Goldberger, A. L. (1992). Loss of "complexity" and aging: Potential applications of fractals and chaos theory to senescence. *Journal of the American Medical Association, 267*, 1806–1809.

Lunney, T. M., Lynn, J., & Hogan, C. (2002). Profiles of older Medicare decedents. *Journal of the American Geriatrics Society, 50*, 1108–1112.

Lunney, J. R., Lynn, J., Foley, D. J., Lipson, S., & Guralnik, J. M. (2003). Patterns of functional decline at the end of life. *Journal of the American Medical Association, 289*, 2387–2392.

Mendonca, J. D., Velamoor, V. R., & Sauve, D. (1996). Key features of maltreatment of the infirm elderly in home settings. *Canadian Journal of Psychiatry, 41*, 107–113.

Mezey, M., & Fulmer, T. (1998). Quality care for the frail elderly. *Nursing Outlook, 46*, 291–292.

Mittleman, M. S., Ferris, S. H., Shulman, E., Steinberg, G., & Levin, B. (1996). A family intervention to delay nursing home placement of patients with Alzheimer's disease: A randomized controlled trial. *Journal of the American Medical Association, 276*, 1725–1731.

Morley, J. E., Baumgartner, R. N., Roubenoff, R., Mayer, J., & Nair, K. S. (2001). Sarcopenia. *Journal of Laboratory and Clinical Medicine, 137*, 231–243.

National Center for Injury Prevention and Control, Centers for Disease Control and Prevention. (2004). *Web-based injury statistics query and reporting system (WISQARS)*. Retrieved on June 3, 2005 from http://www.cdc.gov/ ncipc/wisqars/default.htm

National Institute on Aging. (2003). *Frailty in old age: Pathophysiology and interventions—Program Announcement*. Retrieved June 3, 2005 from http://grants.nih.gov/grants/guide/pa-files/PAS-03-122.html

Office of Statistics and Programming, National Center for Injury Prevention and Control, Center for Disease Control. (2004). *Web-based injury statistics query and reporting system (WISQARS)*. Retrieved June 25, 2005 from http://www.cdc.gov/ncipc/wisqars/default.htm 6-05-2005

O'Keefe, S. & Lavan, J. (1997). The prognostic significance of delirium in older hospitalised patients. *Journal of the American Geriatrics Society, 45*, 247–248.

Paris, B. (2003). Abuse and neglect . . . so prevalent yet so elusive. *Geriatrics, 58*(10), 10.

Parmelee, P. A., Katz, I. R., & Lawton, M. P. (1992). Incidence of depression in long-term care settings. *Journals of Gerontology: Biological and Medical Sciences, 47* (6), M189.

Patten, S. B., & Barbury, C. (2004). Drug-induced depression: A systematic review to inform clinical practice. *Psychotherapy and Psychosomatic, 73*, 207–215.

Raj, A. (2004). Depression in the elderly: Tailoring medical therapy to their needs. *Postgraduate Medicine, 115*(6), 26–42.

Rockwood, K., Hogan, D. B., & MacKnight, C. (2000). Conceptualisation and measurement of frailty in elderly people. *Drugs and Aging, 17*, 295–302.

24 FRAIL OLDER ADULTS

Roubenoff, R. (2003). Sarcopenia: Effects on body composition and function. *Journals of Gerontology A: Biological and Medical Science, 58*, M1012–M1017.
Roubenoff, R., & Hughes, V. A. (2000). Sarcopenia: Current concepts. *Journals of Gerontology A: Biological and Medical Science, 55*, M716–M777.
Rowe, J. W., & Kahn, R. L. (1998). *Successful aging.* New York: Pantheon.
Rubenstein, L. Z., & Josephson, K. R. (2002). The epidemiology of falls and syncope. *Clinics in Geriatric Medicine, 18*, 141–158.
Schuurmans, H., Steverink, N., Lindenberg, S., Frieswijk, N., & Slaets, J. P. J. (2004). Old or frail: What tells us more? *Journals of Gerontology A: Biological and Medical Sciences, 59A*(9), 962–965.
Schneider, D. C., & Mader, S. L (2002). Falls. In R. J. Ham, P. D. Sloane, & G. A. Warshaw (Eds.), *Primary care geriatrics: A case-based approach* (4th ed., pp. 349–359). St. Louis: Mosby.
Schulz, R., & Beach, S. (1999). Caregiving as a risk factor for mortality: The caregiver health effects study. *Journal of the American Medical Association, 282*, 2215–2219.
Shirey, L., & Summer, L. (2000). Caregiving: Helping the elderly with activity limitations. *National Academy On An Aging Society, 7*(5), 1–6.
Sloane P. D. (2002). Normal aging. In R. J. Ham, P. D. Sloane, & G. A. Warshaw (Eds.), *Primary care geriatrics: A case-based approach* (4th ed., pp. 15–28). St. Louis: Mosby.
Stone, R., Cafferata, G. L., & Sangl, J. (1987). Caregivers of the frail elderly: A national profile. *Gerontologist, 27*, 616–626.
Strawbridge, W. J., Shema, S. J., Balfour, J. L., Higby, H. R., & Kaplan, G. A. (1998). Antecedents of frailty over three decades in an older cohort. *Journals of Gerontology B: Psychological and Social Sciences, 53*(1), S9–S16.
Sullivan, G. M., & Korman, L. B. (1993). Drug-associated confusional states in older persons. *Topics in Geriatric Rehabilitation, 8*(4), 4.
Tennstedt, S. L., & McKinley, J. B. (1994). Frailty and its consequences. *Social Science and Medicine, 38*, 863–865.
Tideiksaar, R. (1997). *Falling in Old Age.* New York: Springer Publishing.
U.S. Census Bureau. (2004). *Projected population of the United States, by age and sex: 2000 to 2050.* Retrieved June 5, 2005 from http://www.census.gov/ipc/www/uninterimproj/.
Walston, J. (2004). Frailty—The search for underlying causes. *Science of Aging Knowledge and Environment, 4*, pe4.
Wilson, J. F. (2004). Frailty—and its dangerous effects—might be preventable. *American College of Physicians, 141*, 489–492.
Woodhouse, K. W., & O'Mahoney, M. S. (1997). Frailty and aging. *Age and Ageing, 26*, 245–246.

CHAPTER TWO

Health Care Strategies for Frail Older Adults

J. Stoukides, C. Holzer, J. Ritzau, and P. Burbank

Although frail older adults comprise a minority within their own age cohort, they consume 50% of all hospital care, over 80% of home care services, and occupy over 90% of all nursing home beds in the United States (Mezey & Fulmer, 1998). They require multiple health services that address complex, acute, and long-term care needs. Providing comprehensive care for older adults who are frail is a challenging endeavor that can be greatly rewarding. After considering the many issues and problems associated with frailty, health care providers may be overwhelmed with the complexity of needs of this population. Studies have documented, however, that it may be possible to successfully treat older adults who are frail by slowing or even reversing the progression of frailty. Additionally, as more evidence for biological and physiological precursors becomes available, the potential for preventing and treating frailty grows.

Frail patients have special needs for care beyond simply treating their diseases and accompanying disabilities. Fried, Ferrucci, Darer, Williamson, and Anderson (2004) point out that comorbid diseases, difficulty carrying out activities of daily living (ADLs), and the progressive weakness associated with frailty are three different, but causally interconnected problems for older adults.

In addition to assessment and treatment of underlying diseases, interventions to minimize loss of weight, strength, and muscle mass are needed. These interventions include a regular exercise program including resistance exercise, special attention when encountering stressful conditions and environments such as medical procedures and hospitalization (Fried et al., 2004), careful monitoring of medications, and adequate intake of calories, protein, and micronutrients (Kinney, 2004).

This chapter begins with a discussion of comprehensive geriatric assessment (CGA), including an interdisciplinary team approach, which is necessary for addressing the complex issues of the frail older adults. Frailty assessment tools are also discussed. Then two types of interventions are reviewed: those that address the common areas associated with frailty, such as falls, polypharmacy, depression, delirium, dementia, and caregiver issues; and those that address the syndrome of frailty in general, such as exercise and nutrition.

COMPREHENSIVE GERIATRIC ASSESSMENT

Description

Quality care of frail older adults begins with an accurate multidimensional assessment of four domains of health: physical, psychological, socioenvironmental, and functional. This is best accomplished with CGA, the foundation of the geriatric care system (Rubenstein, 2004). A CGA has been defined as an interdisciplinary approach to the assessment and diagnosis of physical and psychosocial impairments and functional disabilities in frail older adults (Siu, Reuben & Moore, 1994). It consists of three steps: screening of appropriate patients, assessment and developing recommendations, and implementing recommendations as planned (Reuben, 1999).

The need for an interdisciplinary team approach is well established. Interdisciplinary teams, however, do not "just happen" when health care professionals from different disciplines work together. The actual process of interdisciplinary team development requires education and team training on group dynamics, conflict management, and internal team issues. Follow-up team support on advocacy and empowerment within the larger organizational context is also needed for success. Nationally, two programs, the Geriatric Education Centers and the Geriatric Interdisciplinary Team Training programs, have been valuable resources for interdisciplinary team training (Clark, Leinhaus, & Filinson, 2002; Drinka & Clark, 2000).

The typical frail patient seen in CGA usually has multiple and interacting medical and psychosocial impairments. The goal of CGA is to identify these impairments and improve the function and health, quality of life, and possibly survival of the frail older patient. The CGA activities also provide the foundation for interdisciplinary care plans, address previously undiagnosed health and psychosocial problems, stratify risk for future morbidity, and develop appropriate preventive measures. The care plan identifies present or possible limitations of the patient's ability to function in daily life and develops strategies and interventions to improve outcomes. Treatment plans based on such assessment should be developed in conjunction with the patient, the caregiver, or both, and should aim to improve and maintain function, reduce unnecessary use of health care resources, and ultimately increase years of quality life (Laird & Studenski, 1999). These goals are achieved and coordinated through interdisciplinary treatment and rehabilitation (Siu et al., 1994).

The CGA provides the health care team with full knowledge of a patient's coexisting medical problems and their severity, nutritional status, cognitive and emotional function, mobility and continence problems, medication lists, and psychosocial background. The traditional medical examination is supplemented with specific assessments to detect impairments that are particularly prevalent and important in the frail elderly. These include impairments of cognition, mood, mobility, gait, balance, continence, nutrition, vision, and hearing. In some populations of older persons, screening for alcoholism or other selected disorders may be indicated (Siu et al., 1994). The scope of CGA is broad in order to address the medical, sensory, functional, psychologic, and social limitations that can impact the lives of older persons and their caregivers. This baseline information of a patient's mental and physical function becomes critical for the accurate identification of frailty (Fretwell, 1990).

Comprehensive geriatric assessments are carried out in various settings by members of the interdisciplinary health care team. These include inpatient and outpatient settings, in the home and in long-term care arenas. The interdisciplinary team typically includes at least a physician, a nurse or nurse practitioner, and a social worker. However, most programs employ a variety of other disciplines, including physical and occupational therapy, psychology or psychiatry, rehabilitation medicine, audiology, clinical pharmacy, dentistry, podiatry, nutrition, and other medical or surgical subspecialties on a consulting basis (Siu et al., 1994).

One barrier to completion of the CGA is the length of time required to do a complete assessment. In an effort to streamline the assessment, an abbreviated CGA was developed, which used 15 items that were useful in screening for those older adults who would benefit from a full CGA (Overcash, Beckstead, Extermann, & Cobb, 2005).

Outcomes of Comprehensive Geriatric Assessment

Studies on the effectiveness of CGAs document that CGA programs improve patient outcomes. In an early randomized controlled trial (RCT), Rubenstein et al. (1984) found that hospitalized patients in the geriatric evaluation unit receiving CGA had more diagnoses, improved function, reduced nursing home placement, reduced mortality, lower rehospitalization rates, lower costs, and increased survival. Since then, more mixed results have emerged from studies in several countries. Some CGA programs were found to have more benefits than others, especially the inpatient units and in-home assessment teams. A meta-analysis of controlled trials found an 18% reduction in mortality risk, a 25% increased likelihood of living at home, a 41% increased chance of improvement in cognition, and a 12% lowered risk of hospitalization. Functional status was significantly improved only for those in the inpatient geriatric evaluation and management units (Stuck, Siu, Wieland, Adams, & Rubenstein, 1993). A recent review of inpatient CGAs found that hospitalized patients receiving CGA had decreased short-term mortality, a better chance of living at home, one year later, and improved physical and cognitive function. The CGA was not shown to decrease long-term mortality, however (Ellis & Langhorne, 2005).

COMPONENTS OF THE COMPREHENSIVE GERIATRIC ASSESSMENT

History

The CGA should begin with a discussion of the reason for seeking medical attention, stated in both the patient's and the caregiver's words. It should address the specific functional losses that the patient may be experiencing or that the caregiver may be observing, as well as the more traditional medical complaints. At the onset of the CGA it is important to assess that the patient be able to see and hear the examiner, respond to questions, and give an accurate history. If the patient is unable to give an accurate history, the caregiver should be included in the visit.

As part of the history, all medical diagnosis should be listed with a statement of duration and impact on the patient's physical and mental function. Nutritional information should document any changes in weight and appetite. An extensive medication review including prescription and over-the-counter medications is paramount. The medication history should include the duration of use and any adverse drug reactions, as well as a review of the impact of each medication on the patient's physical and mental functions (Fretwell, 1997).

Physical/Functional Assessment

A comprehensive physical examination is performed paying special attention to the neurologic and musculoskeletal systems. Close observation of gait, balance, and range of motion is necessary. Assessment of type and frequency of urinary incontinence is also important. Laboratory evaluation is required to rule out any reversible causes of dementia and disease.

Functional assessment is the foundation of geriatric rehabilitation. It is the key to understanding the impact of medical illness on the older person and family. The items composing functional assessment are the ADLs and the instrumental activities of daily living (IADLs). The ADLs are the functions that are fundamental to independent living, such as bathing, dressing, toileting, transfer, continence, and feeding. The IADLs include more complex daily activities, such as using the telephone, housekeeping, and managing money. A basic schedule to assess ADL is the Katz Index of ADL, which provides a framework for assessing the ability to live independently (Gallo, Fulmer, Paveza, & Reichel, 2000).

Considering the basic ADL items in evaluation of an older person has several important advantages. Focusing on functional abilities allows matching of services to needs. For example, someone who requires only assistance in bathing may be maintained independently with the help of a home health aide to perform the task once a week. Thus, functional assessment can assist the health care provider to focus on the frail elder's capabilities and when there is a change, to enlist the help of appropriate community services (Gallo et al., 2000).

Mental Status Assessment

Mental status assessment is key to evaluating the health of older persons. An accurate medical and social history obtained from an older person is dependent on adequate cognitive functioning. An assessment of the patient's level of consciousness, attention, language, memory, proverb interpretation, similarities calculations, writing, and constructional ability are encompassed in a comprehensive mental status examination (Gallo et al., 2000).

Mini-Mental State Exam (MMSE) (Folstein, Folstein, & McHugh, 1975) is the most widely used screening tool for cognitive dysfunction. Scores of less than 24 (out of a possible 30) are highly correlated with cognitive loss. Many other screening instruments have also been shown to appropriately identify cognitive impairment in older persons. The three-item recall method has shown relatively good sensitivity in comparison with the MMSE. Evaluation of the clock-drawing test has also demonstrated its usefulness in identifying patients likely to develop progressive cognitive loss (Laird & Studenski, 1999). Other common screening tests for cognitive impairment include the Mental Status Questionnaire, the Short Portable Mental Status Questionnaire, the Set Test, the Cognitive Capacity Screening Examination, the Short Test of Mental Status, and the Blessed Information–Memory Concentration Test. These screening instruments have not been as extensively studied as the MMSE, however (Siu et al., 1994). Further evaluation should be performed on patients with a positive screen.

The diagnosis of the etiology of a dementing illness is frequently made on the basis of exclusion. Advances in medical technology have continued to place greater emphasis on imaging studies in an attempt to determine a causative agent for the clinical state. Imaging studies can be helpful in ruling out structural abnormalities but provide little helpful information in adding a definitive diagnosis to the degenerative causes. Laboratory studies also serve an important exclusionary role in determining potentially reversible metabolic abnormalities. Establishing an accurate diagnosis is best accomplished by a thorough interdisciplinary assessment evaluating the patient's history, physical findings, and laboratory values (Dugu, Neugroschl, Sewell, & Marin, 2003).

DEPRESSION

Diagnosing depression in the elderly is often difficult. Rather than having symptoms of depressed mood or crying spells, older persons are likely to have nonspecific somatic complaints such as fatigue, abdominal pain, or headache. Family members may bring the patient to the physician with a presentation of "just not feeling well" (Schneider & Mader, 2002).

A variety of assessment instruments are available to screen for depression. Some instruments have been developed specifically for frail older patients. One of these instruments is the Geriatric Depression Scale (GDS) (Yesavage & Brink, 1983), a 30-item instrument that asks for yes/no responses to a series of questions covering symptoms and the manifestations of depression. Scores of 11 or more on this 30-point instrument substantially increase the probability of depression. Short forms of the Geriatric Depression Scale (15 items and 4 items) have also been tested and validated (Sheikh & Yesavage, 1986). The Cornell Scale for Depression in Dementia (Alexopoulos, Abrams, Young, & Shamoian, 1988) is useful for screening in frail elders who have cognitive impairment. The GDS tends to focus on the psychological symptoms of depression and excludes somatic symptoms. The Cornell Scale excludes symptoms that may be attributed to both depression and dementia.

Suicide ideation should be assessed in depressed older adults. Several studies have found that up to 75% of older adults who die by suicide have visited a primary care physician within a month of their suicide (Katz, Streim, & Parmalee, 1994; Miller, 1978). These findings point to the urgency of improving detection and treatment of depression as a means of reducing suicide risk among older persons.

SOCIAL AND SPIRITUAL ASSESSMENT

The emotional well-being and perceived quality of life of the older patient are significant determinants of functional abilities. A social assessment covers a wide range of issues such as bereavement, isolation, financial matters, caregiver issues, environmental factors such as home and personal safety, and assessment of elder maltreatment (Laird & Studenski, 1999). Further social evaluation includes individual social skills, including marital history; issues of physical and emotional intimacy; a review of family support systems, including numbers of and relationships between potential caretakers; and use of existing community resources. Values about medical treatments such as surgery, feeding tubes, ventilators, cardiopulmonary resuscitation, and documentation of prior directives such as durable power of attorney or living will are also addressed in the social assessment (Fretwell, 1997).

Because of the significant risk associated with the caregiving experience, the assessment of caregiver burden is critical in the assessment of social support. The task of caregiving can be demanding and onerous to the caregiver. Research suggests a link between the caregiving experience and the risk of depression among caregivers. Furthermore, caregiver depression has been linked to increased risk of elder abuse. Thus, it is crucial for the practitioner to carefully assess for caregiver burden (George & Gwyther, 1986).

Religion and spiritual issues may be especially important among frail older adults. Assessment of spiritual well-being, using nursing diagnosis (North American Nursing Diagnosis Association, 1999) criteria involves asking questions of patients about concerns with meaning and purpose in life, disturbances in belief systems, or requests for spiritual assistance (Highfield, 2001).

SCREENING AND IMMUNIZATIONS

Screening tests and examinations often have different recommendations for frail older adults. In a review article summarizing best evidence for screening recommendations, the authors conclude that it is reasonable to screen and treat elderly populations at high risk, such as those with coronary artery disease, cerebrovascular disease, obesity, smoking, or diabetes (Higashi et al., 2004). In the frailest patients, screening and detection may present an unwanted burden from which they may not benefit because of low life expectancy at baseline. In recommending screening procedures, clinicians must look at a patient's anticipated life expectancy, risk of testing and potential for treatment to decide who to refer for additional testing. In most cases, screening for colorectal cancer, routine mammograms, Papanicolaou tests, and prostate cancer screening are generally not recommended for frail older adults (Higashi et al., 2004; U.S. Preventive Task Force, 1996). All screening in older adults should focus on their life expectancy, functional status, personal goals and values, as well as an understanding of current evidence-based recommendations about screening for disease.

Immunizations are an important part of preventive health in frail older persons. It is widely accepted that persons older than 65 years be vaccinated annually for influenza and at least once for pneumococcal infections; however, only 67% of this population received flu shots in 1999 and 45% had never received pneumococcal vaccination (Farr, Johnson, & Cobb, 1995). Many patients decline vaccinations because of fear that they cause illness, but studies do not show any increase in adverse reactions between patients who received the influenza vaccine or placebo (Margolis, Nichol, Poland, & Pluhar, 1990). Some confusion still exists in the population about the pneumococcal vaccine. The vaccine is effective in reducing serious illness, but does not "prevent" pneumonia (Farr et al., 1995). A study by Sisk et al. (1997), however, showed that vaccination of the 23 million unvaccinated adults in 1993 would have resulted in a savings of 194 million dollars and gained 78,000 years of healthy lives.

FRAILTY INDICES

The syndrome of frailty has been defined theoretically by several authors, however, practical tools to identify, assess, and monitor frailty in clinical practice are needed. Strawbridge, Shema, Balfour, Higby, and Kaplan (1998) developed a frailty questionnaire based on identified risk factors in four functional domains: physical, nutritive, cognitive, and sensory. In 2004, Matthews et al. studied the validity and utility of the Strawbridge frailty questionnaire and determined that it was consistent with several single-item measures of functional ability. In addition, frailty on the Strawbridge score correlated with 3-year adverse health outcomes. Clinical assessment of frailty status by the primary care geriatrician was a more powerful predictor of adverse health outcomes than Strawbridge scores, however. It was suggested that perhaps the Strawbridge question-naire over-emphasized the sensory domain (Matthews et al., 2004).

Two other approaches to assess frailty are the Frailty Index (FI), based on a CGA instrument (Jones, Song, & Rockwood, 2004) and the Clinical Global Impression of Change in Physical Frailty (CGIC-PF) instrument (Studenski et al., 2004). The FI assigns scores of 0 (no problem), 1 (minor problem), or 2 (major problem) to each of the 10 standard domains in the CGA: cognitive status, mood and motivation, communication, mo-bility, balance, bowel function, bladder function, IADLs and ADLs, nutrition, and social resources. The advantage of the FI is that it can be calculated from the data already collected in the CGA (Jones et al., 2004). The CGIC-PF assesses six intrinsic domains (mobility, balance, strength, endurance, nutrition, and neuromotor performance) and seven consequences domains (medical complexity, health care utilization, ap-pearance, self-perceived health, ADLs, emotional status and social status). Change is scored on a 7-point scale for clinical indicators within each domain (Studenski et al., 2004). Although initial testing indicates that both of these tools are valid and reliable, the FI was designed to be practical for clinicians, whereas the CGIC-PF was developed for research and studies of outcome measures.

PROBLEM-CENTERED STRATEGIES

Although assessment of these factors is described in the discussion of the CGA, a more detailed discussion of strategies for falls, depression, delirium, polypharmacy, and dementia is included here as they are espe-cially problematic for frail older adults.

Falls

Because falls are usually multifactorial, a multidimensional fall risk assessment is useful to target fall risk factors and individualize treat-ment approaches. (Buckwalter, Katz, & Martin, 2004a) The fall evalu-ation and risk assessment begins with a directed history of the events surrounding the fall. A comprehensive physical examination should be performed with special emphasis on vision, skin, cardiovascular system, neurological status, musculoskeletal system and cognitive evaluation. All older persons who have experienced recurrent falls should undergo laboratory testing to rule out treatable conditions. It is essential that gait be observed as there is strong evidence that balance and gait assess-ment is the single best predictor of individuals at increased risk of falling (Schneider & Mader, 2002).

The goal of treatment is to minimize fall risk and maximize functional independence. Acute illness or new problems that may have contributed to the fall should be treated. Injuries from the fall should be treated, and attention should be paid to the potential psychological consequences. Specific medical factors that have been identified through the fall evaluation as possible causes should be improved through appropriate interventions. Review of all medications should be performed, and an attempt should be made to reduce the number of medications and eliminate high-risk medications (Schneider & Mader, 2002).

Environmental interventions to prevent falls include regular eye examinations, providing proper lighting (use night lights at night); furnishing proper assistive devices such as hip protectors to reduce risk of injury, hand rails, raised toilet seats, and shower benches in bathrooms; eliminating extension cords, throw rugs and other floor clutter; and providing adjustable beds and chairs (Buckwalter, Katz, & Martin, 2004b).

Fall prevention programs should include physical therapy. A physical therapist can instruct the patient in muscle strengthening and balance exercises, evaluate the patient for use of an appropriate ambulatory assistive device and train his/her in its use, provide transfer and gait training, and if possible, perform a home safety evaluation designed to modify and adapt the environment for fall reduction (Tinetti, 1997). There has been much research in fall prevention for older adults resulting in evidence-based recommendations. The Frailty and Injuries: Cooperative Study of Intervention Techniques (FICSIT) tested multiple interventions in a multicenter study with over 2300 subjects. Results from the FICSIT suggested that high-intensity, resistive strength training; certain balance exercise programs such as tai chi; and a multiple risk-factor reduction strategy are all potentially successful approaches to reducing the rate of falls among elderly persons (Schneider & Mader, 2002).

Padding for falls (such as hip protectors) has been shown to significantly decrease the number of hip fractures in institutionalized elders and, in one study, to improve confidence in the ability to perform activities of daily living. Hip fractures were reduced by 80–100% among those who correctly wore their hip protectors. Wearing protective hip pads also improved balance confidence and helped to restore independence (Bloem, Steijns, & Smits-Englesman, 2003).

Polypharmacy

An interdisciplinary approach to drug management is the key to identifying potential drug-induced adverse effects. Comprehensive Functional Assessment can serve to establish an older patient's baseline function.

Any changes noted in the patient's functional status by team members are suspected as a potential adverse drug effect, even if it is not commonly considered a problem based on initial literature review. A comprehensive medication review should be initiated at the start of an episode of care for all frail elderly patients. It is vitally important not to limit the intensity of drug review to the start of the care but to re-evaluate the medication regimen on a daily basis and when additional medications are added to the drug regimen (Higashi et al., 2004).

Assessing compliance issues is extremely important as it can have wide-ranging impact on a frail elder overall quality of care. Unrecognized under-utilization of medication can lead to inappropriate dose escalations or abandonment of an effective therapy without an adequate trial. Also recognition of underutilization is extremely important when a patient enters an environment where compliance is assured, such as a hospital or nursing home. This forced compliance can either suddenly or over time cause wide-ranging adverse events. These events are frequently not attributed to the offending medication due to perceived long-standing safe use at the current dosage. Similarly, unrecognized overutilization can lead to problems with withdrawal reactions, and exacerbation of symptoms that were being treated with a higher dose of medication (Chouinard, 2004).

Suboptimal prescribing by physicians contributes to adverse drug reactions and polypharmacy (Hanlon, Schmader, Ruby, & Weinberger, 2001). A study of outpatient geriatric evaluation and management found that this approach reduced serious adverse drug reactions compared to usual care (Schmader et al., 2004).

Depression

A diagnosis of depression should be considered in all older adults who report somatic symptoms, particularly those who have chronic symptoms that seem to have no conclusive organic basis. Because of the close association between depressive symptoms and many medical illnesses, however, the CGA is especially important to avoid missing a concomitant or causative illness (Schneider & Mader, 2002).

Early treatment of depression with pharmacologic agents is highly recommended for older adults. Successful pharmacotherapy begins with choosing a medication that is compatible with the patient's other medications and has side-effects that are minimally disruptive to the patient. Currently, selective serotonin reuptake inhibitors (SSRIs) are the first choice for treatment of depression in older patients. Patients need to be informed that the medication can take anywhere from 6 to 12 weeks to work.

Effective treatment of depression in the frail elders generally requires an interdisciplinary approach. Treatment is complex in that it involves consideration of the role of comorbid disease, cognitive changes, concomitant medications, and the patient's support systems. The efficacy of pharmacologic therapy appears to be enhanced by also addressing the social support structure of the patient. It may be useful to suggest community support services, such as case management or Meals on Wheels. Many older people with major depression respond well to psychotherapy combined with antidepressant medications (Schneider & Mader, 2002).

Electroconvulsive therapy (ECT) is an effective treatment for older patients with major depression, with success rates approaching 90%. Side effects such as memory loss are more common among older adults, however. Although some believe that ECT is the treatment of choice for older adults, most clinicians reserve ECT for refractory cases or for cases in which a high risk of morbidity or mortality would be associated with waiting as much as 4 to 6 weeks for a significant response to medications. Such high-risk patients include those who are actively suicidal or who are refusing to take adequate nutrition and hydration because of depressive illness (Schneider & Mader, 2002).

Delirium

The diagnosis of delirium is made largely on clinical examination, with the assistance of screening instruments such as the Neecham Confusion Scale (Neelon, Champagne, Carlson, & Funk 1996), the Confusion Assessment Method (Inouye et al., 1990), or portions of the Mini-Mental Status exam (Folstein et al., 1975) that focuses on attention, recall, and orientation. The Neecham Confusion Scale, regarded by some as the best screening instrument for delirium (Milisen, DeGeest, Abraham, & Delooz, 2001), assesses 9 components in 13 areas of cognitive processing, behavior, and physiologic control. It incorporates change in mental status as well as in physiological behavior areas.

An essential component of the history-taking is to establish the patient's baseline mental status to determine if the current state is a departure from their norm. Doing this usually involves a reliable informant, either a relative or a caregiver, such as a primary nurse if the patient is in a long-term care facility. Next, the underlying medical problem causing the delirium must be aggressively sought. Most delirious patients require hospitalization to try to sort out the etiology, and many medically ill patients who get admitted to the hospital become delirious during their hospitalization. Management of delirium in the hospital includes looking for causative agents and good supportive medical care.

Nonpharmacologic therapy for delirious patients includes prompt recognition of the disorder and correction if possible of the underlying disorders, including simplifying the number and dosage of medications. Environmental improvements include providing eyeglasses and hearing aids if they are usually used and bringing familiar items from home. In addition, minimizing abrupt relocations and good sleep hygiene is essential in preventing or improving delirium. Having continuity of nursing staff throughout the patient's stay, as well as frequent reorientation has been shown to decrease the incidence of delirium. (Williams, Campbell, Raynor, Mlynarczyk, & Ward, 1985). Sometimes the best ally to the health care team is a known family member who can stay with the patient, adding a familiar face and decreasing the need for staff to be present at all times to ensure patients' safety. All attempts to minimize invasive tubes and lines should be undertaken. Involvement of physical therapists early in a patient's clinical course can ameliorate some of the deconditioning that occurs as a result of the delirium. Good medical care, including minimizing fall risk, aspiration risk, and prevention of pressure ulcerations cannot be overemphasized, and is best accomplished by an interdisciplinary approach.

Some medications that have been useful in the short-term management of agitation are antipsychotics. Clinicians need to be aware, however, that older patients require much lower doses of these medications than younger patients to avoid adverse outcomes. Routine use of benzodiazepines in older patients, except for those who may be delirious because of ethanol withdrawal, is not recommended.

Although the use of physical restraints has decreased over the past two decades, they continue to be controversial and problematic. Studies have shown that restraints are ineffective in preventing patient removal of medical devices, such as catheters and tubes (Mion, 1996; Mion et al., 2001), nor do they prevent falls or injuries from falls (Braun & Capezuiti, 2000; Capezuti, Strumpf, Evans, Grisso, & Maislin, 1998; Mion et al., 2001). Instead, harmful consequences have been found to be associated with restraint use (Frengley & Mion, 1998). In 2001, JCAHO mandated that all patients must have individual patient orders for restraints and timely assessments by health care providers, changing the standard of practice to nonrestraint except under exceptional circumstances. Alternatives to restraints, such as presence of loved ones, personal alarm devices, consistent staff, employment of sitters, reduction of light at night, noise reduction, and promoting normal sleep patterns should be used whenever possible (O'Connell & Mion, 2003).

Dementia

A review of the interventions available for treating the diseases and cognitive problems associated with dementia is beyond the scope of this chapter. The discussion here focuses on general types of strategies that have been used successfully to improve cognitive functioning or to slow decline or to manage behavioral issues that may accompany cognitive impairment.

At the physiological level, strategies include careful management of comorbid conditions and use of medications to improve cognitive function. Cognitive and psychosocial interventions include memory retraining, learning and problem-solving activities, reminiscence therapy, behavior therapy, and stress reduction. These have been studied and found to improve or slow cognitive decline (Cacchione, 2000). Validation therapy, developed by Feil (1993), is an approach for communicating with elders with dementia in order to improve communication and orientation and reduce problematic behaviors (Benjamin, 1999; Feil, 1993). A structured environment and maintenance of social support are also helpful. Use of the creative arts (music, art therapy, and drama) have also been found to be effective (Sterritt & Pokorny, 1994). Pet therapy studies have also documented numerous positive effects. The creative approaches and programs that have been utilized with frail elders with dementia are too numerous to mention; however, the general goal for all is improvement or maintenance in quality of life (Volicer & Bloom-Charette, 1999).

CAREGIVER ISSUES, ABUSE, AND NEGLECT

Health care providers are uniquely suited to identify and report such cases to the appropriate authorities, and are required by law to do so if they suspect mistreatment. Poor care may be defined broadly as any act that has the potential to harm the patient emotionally, physically, or financially (Schultz & Williamson, 1997). Physical abuse such as hitting a patient, tying someone to a chair, shaking or pinching an older patient is the easiest for a caregiver to recognize. Detecting psychological abuse, such as threatening to put someone in a nursing home, yelling, or locking a patient in a room is more difficult. Physical neglect includes things such as not giving a patient proper nutrition, proper medical care, or adequate supervision, and can be picked up by providers with a careful history and physical examination. Psychological neglect such as not providing a loving environment is very difficult to discern, however. Exploitation includes theft or misuse of an older person's resources (Schultz & Williamson, 1997). If mistreatment is suspected, it is important to interview the patient and the suspected abuser separately, and to provide a safe place for the frail elder if the home environment is deemed too unsafe for them to return. Involvement of the state's Department of Elderly Affairs or Adult Protection Services can provide resources to investigate suspected cases and take proper action when required.

Caregivers are a necessary safety net for many older patients. They merit provider's attention to reduce caregiver stress and burnout so as to go on providing care at the highest quality for the longest amount of time possible with a minimum of impact on the caregiver's health status.

Health care providers focused on the physiological condition may overlook the possibility that therapy has failed as a result of noncompliance with the treatment plan. There may also be a reluctance of the caregivers to admit to the noncompliance due to fear of the legal implications. In addition, the interpersonal relations between the patient and the caregiver may be different when in the physician's office environment, thus not arousing suspicion on the part of the physician. Home visits by nurses, social workers, health aides and other members of the care team can be instrumental in identifying an abusive relationship (Matthias & Benjamin, 2003).

Once suspected or identified the treatment of an abusive situation can be difficult. Concern over the potential legal ramifications frequently leads to under-reporting. Also fear of disrupting a fragile therapeutic relationship can lead to the avoidance of confrontation with caregivers. Consideration of the various factors leading to the problem, and an interdisciplinary approach are essential for a successful resolution of the problem.

SYNDROME-CENTERED STRATEGIES

General health strategies that have multisystem effects (e.g., exercise and nutrition) play a key role in preventing and treating frailty, in addition to having a positive effect on most of the accompanying problems of frailty such as falls, dementia, depression, and comorbid conditions. Of the three types of strategies for treating and preventing frailty—exercise, nutrition, and medications—exercise remains the most widely studied and the most effective (Borst, 2004).

Exercise

Numerous studies have documented the effectiveness of exercise in slowing the functional decline associated with frailty. In 1990, Fiatarone et al. studied high-intensity strength training in frail nursing home residents in their 90s, and found an average increase of 174% in muscle strength along with an increase in muscle size and functional mobility after the 8-week intervention. In a subsequent study in 1994, the effects of high-intensity resistance exercise and nutritional supplements in frail older adults were studied (Fiatarone et al., 1994). Findings showed a 113% increase in muscle strength compared to 3% in nonexercisers, 11.8% improvement in gait velocity (3.6% decline in control group), improved stair climbing ability, and increased level of spontaneous physical activity. The nutritional supplement had no effect on primary outcome measures among nonexercisers but did increase total energy intake among exercisers. This study demonstrated that it is possible, through vigorous resistance exercise, to reverse the functional decline associated with frailty. Other selected RCT studies documenting positive effects of exercise in frail older adults are listed in Table 2.1. Although some studies with shorter interventions, such as Hageman and Thomas (2002) with a 6-week resistance training program fail to show significant improvement in functional measures, most exercise intervention studies do show improvement.

Nutrition

Nutritional factors have been noted to play an important role in frailty; however, fewer studies have addressed nutritional interventions. The term "nutritional frailty" has been used to refer to a sudden accelerated weight loss together with sarcopenia (a loss of muscle mass and strength) (Bales & Ritchie, 2002). Inadequate food intake is common among older adults with estimates of more than 60% of older people ingesting less than the recommended daily allowance for energy and protein (Kinney, 2004). A study comparing low protein with recommended daily protein diets found that older women on low protein diets for 9 weeks had decreased muscle mass, decreased nitrogen balance, and muscle weakness (Castaneda, Charnley, Evans, & Crim, 1995). Thus, it seems that in a short time, protein malnutrition can make a dramatic impact on muscle mass and function (Roubenoff, 2003). Correcting malnutrition is more difficult among frail older adults than among younger people, emphasizing the importance of prevention (Hebuterne, Berman, & Schneider, 2001).

Impaired nutritional status has also been associated with cognitive impairment (Gonzales-Gross, Marcos, & Pietrzik, 2001). Wouters–Wessling et al. (2001) studied the effect of an enriched drink on cognitive function in frail elders and found improvements in two of four tests of cognitive functioning after 6 months. Adequate hydration is also necessary as frail older adults are at high risk of dehydration, which may increase the severity of illness as well as the risk of death (Kleiner, 1999). In general, frail elders should receive at least 1500 cc of fluid per day with adjustments made according to environment factors, although it may sometimes be possible to maintain fluid balance with less (Feinsod et al., 2004).

TABLE 2.1 Summary of Selected Random Controlled Trials of Exercise Interventions with Frail Older Adults

Author	Sample	Results
Binder et al. (2002)	115 community-dwelling men and women with mild-moderate physical frailty, mean age = 83	Intensive 12-month exercise training improved physical function, performance, and VO$_2$ max
Gill et al. (2002)	188 community-dwelling physical frail men and women, aged 75 or more	9-month PT program focusing on improving balance, strength, and transfer ability, reduced functional decline among those with moderate (not severe) frailty
Wolf et al. (2003)	200 community-dwelling frail men and women, mean age = 76.2	15-week tai chi and balance training reduced risk of multiple falls and had a positive effect on biomedical and psychosocial indices of frailty
Lord et al. (2003)	551 self- and intermediate care people in retirement villages in Australia, mean age = 79.5	12-month group exercise program reduced falls, increased stepping reaction time, 6 min. walking distance, and simple reaction time.
Baum et al. (2003)	20 frail nursing home resides aged 75–99	1-year group exercise program with range of motion and strength training, reduced time in Timed Up & Go test, improved physical performance, balance, and cognition.
Brown et al. (2000)	84 frail older adults attending out patient rehab., mean age = 83	3-month low-intensity supervised exercise showed significant improvement in physical performance, increased flexibility, strength gait speed and balance.
Villareal et al. (2003)	28 physically frail women on hormone replacement therapy aged 75 year or more	9-month supervised PT, resistance and endurance exercise increased bone mineral density and muscle strength.

Pharmacotherapy Interventions

Pharmacological interventions are being developed in response to research evidence for biological factors underlying frailty and sarcopenia. Drugs relating to growth factors (such as IGF-1 and nerve growth factors), to hormones (such as testosterone), and nutritional supplements (such as protein powder and creatine) are being examined for their effectiveness in treating frailty (Lynch, 2004). More research will be forthcoming in this area.

SYSTEMS OF CARE

Frail elders, by definition, need assistance with ADLs and IADLs and require supportive care. Internationally, several different systems of care have been developed to meet these needs; however, fewer systems are available in the United States (Johnston & Reifler, 1999). There is a lack of medical and nonmedical care that addresses problems encountered by frail older people. Systems that deliver culturally competent care to frail elders, provide case management services, target at-risk older adults, develop partnerships with families, use telemedicine and assistive technology, and promote healthy aging are needed to address the issues of this population (Young, 2003).

Most frail older adults prefer to remain at home; however, this is dependent on having a willing and able caregiver. Approximately 18% of older people aged 85 years or older reside in nursing homes (National Center for Health Statistics, 2004). Day care centers provide care for people with serious physical and mental disabilities, including dementia, and offer a variety of activities such as exercise, crafts, music, and bathing. These have proliferated in numbers over the past 25 years, however, still fall short of the projected national need (Reifler, 1992). Dementia care units are specialty units that incorporate environmental modifications and are often part of a nursing home. These provide supportive and nursing care to people with dementia who are unsafe to live alone. Although dementia care units do not appear to slow functional decline (Phillips et al., 1997), they do seem to be less costly than traditional nursing home care, and improve resident comfort and satisfaction.

Group living homes have been used successfully for care of demented and frail older adults in Scandinavian countries. These facilities offer 24-hour staffing and have been shown to improve quality of life with less cost than institutional care (Annerstedt, 1997; Malmberg & Zarit, 1993).

Other systems have been developed to provide comprehensive care to frail older adults residing in the community. The Program for All-inclusive

Care for Elderly (PACE), emerging in the 1970s, provides interdisciplinary care, hospital and long-term care, pharmacy services, and specialist services if needed with the goal of providing quality comprehensive care at lower cost (Boult & Pacala, 1999; Mui, 2001). Following its early successes, PACE was designated as a permanent Medicare program in 1997; however, the number of PACE programs has not grown as expected (Gross, Temkin-Greener, Kunitz, & Mukamel, 2004).

Hospital Care

Hospitals are particularly hostile environments for frail elders, frequently triggering a cascade of decline. Moving to a fast-paced, high-tech environment, away from their social supports and usual routines often precipitates delirium and loss of functional capacity (Calkins & Naughton, 1999). Specialized Geriatric Evaluation Units, where interdisciplinary staff assess and give direct care to patients on the unit have been found to decrease subsequent rates of institutionalization, improve 6-month function, and decrease mortality (Applegate et al., 1990).

Acute Care for the Elderly (ACE) units use a biopsychosocial model, provide function-oriented interdisciplinary team interventions, and emphasize fitting the hospital environment to the patient's needs. Study results show that patients receiving care on an ACE unit had improved functional outcomes at discharge at lower cost than the usual hospital care (Covinsky et al., 1998). ACE units, however, are not being widely utilized by hospitals. Given the clinical, functional, and economic benefits, further exploration of barriers to implementation of these types of units is needed (Jayadevappa, Bloom, Raziano, & Lavizzo-Mourey, 2003).

A different hospital-wide approach, the Hospitalized Elder Life Program (HELP), screens patients age 70 or older on admission and targets interventions to identified risk factors using an interdisciplinary team approach. Results of a clinical trial testing HELP indicate that this approach prevents cognitive and functional decline in at-risk elders (Inouye, Bogardus, Baker, Leo-Summers, & Cooney, 2000).

Long-Term Care

Long-term care can be either community- or nursing home-based. Community services such as visiting nurse services, social services, physical therapy, Meals on Wheels, and respite care can support caregivers to maintain their frail family member at home. A health care initiative using nurse and social worker case managers provided traditional hands-on care along with distance-based health care through a telehealth unit in elder's homes. This unit was used for regular in-home physical assessment providing two-way audio and visual communication allowing the nurse to complete a comprehensive physical assessment. Outcomes of this program showed a decrease in emergency room visits, decreased emergency department costs, a decline in hospital admissions, decreased hospital costs, and decreased length of stay in the hospital (Duke, 2005).

The PACE program and small "board and care" homes have also been shown to be less costly community-based alternatives to nursing home care (Ford, 1999). Outcome studies show that community-based long-term care does not increase survival or reduce the rate of decline, however. Some studies show a decrease in unmet needs and improvement in patient and caregiver life satisfaction; however, these satisfaction levels seem to diminish over time (Weissert & Hedrick, 1999). Assisted living environments do not generally offer the level of care usually needed by frail elders.

Nursing-home-based long-term care provides 24-hour skilled nursing care with most of the daily care delivered by nursing assistants with minimal education. The nursing assistants are supervised by LPNs or RNs, who also frequently lack education about older people's special needs. There is wide variation in both quality of care and quality of life in nursing homes; however, a discussion of these issues is beyond the scope of this chapter. There is much literature that addresses these areas (Arling, Kane, Lewis, & Mueller, 2005; Kane, 1981, 2003), and efforts to improve nursing home care are underway. Programs to change the culture of nursing homes such as the Eden Alternative and the Pioneer Network are examples of changes that positively affect both quality of life and quality of care in nursing homes.

Advance Directives

A discussion of care of frail elders would be remiss without addressing issues of advance directives. Advance directives have become an important issue in facility-based health care since the Patient Self-Determination Act, a federal law passed in 1990, which requires that health care facilities ask patients about advance directives upon admission (U.S. Congress, 1990). Despite the majority of the population being in favor of completing living wills, however, only about 20% of the population has completed a living will (Emanuel, Barry, Stoeckle, Ettelson, & Emanuel, 1991; Miles, Koepp, & Weber, 1996). A recent study by Kahana, Dan, Kahana, and Kercher (2004) showed that 18% of caregivers and 73% of primary care physicians for older adults did not know their preferences about end-of-life care. Completing advance directives with elderly frail patients is an important preventive health measure that clinicians must undertake (Happ et al., 2002).

The frail older adult population can greatly benefit by advance directive planning, not only because they have a high mortality rate but also because inherently, they interact with health care systems frequently and in the case of residents of long-term care facilities, live daily with the ability to have aggressive and life-sustaining treatments instituted by trained health care professionals. In addition, as many frail elderly have cognitive impairment that precludes their participating directly in determining their care, an advance directive completed before they became cognitively impaired helps guide their treatment and care in a way they would have wanted before they became ill.

The ideal time to discuss advance directives with a patient is when he or she is well and competent to make decisions for themselves. Unfortunately, health care professionals often find themselves having this discussion at times of crisis, which results in oversimplification and a great deal of burden on families called in at the last minute to make difficult choices. Ideally, an advance directive should start with a discussion of a patients' own set of values rather than a check list of what they do or do not want to be done. For example, a patient may say, "if I cannot take care of myself, I do not wish to become a burden on my family," or "When I can no longer recognize my loved ones, I do not wish to live any more" and these values-based statements can then be applied to real-life situations to complete the check list of what people do and do not want to be done for them (Doukas & McCullough, 1991).

To ensure that the care a patient receives is in keeping with his or her wishes, making a living will as specific as possible is very important. Many legal documents are loosely worded that people not receive "life-sustaining measures" if a patient's condition is "deemed terminal" or in cases of "permanent unconsciousness" (Annas & Glantz, 1986). End-of-life care improves if advance directives can name specific interventions, such as intubation and resuscitation, having a feeding tube, receiving intravenous fluids or antibiotics, receiving dialysis, and being transported back to the hospital. These specifics should be in a written document that is signed by a patient and/or surrogate decision-maker and two witnesses who are not related to the patient or decision maker or physician. Although legal issues vary from state to state, most states will honor a document completed in this fashion.

A very important part of end-of-life conversations is the designation of a surrogate decision maker, a durable power of attorney for health care. This person ideally should act as the patient himself, making decisions in a manner that the patient would have if they were able to. However, in practice, the surrogate often makes decisions as he or she would want the treatment to proceed. A patient's detailed and written advance directive may help guide the surrogate to act in the way the patient would have wanted, and restrict surrogate decisions to specific clinical situations that could not be anticipated when the directive was written (Emanuel & Emanuel, 1989).

The last thing important to consider in advance planning is that at any time, a patient's or family's wishes can change, and reviewing their stated preferences periodically as their health status changes ensures that the document continues to reflect their true preferences (Straton et al., 2004).

SUMMARY

The complex needs of frail older adults challenge health care providers, staff, and family members who care for them. The intensity of care required strains even the most progressive health care systems. As the number of frail older adults increases with the growth of the older population as a whole, demands on the health care system, especially long-term care, become increasingly difficult. The emphasis currently is on treating frailty by improving strategies at the individual and system levels. Developing and testing innovative strategies to meet the frail elders' needs is one approach that merits attention. Educating health care professionals of all kinds and direct caregivers (such as nursing assistants) about the unique needs of this population also holds much promise for improving care. Working to change the acute and long-term care environments to more successfully meet the frail older person's needs also has the potential to improve patient's outcomes. The greatest potential for success however lies in two areas. The current research being done on antecedents and risk factors of frailty offers hope for discovery of underlying biological and physiological factors. There is potential for these factors to then be altered to prevent or limit progression of frailty itself. The second area offering hope requires behavior change on the part of the older person. The single most important action older adults can take to forestall frailty seems to be maintenance of an active lifestyle including regular moderate and vigorous exercise. Lastly, attitude change on the part of older adults, health care providers, and the public in general is essential. No one is surprised when a 90-year-old becomes frail. The expectation of frailty as a part of advanced old age is common as a condition associated with functional decline and death. There are many older adults who do not become frail, however, as evidenced in the centenarian studies. Changing the attitudes of society from one of an expectation of frailty to anticipation of a long, functional life is necessary but will be the greatest challenge.

REFERENCES

Alexopoulos, G. S., Abrams, R. C., Young, R. C., & Shamoian, C. A. (1988). Cornell Scale for Depression in Dementia. *Biological Psychiatry, 23,* 271–284.

Annas, G. J., & Glantz, L. H. (1986). The right of elderly patients to refuse life-sustaining treatment. *Milbank Quarterly, 64*(Suppl. 2), 95–162.

Annerstedt, L. (1997). Group-living care: An alternative for the demented elderly. *Dementia and Geriatric Cognitive Disorders, 8*(2), 136–142.

Applegate, W. B., Miller, S. T., Graney, M. J., Elan, J. T., Burns, R., & Akins, D. E. (1990). A randomized controlled trial in a geriatric assessment unit in a community rehabilitation hospital. *New England Journal of Medicine, 322,* 1572–1578.

Arling, G., Kane, R. L., Lewis, T., & Mueller, C. (2005). Future development of nursing home quality indicators. *Gerontologist, 45*(2), 147–156.

Bales, C. W., & Ritchie, C. S. (2002). Sarcopenia, weight loss, and nutritional frailty in the elderly. *Annual Review of Nutrition, 22,* 309–323.

Baum, E. E., Jarjoura, D., Polen, A.E., Faur, D., & Rutecki, G. (2003). Effectiveness of a group exercise program in a long-term care facility: a randomized pilot trial. *Journal of the American Medical Director's Association, 4*(2), 74–80.

Benjamin, B. J. (1999). Validation: A communication alternative. In L. Volicer & L. Bloom-Charette (Eds.), *Enhancing the Quality of Life in Advanced Dementia* (pp. 107–125). Philadelphia: Brunner/Mazel.

Binder, E. F., Schechtman, K. B., Ehsani, A. A., Steger-May, K., Brown, M., Sinacore, D. R., Yarasheski, K. E., & Holloszy, J. O. (2002). Effects of exercise training on frailty in community-dwelling older adults: results of a randomized, controlled trial. *Journal of the American Geriatric Society, 50,* 1921–1928.

Bloem, B. R., Steijns, J. A., & Smits-Engelsman, B. C. (2003). An update on falls. *Current Opinion in Neurology, 1,* 15–26.

Borst, S. E. (2004). Interventions for sarcopenia and muscle weakness in older people. *Age and Ageing, 33*(6), 548–555.

Boult, C., & Pacala, J. T. (1999). Integrating care. In E. Calkins, C. Boult, D. H. Wagner, & J. T. Pacala (Eds.), *New ways to care for older people: Building systems based on evidence* (pp. 196–209). New York: Springer Publishing.

Braun, J. A., & Capezuti, E. (2000). The legal and medical aspects of physical restraints and bed siderails and their relationships to falls and fall-related injuries in nursing homes. *DePaul Journal of Health Care Law, 4*(1), 1–72.

Brown, M., Sinacore, D. R., Ehsani, A. A., Binder, E. F., Holloszy, J. O., & Kohrt, W. M. (2000). Low-intensity exercise as a modifier of physical frailty in older adults. *Archives of Physical and Medical Rehabilitation, 81,* 960–965.

Buckwalter, K., Katz, I., & Martin, H. (2004a, Winter). Guide to the prevention and management of falls in the elderly part I. *CNS/ LTC, CNS News,* pp. 7–11.

Buckwalter, K., Katz, I., & Martin, H. (2004b, Spring). Guide to the prevention and management of falls in the elderly, part II. *CNS/LTC, CNS News,* pp. 31–36.

Cacchione, P. Z. (2000). Cognitive and neurologic function. In A. G. Lueckenotte (Ed.), *Gerontologic nursing* (2nd ed., pp. 615–654). St. Louis: Mosby.

Calkins, E., & Naughton, B. J. (1999). Care of older people in the hospital. In E. Calkins, C. Boult, D. H. Wagner, & J. T. Pacala (Eds.), *New ways to care for older people: Building systems based on evidence* (pp. 99–111). New York: Springer Publishing.

Capezuti, E., Strumpf, N. E., Evans, L. K., Grisso, J. A., & Maislin, G. (1998). The relationship between physical restraint removal and falls and injuries among nursing home residents. *Journals of Gerontology A Biological and Medical Sciences, 53*(1), M47–M52.

Castaneda, C., Charnley, J. M., Evans, W. J., & Crim, M. C. (1995). Elderly women accommodate to a low-protein diet with losses of body cell mass, muscle function, and immune response. *American Journal of Clinical Nutrition, 62*, 30–39.

Chouinard, G. (2004). Issues in the clinical use of benzodiazepines: Potency, withdrawal, and rebound. *Journal of Clinical Psychiatry, 65*(Suppl. 5), 7–12.

Clark, P. G., Leinhaus, M. M., & Filinson, R. (2002). Developing and evaluating an interdisciplinary clinical team training program: Lessons taught and lessons learned. *Educational Gerontology, 28*(6), 511–529.

Covinsky, K. E., Palmer, R. M., Kresevic, D. M., Kahana, E., Counsell, S. R., Fortinsky, R. H., & Landesfeld, C. S. (1998). Improving functional outcomes in older patients: Lessons from an acute care for elders unit. *Joint Commission Journal on Quality Improvement, 24*(2), 63–76.

Doukas, D. J., & McCullough, L. B. (1991). The values history, the evaluation of the patients values and advance directives. *Journal of Family Practice, 32*(2).145–153.

Drinka, T. J. K., & Clark, P. G. (2000). *Health care teamwork: Interdisciplinary practice and teaching*. Westport, CT: Auburn House.

Dugu, M., Neugroschl, J., Sewell, M., & Marin, D. (2003). Review of dementia. *Mt. Sinai Journal of Medicine, 70*(1), 45–53.

Duke, C. (2005). The frail elderly community-based case management project. *Geriatric Nursing, 26*(2), 122–127.

Ellis, G., & Langhorne, P. (2005). Comprehensive geriatric assessment for older hospital patients. *British Medical Bulletin, 71*, 45–59.

Emanuel, L. L., Barry, M. J., Stoeckle, J. D., Ettelson, L. M., & Emanuel, E. J. (1991). Advance directives for medical care—a case for greater use. *New England Journal of Medicine, 324*, 889–895.

Emanuel, L. L., & Emanuel, E. J. (1989). The medical directive: A new comprehensive advance care document. *Journal of the American Medical Association, 261*, 3288–3293.

Farr, B. M., Johnson, B. L., & Cobb, D. K. (1995). Preventing pneumococcal bacteremia in patients at risk: Results of a matched case-controlled study. *Archives of Internal Medicine, 155*, 2336–2340.

Feil, N. (1993). *The validation breakthrough*. Baltimore: Health Professions Press.

Feinsod, F. M., Levenson, S. A., Rapp, K., Rapp, M. P., Beechinor, E., & Leibmann, L. (2004). Dehydration in frail, older residents in long-term care facilities. *Journal of the American Medical Directors Association, 5*(Suppl. 2), S35–S41.

Fiatarone, M. A., Marks, E. C., Ryan, N. D., Meredith, C. N., Lipsitz, L. A., & Evans, W. J. (1990). High-intensity strength training in nonagenarians. Effects on skeletal muscle. *Journal of the American Medical Association, 263*, 3029–3034.

Fiatarone, M. A., O'Neill, E. F., Ryan, N. D., Clements, K. M., Solares, G. R., Nelson, M. E., Roberts, S. B., Kehayias, J. J., Lipsitz, L. A., & Evans, W. J. (1994). Exercise training and nutritional supplementation for physical frailty in very elderly people. *New England Journal of Medicine, 330*, 1769–1775.

Folstein, M. F., Folstein, S. E., & McHugh, P. R. (1975). Mini-mental state: Practical method for grading the cognitive state of patients for the clinician. *Journal of Psychiatric Research, 12*(3), 189–198.

Ford, A. B. (1999). Overview of community-based long-term care. In E. Calkins, C. Boult, D. H. Wagner, & J. T. Pacala (Eds.), *New ways to care for older people: Building systems based on evidence* (pp. 135–142). New York: Springer Publishing.

Frengley, J. D., & Mion, L. C. (1998). Incidence of physical restraints on acute general medical wards. *Journal of the American Geriatrics Society, 34*, 565–568.

Fretwell, M. D. (1997). Comprehensive geriatric assessment. In F. F. Ferri, M. D. Fretwell, & T. J. Wachtel (Eds.), *Practical guide to the care of the geriatric patient* (2nd ed., pp. 19–25). St. Louis: Mosby.

Fretwell, M. D. (1990). Acute hospital care for frail older patients. In W. R. Hazzard, R. Andres, E. L. Bierman, & J. P. Blass (Eds.), *Principles of geriatric medicine and gerontology* (pp. 247–253). New York: McGraw-Hill.

Fried, L. P., Ferrucci, L., Darer, J., Williamson, J. D., & Anderson, G. (2004). Untangling the concepts of disability, frailty, and comorbidity: Implications for improved targeting and care. *Journals of Gerontology A: Biological and Medical Science, 59*, 255–263.

Gallo, J. J. (2000). Mental status assessment. In J. J. Gallo, T. Fulmer, G. J. Paveza, & W. Reichel (Eds.), *Handbook of geriatric assessment* (3rd ed., pp. 29–100). Gaithersburg, MD: Aspen.

George, L. K., & Gwyther, L. P. (1986). Caregiver well-being: A multidimensional examination of family caregivers of demented adults. *Gerontologist, 26*, 253–259.

Gill, T. M., Baker, D. I., Gottschalk, M., Peduzzi, P. N., Allore, H., & Byers, A. (2002). A program to prevent functional decline in physically frail, elderly persons who live at home. *New England Journal of Medicine, 347*, 1068–1074.

Gonzales-Gross, M., Marcos, A., & Pietrzik, C. (2001). Nutrition and cognitive impairment in the elderly. *British Journal of Nutrition, 86*, 313–321.

Gross, D. L., Temkin-Greener, H., Kunitz, S., & Mukamel, D. B. (2004). The growing pains of integrated health care for the elderly: Lessons from the expansion of PACE. *Milbank Quarterly, 82*(2), 257–282.

Hageman, P. A., & Thomas, V. S. (2002). Gait performance in dementia: The effects of a 6-week resistance training program in an adult day-care setting. *International Journal of Geriatric Psychiatry, 17*, 329–334.

Happ, M. B., Capezuti, E., Strumpf, N. E., Wagner, L., Cunningham, S., Evans, L., & Maislin, G. (2002). Advance care planning and end-of-life care for hospitalized nursing home residents. *Journal of the American Geriatrics Society, 50*, 829–835.

Hebuterne, A., Berman, S., & Schneider, S. M. (2001). Aging and muscle: The effects of malnutrition, re-nutrition, and physical exercise. *Current Opinion in Clinical Nutrition and Metabolic Care, 4*, 295–300.

Higashi, T., Shekelle, P. G., Solomon, D. H., Knight, E. L., Roth, C., Chang, J. T., et al. (2004). The quality of pharmacologic care for vulnerable older patients. *Annals of Internal Medicine, 140*(9), p. 152.

Highfield, M. E. F. (2001). Spiritual and religious care. In T. T. Fulmer, M. D. Foreman, & M. Walker (Eds.), *Critical care nursing of the elderly* (pp. 326–352). New York: Springer Publishing.

Inouye, S. K., Bogardus, S. T. Jr., Baker, D. I., Leo-Summers, L., & Cooney, L. M. Jr. (2000). The Hospital Elder Life Program: A model of care to prevent cognitive and functional decline in older hospitalized patients. *Hospital Elder Life Program. Journal of the American Geriatrics Society, 48*, 1697–1706.

Jayadevappa, R., Bloom, B. S., Raziano, D. B., & Lavizzo-Mourey, R. (2003). Dissemination and characteristics of acute care for elders (ACE) units in the United States. *International Journal of Technology Assessment in Health Care, 19*(1), 220–227.

Johnston, D., & Reifler, B. V. (1999). Comprehensive care of older people with Alzheimer's Disease. In E. Calkins, C. Boult, D. H. Wagner, & J. T. Pacala (Eds.), *New ways to care for older people: Building systems based on evidence* (pp. 158–167). New York: Springer Publishing.

Jones, D. M., Song, X., & Rockwood, K. (2004). Operationalizing a frailty index from a standardized comprehensive geriatric assessment. *Journal of the American Geriatrics Society, 52*, 1929–1933.

Kahana, B., Dan, A., Kahana, E., & Kercher, K. (2004). The personal and social context of planning for end-of-life care. *Journal of the American Geriatrics Society, 52*, 1163–1167.

Kane, R. A. (1981). Assuring quality of care and quality of life in long term care. *Quality Review Bulletin, 7*(10), 3–10.

Kane, R. A. (2003). Definition, measurement, and correlates of quality of life in nursing homes: Toward a reasonable practice, research, and policy agenda. *Gerontologist, 43*(Spec No. 2), 28–36.

Katz, I. R. Streim, J., & Parmalee, P. (1994). Prevention of depression, recurrences, and complications in late life. *Preventive Medicine, 23*, 743–750.

Kinney, J. M. (2004). Nutritional frailty, sarcopenia and falls in the elderly. *Current Opinion in Clinical Nutrition and Metabolic Care, 7*, 15–20.

Kleiner, S. M. (1999). Water: An essential but overlooked nutrient. *Journal of the American Dietetic Association, 99*, 200–206.

Laird, R. D., & Studenski, S. A. (1999). Assessment. In E. L. Cobbs, E. H. Duthie, & J. B. Murphy (Eds.), *Geriatric review syllabus* (4th ed., pp. 75–79). Dubuque, IA: Kendall/Hunt.

Lord, S. R., Castell, S., Corcoran, J., Dayhew, J., Matters, B., Shan, A., & Williams, P. (2003). The effect of group exercise on physical functioning and falls in frail older people living in retirement villages: a randomized, controlled trial. *Journal of the American Geriatrics Society, 51*, 1685–1692.

Lynch, G. S. (2004). Emerging drugs for sarcopenia: Age-related muscle wasting. *Expert Opinion on Emerging Drugs, 9*(2), 345–361.

Malmberg, B., & Zarit, S. H. (1993). Group homes for people with dementia: A Swedish example. *Gerontologist, 33*(5), 682–686.

Margolis, K. L., Nichol, K. L., Poland, G. A., & Pluhar, R. E. (1990). Frequency of diverse reactions to influenza vaccine in the elderly, a randomized placebo-controlled trial. *Journal of the American Medical Association, 264*, 1139–1141.

Matthews, M., Lucas, A., Boland, R., Hirth, V., Odenheimer, G., Wieland, D., Williams, H., & Eleazer, G. P. (2004). Use of a questionnaire to screen for frailty in the elderly: An exploratory study. *Aging Clinical and Experimental Research, 16*(1), 34–40.

Matthias, R. E., & Benjamin, A. E. (2003). Abuse and neglect of clients in agency-based and consumer-directed home care. *Health and Social Work, 28*(3), 174–184.

Mezey, M., & Fulmer, T. (1998). Quality care for the frail elderly. *Nursing Outlook, 46*, 291–292.

Miles, S. H., Koepp, R., & Weber, E. P. (1996). Advance end-of-life treatment planning: A research review. *Archives of Internal Medicine, 156*, 1062–1068.

Milisen, K., DeGeest, S., Abraham, I. L., & Delooz, H. H. (2001). Delirium. In T. T. Fulmer, M. D. Foreman, & M. Walker (Eds.), *Critical care nursing of the elderly* (2nd ed.). New York: Springer Publishing, 41–52.

Miller, M. (1978). Geriatric suicide: The Arizona study. *Gerontologist, 18*(5 Pt. 1), 488–495.

Mion, L. C. (1996). Establishing alternatives to physical restraint in the acute care setting: A conceptual framework to assist nurses' decision making. *AACN Clinical Issues, 7*(4), 592–602.

Mion, L. C., Fogel, J., Sandhu, S., Palmer, R. M., Minnick, A. F., Cranston, T., et al. (2001). Outcomes following physical restraint reduction programs in two acute care hospitals. *Joint Commission Journal on Quality Improvement, 27*(11), 605–618.

Mui, A. C. (2001). The Program of All-Inclusive Care for the Elderly (PACE): An innovative long-term care model in the United States. *Journal of Aging and Social Policy, 13*(2–3), 53–67.

National Center for Health Statistics. (2004). *Health, United States, 2004 with chartbook on trends in the health of Americans.* Washington, DC: U.S. Government Printing Office.

Neelon, V. J., Champagne, M. T., Carlson, J. R., & Funk, S. G. (1996). The NEECHAM Confusion Scale: Construction, validation, and clinical testing. *Nursing Research, 45*(6), 324–330.

North American Nursing Diagnosis Association. (1999). *Nursing diagnoses: Definitions and classification 1999–2000.* Philadelphia: Author.

O'Connell, A. M., & Mion, L .C. (2003). Use of physical restraints in the acute care setting. In M. D. Mezey, T. Fulmer, & I. Abraham (Eds.), *Geriatric nursing protocols for best practice*. New York: Springer Publishing.

Overcash, J. A., Beckstead, J., Extermann, M., & Cobb, S. (2005). The abbreviated comprehensive geriatric assessment (aCGA): A retrospective analysis. *Critical Reviews in Oncology/Hematology, 54*(2), 129–136.

Phillips, C. D., Sloane, P. D., Hawes, C., Koch, G., Han, J., Spry, K., et al. (1997). Effects of residence in Alzheimer's disease special care units on functional outcomes. *Journal of the American Medical Association, 278*, 1340–1344.

Reifler, B. V. (1992). Making something good out of something bad. *Respite Report, 4*, 3.

Reuben, D. B. (1999). Principles of geriatric assessment. In W. R. Hazzard, J. P. Blass, W. H. Ettinger, Jr., J. B. Halter, & J. G. Ouslander (Eds.), *Principles of geriatric medicine and gerontology* (4th ed., pp. 467–481). New York: McGraw-Hill.

Roubenoff, R. (2003). Sarcopenia: Effects on body composition and function. *Journals of Gerontology Biological and Medical Sciences, 58*, M1012–M1017.

Rubenstein, L. Z. (2004). Joseph T. Freeman award lecture—comprehensive geriatric assessment: From miracle to reality. *Journals of Gerontology A: Biological and Medical Sciences, 59*: M473–M477.

Rubenstein, L. Z., Josephson, K. R., Wieland, G. D., English, P. A., Sayre, J. A., & Kane, R. L. (1984). Effectiveness of a geriatric evaluation unit: A randomized control trial. *New England Journal of Medicine, 311*, 1664–1670.

Schmader, K. E., Hanlon, J. T., Pieper, C. F., Ruby, C. M., Francis, S. D., Branch, L. G., Lindblad, C. I., Artz, M., Weinberger, M., Feussner, J. R., & Cohen, H. J. (2004). Effects of geriatric evaluation and management on adverse drug reactions and suboptimal prescribing in the frail elderly. *American Journal of Medicine, 116*, 394–401.

Schneider, D. C., & Mader, S. L. (2002). Falls. In R. J. Ham, P. D. Sloane, & G. A. Warshaw (Eds.), *Primary care geriatrics: A case-based approach* (4th ed., pp. 349–359). St. Louis: Mosby.

Schultz, R., & Williamson, G. M. (1997). The measurement of caregivers outcomes in Alzheimer's disease research. *Alzheimer's Disease and Associated Disorders, 11*(Suppl. 6), 117–124.

Sheikh, J. I., & Yesavage, J. A. (1986). Geriatric Depression Scale (GDS): Recent evidence and development of a shorter version. In T. L. Brink (Ed.), *Clinical gerontology: A guide to assessment and intervention* (pp. 165–174). New York: Hayworth Press.

SHEP Cooperative Research Group. (1991). Prevention of stroke by antihypertensive drug treatment in older persons with isolated systolic hypertension: Final results of the Systolic Hypertension in the Elderly Program (SHEP). *Journal of the American Medical Association, 265*, 3255–3264.

Sisk, J., Moskowitz, A. J., Whang, W., Lin, J. D., Fedson, D. S., McBean, A. M. et al. (1997). Cost-effectiveness of vaccination against pneumococcal bacteremia among elderly people. *Journal of the American Medical Association, 278*, 1333–1339.

Siu, A. L., Reuben, D. B., & Moore, A. A. (1994). Comprehensive geriatric assessment. In W. R. Hazzard, E. L. Bierman, J. P. Blass, Ettinger, W. H., Jr., & Halter, J. B. (Eds.), *Principles of geriatric medicine and gerontology* (3rd ed., pp. 203–211). New York: McGraw-Hill.

Sterritt, P. F., & Pokorny, M. E. (1994). Art activities for patients with Alzheimer's and related disorders. *Geriatric Nursing, 15*, 155–159.

Straton, J. B., Wang, N. Y., Meoni, L. A., Ford, D. E., Klag, M. J., Casarett, D., & Gallo, J. J. (2004). Physical functioning, depression, and preferences for treatment at the end of life: The Johns Hopkins precursors study. *Journal of the American Geriatrics Society, 52*, 577–582.

Strawbridge, W. J., Shema, S. J., Balfour, J. L., Higby, H. R., & Kaplan, G. A. (1998). Antecedents of frailty over three decades in an older cohort. *Journals of Gerontology B: Psychological and Social Sciences, 53*(1), S9–S16.

Stuck, A. E., Siu, A. L., Wieland, G. D., Adams, J., & Rubenstein, L. Z. (1993). Effects of comprehensive geriatric assessment on survival, residence, and function: A meta-analysis of controlled trials. *Lancet, 342*, 1032–1036.

Studenski, S., Hayes, R., Leibowitz, R. Q., Bode, R., Lavery, L., Walston, J., Duncan, P., & Perera, S. (2004). Clinical global impression of change in physical frailty: Development of a measure based on clinical judgment. *Journal of the American Geriatrics Society, 52*, 1560–1566.

Tinetti, M. E (1997). Falls. In C. K. Cassel, H. J. Cohen, & E. B. Larson (Eds.), *Geriatric medicine* (3rd ed.). New York: Springer-Verlag.

U.S. Congress. (1990). *Patient Self-Determination Act. OBRA,* Pub L, 101–508.

U.S. Preventive Task Force. (1996). *Guide to clinical preventive services: Report of the US Preventive Task Force* (2nd ed.). Baltimore: Williams and Wilkins.

Villareal, D. T., Binder, E. F., Yarasheski, K. E., Williams, D. B., Brown, M., Sinacore, D. R., & Kohrt, W. M. (2003). Effects of exercise training added to ongoing hormone replacement therapy on bone mineral density in frail elderly women. *Journal of the American Geriatrics Society, 51*, 985–990.

Volicer, L., & Bloom-Charette, L. (1999). Assessment of quality of life in advanced dementia. In L. Volicer & L. Bloom-Charette (Eds.), *Enhancing the quality of life in advanced dementia* (pp. 3–20). Philadelphia: Brunner/Mazel.

Weissert, W. G., & Hedrick, S. C. (1999). Outcomes and costs of home and community-based long-term care: Implications for research-based practice. In E. Calkins, C. Boult, D. H. Wagner, & J. T. Pacala (Eds.), *New ways to care for older people: Building systems based on evidence* (pp. 143–157). New York: Springer Publishing.

Williams, M. A., Campbell, E. B., Raynor, W. J., Mlynarczyk, S. M., & Ward, S. E. (1985). Reducing acute confusional states in elderly patients with hip fractures. *Research in Nursing and Health, 8*, 329–337.

Wolf, S. L., Barnhart, H. X., Kutner, N. G., McNeely, E., Coogler, C., Xu ,T., & Atlanta FICSIT Group. (2003). Selected as the best paper in the 1990s: Reducing frailty and falls in older persons: an investigation of tai chi and computerized balance training. *Journal of the American Geriatrics Society, 51*, 1794–1803.

Wouters-Wessling, W., Wagenaar, L. W., Rozendaal, M., Deijen, J. B., deGroot, L. C., Bindels, J. G., et al. (2001). Effect of an enriched drink on cognitive function in frail elderly persons. *Journals of Gerontology A: Biological and Medical Sciences, 60A,* 265–270.

Yesavage, J., & Brink, T. L. (1983). Development and validation of a geriatric depression screening scale: A preliminary report. *Journal of Psychiatric Research, 17,* 37–49.

Young, H. (2003). Challenges and solutions for care of frail older adults: *Online Journal of Issues in Nursing* 8:2. Available at www.nursingworld.org/ojin/topic21/tpc21_4.htm

PART II

Aging Prisoners

CHAPTER THREE

Health Issues of Aging Prisoners

T. Smyer and M. Gragert

Aging offenders form a distinct but growing minority of the approximately 2 million people incarcerated in the United States prison system. Older adults who are prisoners are a very heterogeneous population with great variability in health and functional status. In general, they experience multisystem alterations in physiological and psychological functioning that accompany normal aging, in addition to an increased risk of poor health related to socioeconomic status and lifestyle behaviors (Lindquist & Lindquist, 1999; Maruschak & Beck, 2001). The older adult inmates are, on an average, physically 10–11.5 years older than their chronological age related to tobacco use, substance abuse, diet, poverty, and minimal or sporadic health care (Aday, 1994; Edwards, 1998). Add to this the attendant stressors of life in a correctional institution, and it becomes apparent that this is an especially vulnerable population with complex health care needs (Kuhlmann & Ruddell, 2005).

Several studies document the rapidly growing older inmate population and the complex economic and sociopolitical issues surrounding prison health care, making this an important area of concern that must be addressed in an ethical, just, and humane manner (Harrison & Beck, 2005; James, 2004). This predicament, meeting the needs of older prisoners while absorbing the rapidly expanding cost of health care in a correctional system, poses a distinct ethical and moral dilemma. Mara (2004) points out that people may question why attention is being given to health care needs of older inmates when the needs of older adults in the free population are not fully addressed. Ruddell and Tomita (2005) posit that there is a "greater economic hazard by not responding to the health problems within correctional populations" and that incarceration is an ideal time for public health interventions (p. iv).

This chapter presents demographics and background information regarding the general prison environment, including a description of correctional subcultures and categories of older prisoners. A key to understanding the vulnerability of the aging offender is knowledge of the unique environment of the correctional institution. A brief description of changes in sentencing laws is presented to understand the sociopolitical context of aging inmates. The physical and mental health needs of this client group are also described.

THE U.S. CORRECTIONAL SYSTEM

The criminal justice system in the Unites States has multiple and diverse incarceration facilities. There is no centralized system; each state and the federal government have their own systems. Inconsistencies exist across correctional institutions within and between states, causing much confusion. Aging offenders can be found in state and federal prisons, territorial prisons, local jails, U.S. Immigration and Naturalization Service facilities, military facilities, and in Bureau of Indian Affairs or tribal facilities. Additionally, as of mid-year 2003, 6.5% of state and federal inmates were housed in privately operated facilities (U.S. Department of Justice [USDOJ], 2004). Typically, prisons hold inmates with sentences of more than 1 year. Jails are locally operated correctional facilities that confine persons before or after adjudication, and may also incarcerate persons in other categories.

There are approximately 1,500 state, public, and private correctional facilities, 84 federal facilities, and 26 private facilities for federal prisoners (Siegel & Senna, 2004). Based on security concerns, the prisons are classified into maximum, medium, and minimum security (Siegel & Senna, 2004). Additionally, prisons, whether private, federal, or state, all use a system to classify the prisoner's custody/supervision level within the correctional institution (Budd, 1996). These systems vary depending on the correctional institution, however, the principle goal is to accurately identify inmates who are most likely to engage in violent behavior, escape, or have disciplinary problems (Budd, 1996).

Demographics

The total number of incarcerated individuals held in state and federal prisons and jails in 2003 in the United States was 2,085,620 as reported in the Bureau of Justice Statistics Bulletin of November 2004 (USDOJ, 2004). Approximately two thirds of these are in prisons with one third in jails. Texas (166,911), California (164,487), and the federal system (173,059) together held one in every four prisoners in the United States. Approximately half of all prisoners are serving time for violent crimes, followed by 20% for drug offenses and 19% for property offences, such as theft (USDOJ, 2004).

Statistics also indicate that the prison population is aging (USDOJ, 2004). There is growing consensus in the United States in correctional systems about how to define "elderly" with the majority of correctional departments using age of 50 years or older (Aday, 2003; Kuhlmann & Ruddell 2005; Morton, 1992). Researchers, however, use the age of 50 or 55 years in defining the chronological age of elderly inmates, many reporting agencies may still use 55 years as a defining age (Aday, 2003; Kuhlmann & Ruddell, 2005).

The number of offenders aged 55 and older in the state or federal prisons and local jails, in midyear 2003, was 66,200 males and 3,800 females representing 3.4% and 2.1% of the total prison and jail populations, respectively (USDOJ, 2004). The greatest increase (24.4%) in number of inmates sentenced annually between 1995 and 2003 was in the age group of 40–54 years. In the total prison population, inmates in this age group accounted for approximately 46% of the total growth in the U.S. prison population since 1995. In the same time period, population of inmates aged 55 and older increased 85%, more than any other age group. The mean age of sentenced inmates at the time of admission is also increasing. In 2003, the mean age was 33 compared to 31 in 1995 (USDOJ, 2004).

Men are almost 15 times more likely to be incarcerated than women. The lifetime likelihood of going to state or federal prison is estimated to be 1 in every 20 persons (5.1%) with a higher likelihood for men (9%) than for women (1.1%). The rate of incarceration is growing the most for females with a 48% increase; however, the total number of male prisoners has also grown by 29% since 1995. At year end in 2003, state or federal prisons housed 1 in every 1,613 women and 1 in every 103 men in the United States (USDOJ, 2004).

The ethnic proportions found in the criminal justice system do not reflect the overall proportions found in the United States, and to some extent are related to the Sentencing Reform Act of 1984. These federal laws increased the penalties for drug sale and use (Mauer, 1992). Willmott and van Olphen (2005) related that the War On Drugs is the major driver for racial disparities in the correctional system. Although drug use among juveniles is lower for Blacks than for Whites, and only 0.4% higher for Black adults (Substance Abuse and Mental Health Services Administration, SAMSHA, 2004), the majority of those arrested, prosecuted, and given stiff mandatory sentences are Blacks. At the end of the year 2003, there were 3,405 sentenced Black male inmates per 100,000 Black males in the United States compared to 1,231 sentenced Hispanic male inmates per 100,000 Hispanic males and 465 White male inmates per 100,000 White males (USDOJ, 2004). Although Blacks represent only about 12% of the general population, Black inmates represented 44% of all male inmates with sentences greater than 1 year, Hispanics comprised 19%, and Whites 35%. The lifetime likelihood of going to state or federal prison is greater for Blacks and Hispanics than for Whites. Black males have a one in four chance of incarceration, Hispanic males have a one in six chance of incarceration, and White males have a 1 in 23 chance of incarceration (USDOJ, 2004). Although incarceration rates drop with age, the percentage of black males in the age group of 45–54 in prison in 2003 was 3.5%, still considerably higher than the rate for young (25–29 years old) Hispanics (2.6%) and young white males (1.1%).

The overall rate of prison incarceration and length of time served are steadily increasing, now averaging a growth in the prison population of 3.4% per year since 1995. The current U.S. incarceration rate is 715 per 100,000, up from 601 per 100,000 in 1995. The average time served among released inmates was 30 months in 2003 compared to 23 months in 1995 (USDOJ, 2004). This growth is not consistent among prison systems with the federal system growing the most rapidly, by 5.8%, in 2003. Other states with the highest growth are, in order, Texas, Florida, and California along with eight other states. New York, Michigan, and 11 other states had decreases in prison populations, however not enough to offset the increases, resulting in an increase in the total prison population. There are also differences in growth rates by region of the country. Overall, in 2003 the number of inmates incarcerated in the West increased 2.9%, followed by the South (2.2%) and the Midwest (.8%). In the Northeast, the number of inmates declined by 1.5% in the same period of time. State prisons were estimated to be at full capacity to 16% above capacity, while the federal prisons were operating at 39% above capacity (USDOJ, 2004). This steady growth of the prison population in the United States causes an increased strain on an already overburdened prison system. Much of this growth can be attributed to a trend for increase in length of sentence and a sharp increase in time served in prison.

POLITICS OF THE CRIMINAL JUSTICE SYSTEM

It would be remiss to discuss the background of correctional institutions without including the politics of the criminal justice system. The United States, as "the land of the free," now incarcerates a higher percentage of its citizens than any other country (Human Rights Watch, 2003). The two primary goals of incarceration are protection of the public and punishment of offenders. Rehabilitation of prisoners had also been a third goal before the mid-1970s, when prison rehabilitation was criticized on several fronts (Mara, 2004). Politicians have frequently touted being "tough on crime" as a campaign issue. Public policy changes, such as mandatory minimum sentencing, the "three strikes law" (a California law passed in 1994 that mandates life imprisonment for defendants that have three or more prior felony convictions), and decreasing availability of parole or early release have been enacted toward that effort. Rather than protecting the public from serious and violent offenders, however, these policies have instead produced increasingly high rates of confinement of nonviolent offenders. The "War on Drugs," as mentioned previously, has perhaps been the single greatest force behind the growth in the prison population, particularly among women and minorities (Ruddell & Tomita, 2005). Evidence for the lack of success in meeting the goals of protecting the public and rehabilitation of prisoners can be found in such statistics as the high recidivism rate, almost 70% nationally, and the increased incarceration rates of nonviolent offenders (USDOJ, 1994).

Another trend identified by Freely and Simon (1992) is the "new penology" and its emphasis on managing the correctional milieu as a "waste management" system rather than focusing on rehabilitation. Fearn and Parker (2005) stated that this new penology is "more concerned with the actuarial aspects of penology and how to manage efficiently" (p. 6). Those in the dangerous class of criminals are viewed as unredeemable with any investment in this dangerous class seen as futile. The waste management model would entail securing its members at the lowest possible cost (Simon, 1993), placing little emphasis on quality health care for those who are incarcerated.

Finally, when risk factors for criminal behavior are considered, sociopolitical issues again become apparent. Risk factors associated with criminal behavior include male gender, social and economic disadvantage, persistent unemployment, difficult home environment including child abuse and dysfunctional parenting, lack of success in school, and substance abuse (Community Safety and Crime Prevention Council, 1996). Many of these risk factors have their roots in sociopolitical/social justice issues. In addition, the greater percentage of minorities than Whites in prisons may be a reflection of racial disparities, civil rights issues, racial profiling by police, and discrimination beginning with the inequitable treatment of non-White juveniles in the justice system (And Justice for Some, 2000). Thus, the current approach to crime seems to be resulting in a burgeoning, costly, aging prison population without accomplishing two of the three major goals of incarceration.

SUBCULTURES WITHIN THE CORRECTIONAL ENVIRONMENT

Three distinct subcultures emerge when the correctional system is examined: the inmate subculture, the administration subculture, and the health care subculture (Smyer, Gragert, & LaMere, 1997). Each correctional facility varies, however, and will define and have different features that are particular to that system. The older offender is a participant in each of these subcultures. The first two subcultures will be discussed in this chapter, while the health care subculture will be discussed briefly here as well as in greater depth in the following chapter.

Prisoner Subculture

The "inmate subculture" was identified and articulated with the work of Clemmer (1958). His identification of "prisonization" was an important step in understanding the dynamics of change that occur within the individual imprisoned for some time (Siegel & Senna, 2004). The concept of "total institutions" also plays a role in understanding this microcosm of the free world. *Asylums*, a classic work by Erving Goffman (1961), defined total institutions as "places of residence and work where a large number of like-situated individuals, cut off from the wider society for an appreciable period of time, together lead an enclosed, formally administered round of life" (p. xiii). Prisons meet the criteria of total institutions with prison life assuming "batch living" or enforced intimate contact with individuals with whom one would not necessarily choose contact (Goffman, 1961).

The first feature of the total institution and prison is its physical barrier to the outside world. In a confined area, prisoners are cut off from normal social activities and outside contacts become limited. This separation or physical barrier occurs to protect society and acts as punishment for prisoners, or as a setting for rehabilitative measures (LaMere, Smyer, & Gragert, 1996).

Development of a unique way of life is the second feature of a total institution. The free world has certain commonalties of social arrangements, delineations, and expectations. In prison, these may no longer be valid. The "normal" interactions in which most persons in the outside world participate are altered and a new culture is born (LaMere et al., 1996). This culture is an amalgamation of both the formal prison policies and the informal inmate "con code." Although distinct prison subcultures are based on race, prior activities, or interests, these differences serve to contribute to the overall social network of the pervasive prison culture (Goffman, 1961; Sykes, 1970).

"Don't snitch, do your own time, don't show weakness, and maintain respect and dignity" (Irwin, 1980, p. 12) was the old convict code. Group loyalty to the prison population as a whole was part of this code. Siegel and Senna (2004) related that currently correctional systems have strong homogeneous gangs that form along racial lines, and these gangs may have new inmate codes that replace the original code. Siegel and Senna (2004) state that "older, respected inmates could no longer cross racial lines to mediate disputes. Predatory inmates could victimize others without fear of retaliation. Consequently, more inmates than ever are now assigned to protective custody for their own safety" (p. 421). Older offenders believe they are at risk for predation and this adds a stressor to their daily life and interaction (Tartaro, 2002; Vega & Silverman, 1988). Irwin (1980) related that the newer convict code, while incorporating basic tenets of the older code such as "no snitching," has as a central tenet of "toughness" with underlying themes of violence to uphold this persona (Kupers, 2001; Struckman-Johnson & Struckman-Johnson, 2000). The inmate in today's prisons is more prone to violence and will combat threats to reputation or self-concept of "machismo," or if the prisoner feels "disrespected" (Irwin, 1980).

Administrative Subculture

The administrative subculture is made up of correctional officers, clerical workers, social workers, rehabilitation personnel, and other individuals needed to maintain and run the correctional system. Clear and Cole (2000) related that correctional institutions are paramilitary in organization, with ranks of officer, sergeant, lieutenant, and captain. Very clear chains of command as well as lines of communication and responsibility are established.

The role of Correctional Officer is one of the most stressful occupations in society, and second only to a police officer, is the highest risk job in the United States and abroad (Mayhew & Chappell, 2002). There are high incidences of stress-related illnesses such as hypertension and alcoholism, with twice the divorce rate compared with other blue- and white-collar workers. Siegel and Senna (2004) stated that correctional officers are no longer just "guards" but are responsible for diverse and complex role orientation, "and the greatest problem faced by correctional officers is the duality of their role: maintainers of order and security and advocates of treatment and rehabilitation" (p. 433).

Similar to nurses in hospitals, correctional officers have the maximum contact with inmates and are required to counsel, supervise, protect, and process inmates in their care (Smyer et al.,1997). The need for more training for correctional personnel about issues related to aging has been called for (Aday, 1994; Morton, 1992). Knapp and Elder, in a 1998 study, assessed Oklahoma prison personnel ($N = 127$) using Palmore's Facts on Aging Quizzes I and II. Three categories of correctional personnel were identified as particularly in need of training about aging issues: younger personnel, those with less formal education, and those with greater contact with the inmates. Conclusions were that additional training regarding aging and health problems of older adults was needed for prison personnel.

Health Care Subculture

The health care subculture is made up of physicians, nurses, technicians, psychologists, dentists and anyone directly involved in provision of health care to prisoners. Since the 1970s, lawsuits by inmates have changed the face of correctional health care. Schlanger (2003) related that inmate health care was the leading cause of lawsuits in jails and prisons in a recent study.

The offenders' right to health care was mandated in 1976 when violation of the 8th amendment was cited in the landmark Texas case *Estelle v. Gamble* 429 US 97 (1976), and the U.S. Supreme Court ruled that "deliberate indifference to the serious medical needs of prisoners constitutes the unnecessary and wanton infliction of pain" (Siegel & Senna, 2004). From this case, it was determined that the inmate has three basic constitutional rights to health care: the right of access to care, the right to care that is ordered, and the right to a professional medical judgment. Of the seven identified substantive rights of prisoners, three of them relate to health care: medical rights, freedom from cruel and unusual punishment, and the right to minimal conditions necessary for survival, such as medical care (see Table 3.1). Additionally, Rold (1998) related that the Americans with Disabilities Act requires that "correctional officials will have to make substantial efforts to make

TABLE 3.1 Substantive Rights

Access to courts, legal services, and materials
Freedom of the press and expression
Freedom of religion
Medical rights
Freedom from cruel and unusual punishment
Right to the minimal conditions necessary for human survival, such as food, clothing, shelter, and medical care

Adapted from Siegel and Senna (2004).

their services, programs, and activities available to inmates suffering from paralysis, deafness, blindness, and other actual and perceived physical or mental handicaps" (p. 351).

PROFILE OF THE AGING OFFENDER

Aday (2003) identified three types of older offenders: the first-time offender, the habitual or chronic offender, and the aging offender. Goetting (1983) described this third category as "old timers," the offender who has been sentenced at a young age to life in prison without parole.

The first-time offender is usually over age 60 and comprises approximately 40–45% of the older adults imprisoned (Aday, 2003). His/her crimes usually consist of family violence, fraud, drug sales, sex offences, or alcohol-related crimes (Aday, 1994; Fry, 1988). First-time offenders are subject to adjustment problems, as well as predatory behavior from other inmates if placed in the general prison population. The skills needed to survive in prison often are antithetical to the survival skills of the outside world. Fortunately, because of family and community ties, these inmates have a better prognosis for placement in community prerelease programs or prison early release programs (Morton, 1992). The health status of these individuals is likely to reflect the normal decrements and diseases of aging.

The second type, the chronic offender, has participated in criminal activity for most of his or her life. He or she usually adjusts more quickly to the prison environment and routine as a result of multiple past incarcerations. Community release, however, poses a problem, as family and community ties may be tenuous at best (Morton, 1992). The chronic offender's health status is usually poor due to the fact that alcohol, drug abuse, and personality disorders are frequently associated with this type of aged offender (Morton, 1992). Because of poor or nonexistent medical follow-up, chronic conditions usually are well established.

Those who have aged in place comprise the third type of aging offender. Incarcerated as young offenders, usually for an abhorrent criminal act, they have received long sentences. Much of this time may have been spent in maximum-security arrangements with minimal socialization. Community release poses a very difficult problem for this type of offender. The lifetime of aging within the prison system has not prepared the inmate for community release programs. Family and community ties usually have been severed long before release becomes an option (Smyer et al., 1997). The unique culture of prison life results in a loss of autonomy. Inmates become incapable of managing life outside of the structure of prison because of the lost opportunity to develop traditional adult behavioral roles. The inmate may actually view life outside of prison with great trepidation because of the social disconnection between prison life and the unpredictable world outside of prison. Few of the landmarks of adult rites of passage are available to the older inmate. The aged inmate is also unable to measure success or life milestones in material items, such as homes, cars, or other personal possessions. This has the potential to produce a sense of social disconnection involving losses of traditional adult roles and comprises a battery of challenges to the self-concept of the aging prisoner. The health status of this type of prisoner reflects the priorities of health care delivery in his or her prison (LaMere et al., 1996).

HEALTH PROBLEMS OF THE AGED OFFENDER

There is a paucity of research on health needs of prisoners in general and even less on the needs of older prisoners (Lemieux, Dyson, & Castiglione, 2002). It is known, however, that all categories of aged offenders have more health problems than older adults in the general population (McGuire, 2005; National Commission on Correctional Health Care (NCCHC), 2002). Physical decrements associated with the aged offender mirror those in the free world; however, because of physiological factors related to lifestyle in and out of prison and the concomitant increased risk factors, approximately 10–11.5 years may be added chronologically to the age of a prisoner as stated earlier (Aday, 1994; Edwards, 1998). Limited education, poverty, minority status, and unemployment, along with factors such as high-risk behaviors, nutritional deficiencies, substance abuse, or homelessness, add to the compromised overall health status of many older prisoners (Aday 2003; Goldkuhle, 1999).

Approximately one third of state inmates and one fourth of federal inmates of all ages report having a mental condition or physical impairment. Among those aged 45 or older, 48% of state inmates and 39% of federal inmates stated they had a physical impairment or mental condition. Of these, 15.7% of state and 17.7% of federal inmates required surgery for their conditions. Older inmates were also more likely than younger inmates to report difficulty in hearing (13%) and seeing (20%) (USDOJ, 1997). Many inmates in the United States reported having multiple impairments (25% of state and 21% of federal) or that their impairment limited the kind or amount of work they could do. Medical problems were more prevalent among prisoners who were homeless or unemployed at the time of their arrest. On the positive side, fewer older inmates reported being injured either in an accident or in a fight since admission (USDOJ, 1997).

TABLE 3.2   Medical Problems of State and Federal Inmates

Medical problem	Percentage of state inmates(%)	Percentage of federal inmates(%)
Skeletal	2.6	3.1
Circulatory (other than heart)	2.4	2.4
Heart problems	1.1	1.3
Diabetes	0.9	1.5
HIV/AIDS	1.7	0.5
Kidney/liver	0.9	1.4
Respiratory	1.4	1.2
Neurological	0.7	0.4
Cancer	0.2	0.3

From USDOJ (1997).

In a 1997 survey, inmates in state and federal correctional facilities were asked to specify medical problems that they have had since admission to prison. The most commonly reported problems across all age groups were skeletal, circulatory other than heart, heart problems, cancer, diabetes, HIV/AIDS, kidney/liver problems, respiratory problems, and neurological problems. Table 3.2 lists these problems along with the percentages of state and federal inmates reporting each problem.

Aday (2003) compared chronic illnesses of older inmates across studies of older offenders in four state systems (total $N = 618$). Although the percentages varied, he found that almost 40% of older inmates reported having problems with arthritis, with 39% reporting having high blood pressure. Other problems, each affecting about 20% of the older inmates, were heart problems, emphysema, stomach ulcers, and prostate problems. Urinary tract problems, diabetes, and asthma were reported as problems for 9–17% of older inmates responding. Related to functional status, Aday (2001) reported ranges from 17.5% of the sample of inmates needing at least some help with ADLs to 98.7% reported by Douglass (1991).

A study of health issues among older male prisoners in Great Britain also found that 85% of older prisoners had one or more major illnesses, the most common being psychiatric, cardiovascular, musculoskeletal, and respiratory (Fazel, Macmillan, & O'Donnell, 2002). The aging prisoner, along with his or her free world counterpart, may experience frailty and dependence, loss of control, and powerlessness requiring both emotional and spiritual adjustment (Mara, 2004).

May and Lambert (1998) identified HIV, violence, and smoking-related illnesses as the three leading causes of morbidity and mortality in the correctional population in general. In a study of 119 aging prisoners, Colsher, Wallace, Loeffelholz, and Sales, (1992) reported increased rates of incontinence, sensory impairment, and flexibility impairment. Missing teeth were found in 97%, 42% had gross physical functional impairments, and 79% smoked tobacco. Forty percent of these prisoners had histories of hypertension, 19% with previous myocardial infarction, and 18% with emphysema. These studies document the increased physical health problems and corresponding health care needs of older inmates.

Substance abuse is a problem all too familiar to the correctional population. Peters, Greenbaum, Edens, Carter, and Ortiz, (1998) found that out of 400 inmates incarcerated in a Texas prison, approximately 75% had a substance abuse or dependence disorder. Medical problems of all kinds were more common among inmates who had used a needle to inject drugs and among those who were alcohol dependent based on the CAGE diagnostic assessment tool (USDOJ, 1997).

Incarcerated individuals are also underimmunized, with higher rates of hepatitis virus infection (A, B, and C), sexually transmitted diseases, and tuberculosis infection (Askins, Malecki, & Thomas, 2005; Bureau of Justice Statistics, 2002; McGuire, 2005). Other common types of infections encountered in correctional facilities are pneumonia, HIV/AIDS and accompanying opportunistic infections, soft-tissue infection such as cellulitis, and febrile neutrogena (Piliero, Curtin, Szebenyi, & Remick, 1998). Older adults often have weaker immune systems making them more vulnerable to infectious diseases. The chronic stress experienced by older offenders may further weaken immune system functioning.

Mental health issues are a widespread problem within the correctional population as well. Kupers (2001) related that the jails and prisons have become the largest psychiatric facilities in the United States. With deinstitutionalization of the mentally ill population from state hospitals in the 1970s in the United States, a phenomenon known as transinstitutionalization has occurred that documents movement from the state hospitals to nursing homes and correctional institutions (Stein & Alaimo, 1998). This has resulted in a documented increase in percentages of inmates with mental illness in 25 states (National Institute of Corrections, 2001). In a national survey, Ditton (1999) found that just over 15% of inmates aged 55 and over in state prisons and 9% in federal prisons showed signs of frequent mental illness. The highest rates of mental illness were among White females with an estimated 29% identified as mentally ill compared to 20% of Black females and 22% of Hispanic females. A small study of inmates in a U.S. federal correction facility found that 53.7% met criteria for psychiatric disorder (Koenig, et al., 1995). In a recent 12-country study of prisoners, Siegel and Senna (2004) report that 4% were psychotic, 10% had major depression, and 65% had personality disorders with 47% diagnosed with antisocial personality disorder. These studies show that mental health issues are indeed a significant problem for older inmates nationally.

Depression is one of the most common mental health disorders in older adults and the aged prisoner is also at high risk. Depression may be caused by medical illness, chronic pain, polypharmacy, sleep disturbances, and selected stressors (Shua-Haim, Sabo, Comsti, & Gross, 1997; Smyer & Graham, 2003). Older adults may complain of somatic or cognitive symptoms rather than feelings of sadness. They may present in a "manic defense" mode and may appear to be cheerful yet overly "busy." Significant indicators may be changes in sleep patterns, increased or decreased appetite, physical complaints, psychomotor retardation or agitation, lack of energy, as well as cognitive impairments (Shua-Haim et al., 1997; Smyer & Graham, 2003).

The prison culture reflects turbulent and unpredictable levels of violence (Human Rights Watch, 2001; Kuhlmann & Ruddell, 2005). Violence is an identified stressor affecting the older adult prisoner. This enduring stressor can contribute to physical deterioration, particularly in the inmate with chronic illness. The convict in today's prison will use extremes of violence to combat threats to their reputation or self-concept of "machismo" or if the inmate feels "disrespected." The aged prisoner may have chronic pervasive stress levels disguised under a tough veneer and be more prone to self-harm or suicide (Kuhlmann & Ruddell, 2005).

The conditions of persistent stress inherent in a correctional setting impose continual wear and tear on individuals and contribute to the aging process and ill health (Smyer et al., 1997). The decreased adaptive capacity of the aging prisoner makes maintenance of homeostasis more difficult and can contribute to increased mortality and morbidity in this population. Decreased adaptive capacity may manifest as sleep, appetite, and somatic complaints in response to stress or depressive disturbance. McGuire and Pastore (2005) reported that in a recent federal study of state and federal prisons, inmates were three times as likely to commit suicide than to die in an assault.

Cognitive changes due to alcohol and substance misuse may take place in the younger inmate as well as the aging inmate; however, dementia of Alzheimer's type (DAT) is more prevalent with increasing age. Vascular dementia as well as amnestic disorder may also occur in this population and may reflect poor lifestyle choices. Although no documentation on prevalence rates of cognitive impairment among older inmates could be found, one study reported diagnoses of 55 defendants aged 62–88 who were referred for assessment of competence to stand trial. Among this group, 19% were diagnosed with severe dementia (Rosner, Wiederlight, Harmon, & Cahan, 1991). Those caring for older prisoners must be alert to signs of cognitive decline and the many possible causes of cognitive or behavioral changes. Ethical implications arise regarding the continuing incarceration of those with advanced dementia (Fazel et al., 2002).

SUMMARY

The prison population in the United States is growing annually with the over 55-year-old age group increasing most rapidly. Although older adult inmates form a small minority in the U.S. prison population, their numbers are expected to increase continuously. The older prisoners consist of three types: first-time offenders, chronic offenders, and those who have "aged in place." Forty to forty-five percent of older prisoners are first-time offenders, which makes adjustment to the prison role much more difficult and dangerous. Black and Hispanic older and younger offenders represent a disproportionately higher percent of the prison population. The female prison population is growing at an even more rapid rate than the incarcerated male population. The use of drugs and alcohol has substantially contributed to reasons for incarceration. Physical and mental health problems within the older prison population are numerous and add to the cost of caring for these individuals. Major physical health problems include skeletal, circulatory and heart problems, cancer, diabetes, HIV/AIDS, kidney/liver problems, respiratory, and neurological problems. Depression, stress-related disorders, and personality disorders are common mental health issues.

Although health care, costs, and housing have taken center stage in the care of the aging inmate, there is much work to be done by researchers in diverse disciplines to explicate the true nature of the older offender in prison. Lemieux et al. (2002) suggest that much of the literature available about the elder inmate is not supported by robust research studies. Research priorities for older inmates that include a typology of older inmates, a representative survey of health status, and a systematic evaluation of existing programs are needed. Once a clear picture emerges of the health status of aging offenders, strategies can be designed that will be more effective in meeting their many health needs within the constraints of the prison system.

REFERENCES

Aday, R. (1994). Aging in prison: A case study of new elderly offenders. *International Journal of Offender Therapy and Comparative Criminology, 38(1)*, 79–81.

Aday, R. (2001). *A comprehensive health assessment of aged and infirm inmates.* Nashville, TN: Tennessee Department of Correction.

Aday, R. (2003). *Aging prisoners crisis in American corrections.* Westport, CT: Praeger.

And Justice for Some report. (2000). Retrieved May 20, 2005 from http://www.buildingblocksforyouth.org/justiceforsome/jfs.html

Askins, D., Malecki, J., & Thomas, D. (2005). Tuberculosis outbreak among staff in correctional facilities, Florida, 2001–2004; Lessons re-learned. *Infectious Disease in Corrections Report, 8*, 1–5.

Budd, M. (1996). *Montana state prison inmate classification overview.* Deer Lodge, MT: Department of Corrections.

Bureau of Justice Statistics. (2004) Retrieved September 29, 2004 from http://www.ojp.usdoj.gov/bjs/

Clear, T., & Cole, G. (2000). *American corrections* (2nd ed.). Belmont, CA: Wadsworth.

Clemmer, D. (1958). *The prison community.* New York: Holt Rinehart & Winston

Colsher, P., Wallace, R., Loeffelholz, P., & Sales, M. (1992). Health status of older male prisoners: A comprehensive survey. *American Journal of Public Health, 82*, 881–884.

Community Safety and Crime Prevention Council. (1996). Root causes of crime. Waterloo, CT: Community Safety and Crime Prevention Council. Retrieved July, 15, 2005 from www.preventingcrime.net/library/Causese_of_Crime.pdf

Ditton, P. (1999) *Mental health and treatment of inmates and probationers* (NCH 174463). Washington, DC: Department of Justice, Bureau of Justice Statistics.

Douglass, R. L. (1991). *Oldtimers: Michigan's elderly prisoners.* Lansing, MI: Michigan Department of Corrections.

Edwards, T. (1998). *Aging inmate population.* Atlanta, GA: Southern Legislative Council of the Council of State Government.

Fazel, S., McMillan, J., & O'Donnell, I. (2002). Dementia in prison: Ethical and legal implications. *Ethics, Law, & Medicine, 28*, 156–159.

Fearn, N., & Parker K. (2005). Health care for women inmates: Issues, perceptions and policy considerations. *California Journal of Health Promotion, 3* (2), 1–23.

Freely, M., & Simon, J. (1992). The new penology: Notes on the emerging strategy of corrections and its implications. *Criminology, 30*, 449–474.

Fry, L. (1988). The concerns of older inmates in a minimum security prison setting. In B. McCarthy & R. Langworthy (Eds.), *Older offenders perspectives in criminology and criminal justice.* New York: Praeger.

Goetting, A. (1983). The elderly in prison: Issues and perspectives. *Journal of Research in Crime and Delinquency, 20*, 291–309.

Goffman, E. (1961). *Asylums: Essays on the social situation of mental patients and other inmates.* Chicago: Aldine.

Goldkuhle, U. (1999). Health service utilization by women in prison: Health needs indicators and response effects. *Journal of Correctional Health Care, 1*, 63–83.

Harrison, P., & Beck, A (2005) *Prisoners at midyear 2004.* Washington, DC: Bureau of Justice Statistics.

Human Rights Watch (2003). *Incarcerated America.* Retrieved 2/4/06 http://www.hrw.org/backgrounder.

Irwin, J. (1980). *Prisons in turmoil.* Boston, MA: Little, Brown.

James, D. (2004). *Profile of jail inmates, 2002.* Washington, DC: Bureau of Justice Statistics.

Knapp, J. L., & Elder, K. B. (1998). Assessing prison personnel's knowledge of the aging process. *Journal of the Oklahoma Criminal Justice Research Consortium, 4*, 1997–1998. Retrieved July 15, 2005 from https//www.doc.state.ok.US/DOCS/OCJRC/OCJRC 97–98/1997_research.htm.

Koenig, H. G., Johnson, S., Bellard, J., Denker, M., & Fenlon, R. (1995). Depression and anxiety disorder among older male inmates at a federal correctional facility. *Psychiatric Services, 46*, 399–401.

Kuhlmann, R., & Ruddell, R. (2005). Elderly jail inmates: Problems, prevalence, and public health. *California Journal of Health Promotion, 3*(2), 49–60.

Kupers, T. (2001). *Prison madness: The mental health crisis behind bars and what we must do about it.* San Francisco: Jossey-Bass.

Lamere, S., Smyer, T., & Gragert, M. (1996). The aging inmate. *Journal of Psychosocial Nursing, 34*(4), 25–29.

Lemieux, C., Dyson, T., & Castiglione, B. (2002). Revisiting the literature on prisoners who are older: Are we wiser. *Prison Journal, 82*, 440–458.

Lindquist, C. H., & Lindquist, C. A. (1999). Health behind bars: Utilization and evaluation of medical care among jail inmates. *Journal of Community Health, 24*, 285–303.

Mauer, M. (1992). Men in American prisons: Trends, causes and issues. *Men's Studies Review, 9*, 10–12.

May, J. P., & Lambert, W. E. (1998). Medical ethics and correctional health care. In M. Puisis (Ed.) *Clinical practice in correctional medicine.* St. Louis: Mosby.

Mayhew, C., & Chappell, D. (2002). An overview of occupational violence. *Australian Nursing Journal, 9*, 34–35.

Mara, C. (2004). Chronic illness, disability, and long-term care in the prison setting. In P. R. Katz, M. D.Mezey, & M. B. Knapp, (Eds.), *Vulnerable populations in the long-term care continuum* (pp. 39–56). New York: Springer.

Maruschak, L., & Beck, A. (2001). *Bureau of Justice Statistics special report: Medical problems of inmates, 1997.* Washington, DC: U.S. Department of Justice, Office of Justice Programs.

McGuire, M. (2005). The impact of prison rape on public health. *California Journal of Health Promotion, 3*(2), 72–83.

McGuire, K., & Pastore, A. (2005). Sourcebook of criminal justice statistics. Retrieved October 6, 2005, from http://www.albany.edu/sourcebook/pdf/ t60001.pdf

Morton, J. (1992). *An administrative overview of the older inmate.* Washington, DC: U.S. Department of Justice and National Institute of Corrections.

National Commission on Correctional Health Care. Standards for Health Services. (2002). Retrieved May 24, 2005 from http://www.ncchc.org/

National Institute of Corrections. (2001). Provision of mental health care in prisons. Washington, DC: National Institute of Corrections, February, 2001. Retrieved December 17, 2005 from http://www.nicic.org/pubs/2001/016724.pdf

Peters, R., Greenbaum, P., Edens, J., Carter, C., & Ortiz, M. (1998). Prevalence of *DSM IV* substance abuse and dependence disorders among prison inmates. *American Journal of Drug and Alcohol Abuse, 24,* 573–580.

Piliero, P. P., Curtin, J. P. Szebenyi, S., & Remick, S. C. (1998). Management of serious infections in correctional facilities. *Infections in Medicine, 15*(3), 179–183, 187–191.

Rold, W. J. (1998). Medical ethics and correctional health care. In M. Puisis (Ed.), *Clinical practice in correctional medicine.* St. Louis: Mosby.

Rosner, R., Wiederlight, M., Harmon, R. B., & Cahan, D. J. (1991). Geriatric offenders examined at a forensic psychiatry clinic. *Journal of Forensic Sciences, 36,* 1722–1731.

Ruddell, R., & Tomita, M. (2005). Opportunities for change in correctional and community health. *California Journal of Health Promotion, 3*(2), iv–x.

Schlanger, M. (2003). Inmate litigation. *Harvard Law Review, 116,* 1555–1706.

Shua-Haim, J., Sabo, M., Comsti, E., & Gross, J. (1997). Depression in the elderly. *Hospital Medicine, 33*(7), 45–48.

Siegel, L. J., & Senna, J. J. (2004). *Introduction to Criminal Justice.* Stamford, CT: Wadsworth.

Simon, J. (1993). *Poor discipline: Parole and the social control of the underclass, 1890-1990.* Chicago: University of Chicago Press.

Smyer, T., & Graham, M. (2003). Mental health. In C. Uphold & M. Graham, (Eds.), *Clinical guidelines in family practice.* Gainesville, FL: Barmarrae.

Smyer, T., Gragert, M., & LaMere, S. (1997). Stay safe! Stay healthy! Surviving old age in prison. *Journal of Psychosocial Nursing and Mental Health Services, 35*(9), 10–17.

Stein, L., & Alaimo, C. (1998). Medical ethics and correctional health care. In M. Puisis(Ed.), *Clinical practice in correctional medicine.* St. Louis: Mosby.

Struckman-Johnson, C., & Struckman-Johnson, D. (2000). Sexual coercion rates in seven midwestern prison facilities for men. *Prison Journal, 80,* 379–390.

Substance Abuse and Mental Health Services Administration (SAMSHA). (2004). *Results from the 2003 National Survey on Drug Use and Health: National findings* (Office of Applied Studies, NSDUH Series H-25, DHHS Publication No. SMA 04-3964). Rockville, MD: US Government Printing Office.

Sykes, G. (1970). *The society of captives: A study of maximum security prison.* New York: Athenaeum.

Tartaro, C. (2002). The impact of density on jail violence. *Journal of Criminal Justice, 30*, 499–510.

U. S. Department of Justic. (2004) *Bureau of Justice Statistics Bulletin: Prisoners in 2003*. Retrieved June 3, 2005 from www.ojp.usdoj.gov/bjs/pub/pdf/p03.pdf

U. S. Department of Justice. (1997). Medical problems of inmates, 1997. *Special Report: Bureau of Justice Statistics*. Washington, DC: Author.

Willmott, D., & van Olphen, J. (2005). Challenging the health impacts of incarceration: the role for community health workers. *California Journal of Health Promotion, 3*(2), 3–48.

CHAPTER FOUR

Aging Prisoners: Strategies for Health Care

T. Smyer, M. Gragert, and D. C. Martins

Older prisoners have health care needs that are distinct from younger inmates (Watson, Stimpson, & Hostick, 2004) and present unique challenges in programming, custody, medical treatment, and postrelease placement (Older Offenders Initiative Work Group (OOIWG), 1997). As they age, inmates may become ill with physical and/or mental illnesses, their illnesses may exacerbate, they may develop functional limitations, and they may die, all while in prison. This population has an increased rate of physical and psychological problems as they have the common diseases of aging exacerbated by the additional problems associated with the offender's lifestyle and incarceration. These problems are compounded by the fact that many of the older inmates have been without health care for much of their lives. Consequently, by the time they present for medical care, they have a higher rate of late-stage chronic illnesses, infectious diseases, and addictions (Stanford University, 2002). Hutchinson (1998) pointed out that incarceration is an ideal time to provide needed health care services that have been neglected by this population and an opportunity to treat infectious diseases.

As discussed in the previous chapter, the constitutional right to health care for prison inmates was established in *Estelle v. Gamble* (1976) (Vaughn & Carroll, 1998). The U.S. Supreme Court determined that medical care for the imprisoned was an obligation of the government. Based on this ruling, prison personnel are required to provide inmates with the same medical care they would receive in the community, including surgery, hospital care, medications, and special services, such as dialysis if needed.

The older inmate population is experiencing significant growth, nearly quadrupling between 1990 and 2002 (Aday, 2003; Harrison & Beck, 2005). This growth of the older prison population and increased demand for health services are causing a crisis in prison health care. As a result, health care costs are increasing dramatically, placing great strain on prison budgets and taxing their resources.

Older inmates need other services in addition to quality medical care. There is a perception by many that older inmates are simply sitting in prison waiting to die. This, however, is not true of the current situation. Most of the older offenders in prison will be released at some point. This highlights the need for a range of services for older inmates, including the opportunity to learn skills to help them be productive citizens upon release and a place to go when released (OOIWG, 1997). This is especially important as the inmate who is released as older adults may have complex health problems and functional limitations that limit their ability to access resources and manage successfully in the outside community.

The United States is not alone with issues related to aging prisoners. A British Report from the Prison Reform Trust states that prisoners over 60 years of age are being neglected, and that the prison services are not meeting their special health, social, and rehabilitative needs (Howse, 2003). According to the report, the health care of older prisoners was worse than that of the older people in the community. Over 80% of the older prisoners had chronic health problems or disability, and over half of the older prisoners living with mental disorders and depression. Carcach and Grant (1999), in a study from the Australian Institute of Criminology, documents many of the same issues regarding the elderly inmate. Robert (2004) described the increasing numbers of aging offenders as well as the multiple and complex health issues they bring to the correctional health system in a study related to Canadian penitentiaries.

In this chapter, traditional health care of the aging offender within correctional facilities is reviewed along with issues of the rising cost of care. The conflict of goals and values between prison administration and correctional health care providers will also be described. Primary prevention programs, specialty units, long-term care, and hospice programs are discussed as necessary to meet the health care needs of older inmates. Finally, an overview of current programs, such as early release and telemedicine to meet the needs of this vulnerable population is presented, along with suggestions for improvement of care of this vulnerable population.

PRISON HEALTH CARE COSTS

Health care costs are posing a major problem for correctional facilities (Adams, 1995; American Correctional Association, 2004. There is wide variation across states in the overall amounts spent on health care for prisoners. A study of state prison health care costs commissioned by the Federal Bureau of Prisons (Lamb-Mechanik & Nelson, 2000) reported that Alabama had the lowest average daily spending on health care at $2.74 per day for each inmate. Health care expenditures in Massachusetts were the highest at $11.96 per day per inmate, with costs for the other states falling between these two figures.

Costs of caring for older prisoners have increased dramatically. In 1995, the National Correctional Industries Association (NCIA) determined that the confinement of inmates over 55 costs state and federal governments $2.1 billion annually, amounting to an average yearly cost of $69,000 for confining an older prisoner (NCIA, 1996). This is more than three times the amount spent to incarcerate younger inmates. The reason for these increased costs can be seen by examining statistics, such as those for Florida where older inmates represented 9% of the prison population but accounted for 25% of hospital bills, 33% of ambulatory surgery, 26% of ancillary care, and 30% of emergency care (Florida Corrections Commission, 2002). Studies indicate that the costs of imprisoning older felons are approximately three times as high as the average inmate cost with little or no benefit to the general public (Stanford University, 1994).

Cost-containment efforts in the past have resulted in privatization of health care for over 30 prison systems with mixed results. At least 37 states have implemented inmate copayments for medical services, requiring a small fee to be taken from the inmate's commissary fund (Lamb-Mechanik & Nelson, 2000). Medicare-based caps on payments to hospitals that treat inmates have also been established. Other cost reduction measures include restructuring medical staffing, obtaining discounts through bulk purchases, and leveraging resources through cooperative efforts with other government organizations (Stana, 2000). Clearly, new measures to reduce health care costs in correctional facilities while delivering quality health care must be considered.

CONFLICT IN GOALS AND VALUES

Health care professionals and prison administrators including correctional officers often have opposing philosophies and values relating to treatment of prisoners. Much has been written about this "clash of

TABLE 4.1   Comparison of Prison Administrative Subculture and Health Care Subculture

Prison health care	Prison administrative
Caring	Non-caring, distant
Touch	No touch
Belief in patients	Disbelief of inmates
Uniforms	Uniforms
Frequently alone	Never alone—security risk
Trust and respect	No trust
Softness and acceptance	Tough attitude
Kindness is expected by provider	Kindness leads to a "setup" and being taken advantage of

Adapted from Stevens (1993).

cultures" related to health care in correctional facilities. This is illustrated by Stevens's (1993) comparison of elements of the prison administration and health care subcultures (See Table 4.1). Stevens's suggests that the health care personnel in the prison system has a culture that is in direct opposition to the prison administration, creating a tension between "care and custody." The culture of the health care workers includes a caring attitude, touch, belief in patients, often being alone with patients, emphasis on a trusting relationship, acceptance, and kindness. In contrast, the administration's culture is characterized by a noncaring distant approach, no touching, disbelief, not trusting, a tough attitude, and avoidance of being taken advantage of by being too kind. This culture "clash" impacts the working relationship between prison health care providers and prison administration and correctional officers.

Mezey, Dubler, Mitty, and Brody (2002) pointed out that no prison system had achieved the goal of patient-centered care, adding that this approach was antithetical to corrections philosophies and systems. At times, however, prison health care providers also share the view and values of prison administration. In a study of older women in prisons, Wahidin (2004) noted that many of the older women in her sample feared becoming ill because of inadequate medical care and negative attitudes toward them by prison doctors. They reported having their illnesses trivialized and frequently felt humiliated, infantilized, and frustrated with trying to obtain adequate health care. By adopting the philosophy and approach of their employers, health care professionals may reduce the conflict between their values and that of the prison administration.

Droes (1994) discussed the attitudes of nonhealth care workers toward health care as being based on a "continuum of toleration" within correctional facilities. At one end was the "contentious toleration" of health care or where "custody staff accepted inmate health care grudgingly and viewed it as a distraction and interference with the performance of their own work" (p. 203). "Considered toleration" was at the other end of the continuum and was represented by "situations in which custody staff evaluated health care as not only benefiting inmates but also assisting in the performance of their own work" (p. 203). In the "considered toleration" view, inmates would be sent for health care if the medical condition was problematic to work performance, such as gastrointestinal symptoms or a fractured hand. Medical conditions, such as hypoglycemia with a diabetic inmate may not be noticed or referred until work performance is interrupted, however. The quality of the relationship between health care workers, correctional officers, and administration directly affects how health care is delivered and can either deter or facilitate quality health care for older inmates.

PRISON HEALTH SERVICES

Traditional Approach

Much of prison health care is based on an antiquated system originally designed to treat common illnesses like the flu (Greco, 2004) where doctors and nurses see dozens of patients in an hour. The focus has been on physical illnesses and primarily tertiary prevention. It is not designed to serve the large number of prisoners who are chronically, acutely, or terminally ill. Although this traditional approach may have worked with fewer numbers of older inmates, there are many signs that the present system is overloaded and not meeting the needs of older offenders. In addition, there are multiple barriers to health care for prisoners including a maze of paperwork obstacles, not being allowed by guards to seek health care when needed, waiting in long lines for medications, lack of privacy and confidentiality, and lack of primary preventive care (Stanford University, 2002). The increased numbers of older inmates coupled with increased costs, conflict between health care providers and prison administration, and the focus on physical illness and tertiary prevention all contribute to a reduction in quality health care (see Figure 4.1).

The range of health services provided varies widely among prison systems. Smaller prison units may only provide emergency referral, consultation, medication management, and health screening services. Larger facilities may offer these services along with primary care, mental health care, dental care, comprehensive inpatient skilled nursing infirmary, outpatient health care services, long-term care and hospice units, and limited specialty services, such as hemodialysis. Older inmates who need

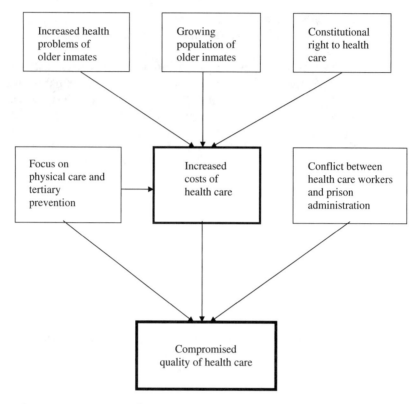

FIGURE 4.1 Factors influencing quality health care for older inmates.

care and are incarcerated in a facility with limited services may be transferred to a larger prison that offers the needed services if space is available. This often increases the inmate's isolation as they are moved away from family and friends who may visit (Dubler, 1998). For services not provided by the correctional facility, inmates may also be transported out to health care on the "outside" at a much higher cost.

Prison health care services traditionally begin upon entry to the correctional facility. Upon admission, the inmate receives a history and physical exam including laboratory tests and tests for infectious diseases. There are standardized procedures for evaluating tuberculosis, human immunodeficiency virus (HIV), and other infectious diseases that may be caused by casual contact (Center of Disease Control, 2001). A medical record including medical, dental, vision, and psychological documentation is started and follows the inmate through their incarceration. The inmate should receive a vision test and glasses should be provided if needed. A dental exam including x-rays should also be done with a plan for dental care. Medications are provided if needed for the offender's medical condition.

Admission care does not always occur as recommended. According to the Bureau of Justice Statistics (USDOJ, 1997), more than 8 out of 10 inmates surveyed reported having a medical exam since being admitted to prison. Nearly 60% reported being checked by staff to see if they were sick, injured, or intoxicated at the time of admission. Approximately 82% were asked questions about their health or medical history. After admission 96.2% reported that they received a skin test for tuberculosis, 86.7% had blood drawn, and 85% had a medical exam (USDOJ, 1997). With older prisoners, who have increased prevalence of acute and chronic illnesses, admission histories and physical exams are imperative.

Most of the traditional prison health system focuses on physical health problems, with fewer services for mental health issues and substance abuse issues. According to Linder, Enders, Craig, Richardson, and Meyers (2002), because inmates are more likely to have a history of alcohol abuse, substance abuse or addiction, and sex industry work, mental health and substance abuse services are needed. Older adults need more programs to address alcohol-related health issues and more than two thirds of older inmates could benefit from substance abuse treatment programs (Arndt, Turvey, & Flaum, 2002).

The most frequently occurring mental health issues among older adults in general are depression, anxiety, delirium, and dementia. Nearly all state correctional facilities screen inmates for mental health problems and provide some kind of treatment. In 2000, one in eight inmates of all ages in state prisons was receiving some mental health therapy, with approximately 20% receiving psychotropic medications, and 2% housed in in-patient psychiatric facilities (USDOJ, 2001). All prison systems care for inmates using a psychopharmacologic approach with inmates who have nonacute mental illness receiving varying amounts of counseling as well. Some departments of corrections manage mental illness in inmates by assigning them to separate housing, whereas others attempt to mainstream them when possible. All but 13 state prison systems provide special mental health care to substance abusers with mental illness (National Institute of Corrections, 2001).

Treatment of Infectious Diseases

Assessment and treatment of infectious diseases present unique challenges to prison health care (Glaser, Warchol, D'Angelo, & Guterman, 1990). Older adults are particularly at risk of contracting infectious diseases because of the reduced efficiency of their immune system, occurring as an age-related change. Among infectious diseases affecting this population, hepatitis is an especially difficult problem. The Center of Disease Control (2002) reports that in California, half of incoming women and one third of incoming men tested positive for hepatitis B virus infection. Viral hepatitis prevention measures, including screening, immunization, and treatment, are expensive. Variable length of sentences and movement of inmates within and between facilities makes complete immunization, monitoring chronic infections, and carrying out treatment difficult. Antiviral therapy for chronic hepatitis B and chronic hepatitis C is complicated and is not appropriate for everyone. Facilities that have instituted viral hepatitis treatment programs have found that periodic training and updates for correctional health and pharmacy staff are needed for successful programs. Successful HIV/AIDS treatment programs in correctional facilities also may provide some useful lessons learned (CDC, 2002). Many inmates with hepatitis also have other illnesses, such as HIV, tuberculosis, diabetes, or mental illness. Treatment of an inmate's hepatitis B or hepatitis C may not be the highest priority for the correctional health staff if a beneficial outcome is uncertain; however, it becomes a public health problem if the prisoner is released back into society.

National Standards and Guidelines

Prison health care is guided by national standards. These national health standards for correctional facilities were first published in 1976 by the American Public Health Association to establish guidelines to improve and standardize health care delivery in the prison setting (Jails and Prisons Task Force, 1976). Since then, the National Commission on Correctional Health Care (NCCHC) (2003) has developed guidelines for health services in prison based on recommendations by the US Congress in 2002. Specific guidelines for care have been written for those with chronic illnesses (e.g., diabetes and hypertension), communicable diseases (e.g., HIV), physical handicaps, frail older adults, terminally ill, mentally ill, and developmentally disabled. The guidelines are a series of written treatment plans with a course of therapy that is multidisciplinary and is based on the inmates needs. These plans have short- and long-term goals and are problem oriented (Paris, 1998). They encourage total disease management with clear indicators of control of the patient's disease and with distinction as to whether the condition is stable, improving, or deteriorating. The guidelines also alert the health care provider about barriers to appropriate treatment commonly found in correctional facilities. The NCCHC (2003) warns that the guidelines cannot and do not substitute for individual clinical professional judgment based upon a specific patient's presentation.

The NCCHC also offers a voluntary accreditation program for prison health services, educational programs, and a certification examination so that health care providers can be recognized as Certified Correctional Health Professionals (CCHP). This credential identifies the provider as one who has demonstrated mastery of national standards and the knowledge expected of leaders working in correctional health care. Accreditation through a peer-review process validates that the standards for health care are being met in the particular prison system. More than 450 prisons and jails nationwide have been accredited.

APPROACHES FOR IMPROVING HEALTH CARE FOR OLDER INMATES

Primary Prevention Programs

Traditional health care in prison systems tends to be not only physically oriented but also crisis or tertiary care oriented, with little attention to primary prevention. In some prison systems, officials are beginning to focus on prevention by changing diets to low-fat, low-salt, and high-fiber meals; introducing exercise programs; and providing health education to inmates. Prevention strategies need to be implemented earlier and more aggressively across all prisons systems, however. Primary prevention measures for inmates may decrease costs through improvement of general health of inmates and decreasing needs for more expensive health care services for older prisoners.

Women's health programs are needed to address the growing number of women who are aging in prison (Lindquist & Lindquist, 1999; Reviere & Young, 2004). According to the California Coalition for Woman Prisoners (2001), older women prisoners experience a uniquely difficult time in prison. The staff and prisoners are often insensitive to the needs of older women. There are routine tests and procedures needed annually by older women, such as pelvic examinations, vision and hearing exams, breast exams, skin cancer checks, and rectal exams. Dental exams should be conducted every 6 months. Proper nutrition and regular exercise are also important to help in decreasing the number of chronic illnesses among the older adult women in prison (California Coalition for Women Prisoners, 2001). Programs such as these for older women may decrease costs and improve overall health status.

Preventive health care measures are especially important for older prisoners (Greco, 2004). Health education and preventative care are necessary to counteract the effects of debilitating lifestyles many older inmates had prior to their imprisonment. Primary health care programs for older adults in the prison system may reduce the severity of many long-term chronic illnesses. In one example, in Ohio, a position for a co-ordinator responsible for specialized populations for older and youthful offenders was developed to help plan, develop, and implement initiatives dealing with the older and younger offenders, both incarcerated and under community supervision (personal communication, J. Lyon, May 24, 2005; Older Offenders Initiative Work Group, 1997). Suggested programs included a "wellness" program and vocational training for older offenders who needed to work upon release. More emphasis would be placed on preparing the older offender for release with an increase in the number of community placement options. Plans would be devised for meeting the specialized medical needs of older offenders. As the older offender population continues to grow, the initiative would also support the addition of more assisted living beds. All staff who dealt extensively with older offenders would be required to attend a 40-hour training program which addressed how to effectively deal with the older inmate population. Programs such as this can have a great impact on improving the health and quality of life of older inmates, both inside prison systems and upon release.

In 1986, the World Health Organization's *Ottawa Charter for Health Promotion* provided the catalyst for the Health in Prisons Project (Whitehead, 2006). Although this is a worldwide effort, the HIPP currently has 25 European members including several from former Eastern Bloc countries. The HIPP project focuses on creating Health Promoting Prisons that are committed to a management structure where planning, implementing, and evaluating health promotion initiatives can take place. Basic principles of the programs should include an internal health promotion steering committee supported by management; active involvement of the targeted audience in program planning; commitment of resources, staff, and training; utilization of a range of health-related approaches; achievable goals and method of evaluation; and a long-term commitment (3 to 5 years) to set up programs (Whitehead, 2006). Although health promotion activities in prisons will never be easy to accomplish, they hold great potential for improvement of health of older inmates, as well as reduction in health care costs over time.

Specialty Units for Older Inmates

Geriatric care and programming are necessities for the immediate future in prison health. The older offender requires an environment that is more slowly paced as well as specialized programming and medical services.

Similarly, more people will be dying in prison, not only due to longer sentences, but also because of diseases such as AIDS and drug-resistant tuberculosis. The development of "theme" units for those special needs may be the model of choice. According to the U.S. Department of Justice by 1985, the National Institute of Corrections had 11 agencies with special units for older inmates. In 1990, a study of 19 state systems and the federal system found that 6% of inmates of age 50 years and older were housed in special units, with 1.2% of that group located in an infirmary setting (Hall, 1990). At least 16 states maintain special facilities to house older inmates (McMahon, 2003). Identification and placement needs of older prisoners as well as security issues are specifically identified by the prison in accordance with the NCCHC standards (if they are an accredited correctional facility).

Aday (2003) described the issues related to facilities and programs for the aging inmate within the context of environmental press theory and pays particular attention to specialized versus mainstream housing Aday (2003 p. 148). Environmental press is defined as "the demands that the social and physical environments make on the individual to adapt, respond, or change" (p. 148). Prisons were made for younger, noisier, more active and more violent offenders, and this physical environment is not conducive to the frail older adult inmate (Aday, 2003). Physical mobility and a sense of safety and security are two issues with which the older inmate has to adapt and cope. Specialty units target these two issues in the prison environment and reduce the demands on the older inmates.

In specialty units, medical care is designed to meet the needs of older inmates with a dual goal of cost containment and humane treatment. Interventions in this setting with the older prisoner include a thorough physical and cognitive assessment including signs and symptoms of depression or stress related to environment disturbances (Smyer, Gragert, & LaMere, 1997). Selye (1978) theorized that conditions of chronic, persistent stress impose continual wear and tear on individuals and contribute to the aging process. The issues of environmental stress as it relates to separate housing (vs. mainstreaming) must be considered in plans for care of older inmates, taking as well as specific programming needs for this population. Concerns for security and safety, as well as physical mobility, are paramount in decision-making. Placement of the older inmate is decided based on these issues, taking into consideration of the number of aged inmates within the system, existing physical features of the prison and potential for remodeling to meet aged prisoner's needs, existing medical services and access, and financial concerns within each system (Word, 2004).

The assessment and treatment of geriatric health problems is an ongoing need that can be readily met on these specialty units or older adult pods (Lipson, 1990). Moore (1989) found that, when pods were designed or modified to meet the needs of aged offenders, the inmates' overall levels of well-being and satisfaction improved. This study also found that specialty pods offered older adults more privacy, minimum security, and more control over their environment. The older prisoners had the opportunity to control their own temperature and lighting in the specialty units, for instance (Morton, 1992). Another concern addressed by the specialty pods was accessibility for those using wheelchairs and the uniform availability of other accommodations that would enable all older inmates to function at the highest level possible (Morton, 1992). Bathrooms accessible to wheelchairs provide better hygiene and allow older inmates to be more independent to carry out the routine activities of daily living. In fact, the lack of specialty pods might place prison facilities in noncompliance with federal law, such as the Americans with Disabilities Act. Legislation mandates that disabled inmates receive the same or comparable services as other inmates.

The specialty units would also have frequent and readily accessible health care, physical accommodations to promote independence (handrails, elevated toilets, and wheelchair accessible sites), and programming for mental health groups as well as gardening, volunteer work, or active participation in a recreation program (Aday, 2003). Programming for these units is an extremely important aspect of the separate unit. Simply grouping the older inmates with no scheduled programming can promote depression and isolation, which contribute to further decline in health status and increased care needs.

Prison-Based Long-Term Care

Among the facilities that are increasingly used with older inmates are secure nursing homes, special needs facilities, and geriatric-assisted living units. North and South Carolina have been leaders in special care geriatric facilities (Aday, 2003). They are best known for their free-standing secure geriatric units at McCain Correctional Hospital and State Park, respectively, although South Carolina also has expanded units throughout the state. Other states are beginning to incorporate skilled nursing facilities within the prison walls in designated sections of the prison facility.

Renovations to unused facilities such as military institutions or state psychiatric centers, can be used to meet the needs of the aging prisoners. These facilities could be modified to provide geriatric specialty care, geriatric dormitories, wheelchair access, and protection from young and violent inmates (Greco, 2004). For the long-term care of older inmates, the Older Offenders Initiative Work Group (1997) in

Ohio recommended 100 assisted living beds for every 1,500–2,000 inmates in the age group of 50–59. The group also recommended caseworker services that would negotiate geriatric beds, geriatric chairs, walkers, hearing aids, dentures, eye glasses, and supportive shoes for those in need.

Mara (2002, 2004) discussed the increased need for long-term care in prison populations. In exploring alternatives for delivery of care to the older prisoners, the use of prison nursing homes and protected environments as well as parole or early release to nursing homes has been considered. Aday (2003) related that in correctional institutions, "special diets, around-the-clock nursing care, building new facilities or remodeling old ones, and restructuring institutional activities are becoming more frequent topics of discussion" (p. 143). As an alternative to prison-based long-term care, aged inmates could be released from prison and re-institutionalized in long-term care facilities in general society (Greco, 2004).

According to Fazel, McMillan, and O'Donnell (2002), caring for older adults with dementia in prison has strong ethical and legal implications, both of which necessitate the use of dementia units or early release. This type of diagnosis increases the older adult's vulnerability and eliminates the "punishment" aspect of prison life from the prisoner's cognitive perspective. It seems that a poor performance on the Mini Mental State Exam (MMSE) and documentation of cognitive impairment should necessitate removal of the affected prisoner from danger in the general prison environment.

Hospice and End-of-Life Care

Incarceration of the terminally ill is controversial; however, with tougher parole and different sentencing guidelines, more people are dying in prisons. The development of hospice programs for end-of life-care in prisons is increasingly the preferred response to the health and care needs of terminally ill inmates (Linder et al., 2002).

According to the National Prison Hospice Association (2005), "hospice" is interdisciplinary comfort-oriented care that allows seriously ill and dying patients to die with dignity and humanity with as little pain as possible in an environment where they have mental and spiritual preparation for the natural process of dying. Many prisons are now offering hospice care (Word, 2004), often developing their own formal hospice programs to enhance the quality of life for dying inmates (USDOJ, 1998). Nonprison-based hospice programs are also available to prisons and the National Prison Hospice Association advocates for the dying patient regardless of setting. Hospice care is a cost-effective alternative as the expense of hospice care is far less than that of traditional treatment in a hospital setting.

The types of hospice service offered in prisons vary from none at all, hospice being considered or developed, some palliative care available, to formal prison-based hospice services (U.S. Department of Justice, 1998). Some prisons provide special privileges for terminally ill inmates to make them more comfortable. These privileges may include relaxed visitation policies, more personal items, special dietary preferences, smoking opportunities, and the service of clergy to help plan memorial services.

End-of-life care in prisons presents special challenges. At an individual level, pain and other troublesome symptoms are often not well managed. Pain management is difficult because of the lack of analgesics allowed to be brought into prisons (Mezey et al., 2002). Additionally, inmates with a history of drug abuse tend to be disbelieved when they report pain, even if they have a progressive chronic illness (Dubler, 1998). Meeting the dying inmates food and hydration needs is also challenging for prison health care staff. Food availability is limited, and prison kitchens lack the resources, flexibility, and inclination to prepare meals for special diets (Dubler, 1998). Few standards for nutrition and hydration for dying inmates are followed by prison systems (Mezey et al., 2002).

In the free world, advance directives are integral to managing terminal care; however, executing advance directives can be difficult in a prison setting. Both a living will or health care proxy can legally be executed in the prison setting; however, they may not necessarily be followed if the dying prisoners wishes conflict with issues of efficient management of the system (Mezey et al., 2002). The Volunteers of America GRACE (Guiding Responsive Action in Corrections at End-of-life) project is developing standards for end-of-life care in prisons. Their GRACE project in jails offers a model of how community-based organizations can partner with local detention centers to provide access to quality end-of-life care for the over 3,000 inmates who die in prisons each year. Resources produced by this group include a handbook, *End of Life Care in Corrections* for caregivers and managers, and a training and video guide on caring for terminally ill inmates (Volunteers of America GRACE Project, 2004).

Hospice care requires interdisciplinary team management. Most teams include security staff, chaplains, mental health staff, and medical personnel. Some teams also include nutritionists, social workers, pharmacists, occupational and recreational therapists (U.S. Department of Justice, 1998). This approach provides an improved dying experience, improved health care, benefits to staff and inmate's morale, better family relationships, and lower cost to the prison and the taxpayers.

Establishing a long-term care and hospice nursing facility in a correctional facility requires administrative support, vision and long-range assessment, and planning and evaluation of outcomes (Chow, 2002). Chow developed a program to serve geriatric inmates with long-term care and a hospice program. This program began with an institutional hospice committee. After a long collaborative effort, the nation's second federal inmate-to-inmate hospice program was established, modeled after the Missouri federal prison program. Inmate hospice volunteers were trained; standards, policies, and procedures for the hospice program were developed. The local community's hospice experts educated the initial volunteers about palliative medicine and medically directed compassionate care. Topics for the in-service included pain management, universal precautions, death concepts, medical conditions, spiritual and psychosocial considerations with dying, hospice standards, and ethical issues. The nurse, chaplain, and social worker counseled the volunteers weekly. Interdisciplinary care planning conferences were also organized to discuss inmate cases, pain management, and eligibility for the hospice program (Chow). Programs such as this exemplify effective use of resources for improvement of long-term and end-of-life care among older inmates.

Early Release and Compassionate Release Programs

In an effort to reduce costs, several states are granting early release to nonviolent prisoners, especially older adult prisoners (McMahon, 2003). State officials, experts in gerontology, and correction facility representatives need to closely examine the aging population in prison and investigate alternatives to incarceration. The question whether more older prisoners should be released before they have served their full sentences is being debated throughout the country. In comparison, probation and electronic monitoring cost much less. The central argument for releasing older inmates is that society cannot afford the medical and personal care they require. If they are physically impaired, they are not a threat to society and should be released to a less costly type of care.

Early release programs are also supported by the fact that recidivism decreases with age. Recidivism studies indicate that older inmates are far less likely than their younger counterparts to continue to commit crimes after release. Additionally, most older prisoners are serving time for nonviolent offenses. The chance of committing crimes declines with age regardless of sex, race, country of origin, ethnicity, or offense. According to a federal study of state recidivism statistics, older parolees and probationers are re-incarcerated infrequently (National Center on Institutions and Alternatives, 1998).

It is recommended that, with these factors in mind, it is sound penal and social policy to provide structured supervised release for prisoners who: (a) are 65 years of age or older, (b) have committed a nonviolent offense, (c) have served a substantial part of their sentence (one third or more), and (d) are deemed to not present a significant risk to the community (National Center on Institutions and Alternatives, 1998). Alternatives such as the Project for Older Prisoners (POPS) can be instituted to combat prison overcrowding and assist aging and disadvantaged prisoners. The POPS is a program in which law students, supervised by faculty, evaluate low-risk older inmates to assist them in obtaining parole or other forms of release from incarceration. Prisoners suitable for POPS are selected based on their age or medical condition. A student is then assigned to the inmate and visits to discuss parole or other options, such as prison health care facilities. The student conducts an extensive background analysis to determine the inmate's likelihood of recidivism. If the prisoner is considered a low-risk inmate, the student assists the inmate in determining where they would live and how they would support themselves upon release. For higher-risk prisoners, students consider what prison nursing home facilities may be available to them. One POPS program option sets up an electronic home-detention system for old and frail parolees who are no longer threats to society (Greco, 2004).

Job training, re-socialization programs, community placements, and continued health service program availability with the prison system are needed so that the older adult is not discharged into the streets with no resources. Some states have used the early release program hastily, which only compounds the problem of older adults who are homeless living on the streets.

Compassionate release of inmates who are extremely ill and dying is both humane and cost-effective (Gillenkirk, 2004). Thirty-three states and the Federal Bureau of Prisons have developed procedures for granting compassionate release of dying prisoners (Volunteers of America GRACE Project, 2001). The release of terminally ill and medically incapacitated prisoners who can no longer pose a threat to the public can save the state taxpayers hundreds of thousands of dollars and provide these men and women with appropriate end-stage medical and palliative care. Unfortunately, compassionate release programs are very limited, with few inmates actually paroled through this mechanism. Eligibility requirements are stringent and the review process is often slow with many inmates dying in prison before the review process is complete. Perhaps the Medical Parole Law should be revised to make the process more efficient without putting the public at risk.

Telemedicine

Some states have been able to keep costs lower through innovative programs such as telemedicine, in which inmates are examined and talk to physicians at a distance by videoconferencing. The use of telemedicine has saved the Texas prison systems between $2.2 and $11 million in 1999, or an estimated $5000 each time telemedicine is used in place of a trip outside the prison (Stein, 2000). Telemedicine fosters faster responses to outbreaks of infectious diseases and makes it easier for specialists to manage treatment to inmates with complex diseases such as HIV or cancer. Telemedicine also seems to positively influence health care outcomes as inmate deaths in the Texas system have decreased by 34% between 1997 and 2000 following the introduction of the telemedicine program (Stein, 2000).

A telemedicine demonstration project linked three federal prisons in Pennsylvania and one federal prison medical center in Kentucky with the Veterans Affairs Medical Center in Kentucky. The goal of the project was to design, install, and utilize a telemedicine system followed by evaluation of outcomes. Findings showed significant cost savings and benefits with decreased in-prison consultations, trips to local providers, and fewer transfers to Federal Medical Centers. This project also projected that the initial costs for purchasing telemedicine equipment would be recovered in less than two years. Additional nonfinancial benefits were that prisoners' waiting time to see specialists decreased, new services became available, such as specialized HIV/AIDS care, and anecdotal evidence showed that the quality of care, especially psychiatric care improved (McDonald, Hassol, & Carlson, 1999). Clearly, telemedicine shows much promise for improving quality health care and reducing costs of correctional health.

Joining Correctional Systems and Academic Institutions

The Texas prison system is one of the largest correctional facilities in the Western world (Raimer & Stobo, 2004). The older adult prisoner represents 5.1% of this prison population. The number of inmates 55 years or older increased by 148% between 1994 and 2002 in this system. Texas implemented a correctional managed care program to correct the fragmented and inadequate health care of the prisoners (Newton & Kendig, 2004; Raimer & Stobo, 2004). To do this, a strategic partnership was developed between the Texas Department of Criminal Justice, the University of Texas Medical Branch at Galveston, and Texas Tech University Health Sciences Center. The two medical schools provide all medical, dental, and psychiatric care for over 125,000 inmates. The

program is staffed by physicians, physician assistants, nurse practitioners, registered nurses, and licensed practical nurses. The health care
provided includes primary ambulatory care in each prison unit, infirma-
ries, regional medical facilities, telemedicine (as discussed earlier) and a
dedicated prison hospital. Specialized programs have been developed for
chronic conditions in hypertension, diabetes, psychiatric disorders, hepatitis, and HIV/AIDS. The program both promotes the public health and
protects public safety through the early detection and treatment of infectious illnesses. It also provides for early treatment with medications that
may reduce morbidity in illnesses, such as hypertension and diabetes.

Direct university involvement in correctional health care resulted
in a more structured delivery of health care, improved outcomes with
chronic illnesses, and cost savings for the state (Newton & Kendig,
2004). Research universities involved in working with vulnerable populations in the prison setting must be certain to provide the same standard
of ethical care as when working with clients outside the prison system.

Geriatric Education for Prison Health Providers

Educational training for correctional staff about age-specific developmental change is necessary (Older Offenders Initiative Work Group, 1997;
Mara, 2004; Smyer et al., 1997). Most of the health providers have little
knowledge of age-related changes (Knapp & Elder, 1998) and little training
or experience in treating illnesses commonly associated with aging. Greco
(2004) reports that few, if any, correctional systems require continuing
education of their medical staffs. Given the rapid increase in aged prisoners,
geriatric and gerontological education and services should be provided.

Health care providers need to be educated to identify age-related
changes to be considered when performing physical assessments with
older adults. Education for prison-based health providers also needs to
address cultural competence. Teaching correctional health workers
about the diverse needs of different cultural groups would assist them to
provide sensitive and appropriate care to prisoners regardless of social
class, race/ethnicity, or political and religious backgrounds (Stanford
University, 2002). The American Correctional Health Service Association and the National Commission on Correctional Health Care offer
both educational programs and conferences for health care workers in
the prison setting.

Interdisciplinary Teams

The inherent complexities of prison health care would suggest that health
care professionals should have a trained specialty in the area. Prison

nurses have been developing and promoting their work to bring correctional health forward as a specialty. Historically, correctional nursing
has not been recognized as a specialty but with the increasing numbers of
aging prisoners this may need to be addressed (Hesketh, 2001; Norman
& Parrish, 1999). Emphasis on an interdisciplinary approach to care
would be essential for the emerging specialty of correctional health
nursing.

An interdisciplinary team approach is especially necessary in prisons,
considering the special needs of the older inmate. Aday (2003) suggested
that aging inmates "require a case management approach and coordinated care" (p. 167). Interdisciplinary teams focus on health and disease,
clinical outcomes, patient safety, patient education, and the role of the
patient in decision making (Newton & Kendig, 2004; Raimer & Stobo,
2004). Due to the complexity of the older prisoner's health issues, the
interdisciplinary team members might include medicine, nursing, dental,
psychiatry and social work, pharmacy, physical and occupational therapy, and correctional officers. The cost of such a team approach may
be offset by the savings in care through improvement in the functional
status of inmates, thus decreasing the costs of care management.

SUMMARY

The aging prisoner is at a great disadvantage in a prison system. Although improvements are being made, most prisons do not have specific
health care programs in place for older adults who are incarcerated.
Older prisoners need physical, cognitive, and psychological assessment
to determine their health care needs as well as programmatic strategies
to meet these complex needs. Health care programs need to be carefully
designed with the older prisoner's special needs, safety, and well-being in
mind. As numbers of older adults in prisons increase, health care needs
rise and costs for prisons and taxpayers escalate. Creative ways of delivering quality, cost-effective care are imperative.

The conflict in goals and values between health care providers and
prison administration must also be addressed. This conflict in approach
to prisoners is made more contentious by the added stress of the increasing cost of health care and continual efforts to reduce costs. Such conflict jeopardizes the delivery of quality health care. Although it may not
be possible to resolve this conflict, an understanding of the roots of the
conflict and increased communication between health care providers
and prison administration may enable both parties to carry out their
functions more effectively with mutual trust and respect, resulting in improved quality of health care.

Educational training for the correctional staff to address specialization in geriatric education, interdisciplinary team development, and cultural competence is necessary. Partnerships to enhance education and health care must be developed with community, state, and national organizations. Primary prevention programs need to be developed to promote healthy living for older adults with both nutrition and exercise programs. Specialty units may better meet the needs of older adult prisoners for hospice care, dementia care, and long-term care.

Discharge programs need to be considered including early release and compassionate release programs. Older adult advocacy and sensitivity is paramount. Policy initiatives that inhibit the prison system and states from discharging the older prisoners to the streets with no resources in place are imperative. Prison administrations will need to work carefully with outside agencies in order to help these prisoners resettle into the community. Prison health care strategies must incorporate a balance between humanitarian efforts, ethical considerations, cost containment, quality health care, positive health outcomes, and social justice. Further research on the health care needs of older adults in prisons and evaluation of programs designed to meet their needs is important. Clear data are needed to progress toward the goal of quality health care at affordable costs for older prisoners.

REFERENCES

Adams, W. (1995). The incarceration of older criminals: Balancing safety, cost, and humanitarian concerns. *Nova Law Review, 19*, 465–486.

Aday, R. (2003). *Aging prisoners: Crisis in American corrections*. Westport, CT: Praeger.

American Correctional Association (2004). Inmate health care. *Corrections Compendium, 29*, 10–20.

Arndt, S., Turvey, C., & Flaum, M. (2002). Older offenders, substance abuse, and treatment. *American Journal of Geriatric Psychiatry, 10*(6), 733–740.

California Coalition for Women Prisoners. (2001). *Legal corner: Growing old in prison–What will it mean?* Staff Attorney, Legal Services for Prisoners with Children. Retrieved May 24, 2005 http://www.womenprisoners.org/fire/000212.html

Carach, C., & Grant, A. (1999). Imprisonment in Australia: *Trends in prison populations and imprisonment rates 1982–1998* ; 28th annual report at the Australian Institute of Criminology. Canberra, Australia: Australian Institute of Criminology.

Center for Disease Control. (2001, January). Federal bureau of prisons report on infectious disease management. Atlanta, GA: National Center on STD, HIV and TB Prevention. Retrieved May 24, 2005 from http://www.nicic.org/pubs/2001/016669.pdf

Center for Disease Control. (2002). Viral hepatitis and the criminal justice system. Prevention Among Injection Drug Users. Retrieved May 24, 2005 from http://www.cdc.gov/idu/hepatitis/viralhep_crimhal_just.htm

Chow, R. (2002). Initiating a long-term care nursing service for aging inmates. *Geriatric Nursing, 23*(1), 24–27.

Correctional Services of Canada. (2005). Programs that word with and treats elderly and infirm offenders in the pacific region, Canada. Retrieved April 1, 2005 at http://nicic.org/Misc/URLShell.aspx?SRC=Catalog&REFF=http://nicic.org/Library/016561&ID=016561&TYPE=HTML&URL=http://www.apcca.org/Pubs/news11/#item15

Droes, N. S. (1994). Correctional nursing practice. *Journal of Community Health Nursing, 11*, 201–210.

Dubler, N. (1998). The collision of confinement and care: End of Life care in prison and jails. *Journal of Law, Medicine and Ethics, 26*, 149–156.

Fazel, S., McMillan, J., & O'Donnell, I. (2002). Dementia in prison: ethical and legal.

Florida Corrections Commission. (2002). Data on Florida's aging prison population. Retrieved February 7, 2005 from www.angelfire.com/f13/starke/elderlydata.html

Gillenkirk, J. (2004). Compassionate release long overdue. ACLU News: The Newspaper of the ACLU of Northern California. Retrieved May 24, 2005 from http://www.aclunc.org/aclunews/news0407/compassionate.html

Glaser, J., Warchol, A., D'Angelo, D., & Guterman, H. (1990). Infectious diseases of geriatric inmates. *Review of Infectious Diseases, 12*, 683–692.

Greco, R. (2004). *Older prisoners.* New York: New York State Office for the Aging.

Hall, M. (1990). *Special needs inmates: A survey of state correctional systems.* Technical Assistance Report # 90A1064. Boulder, CO: National Institute of Corrections Information Center.

Harrison, P., & Beck, A. (2005). *Prisoners at midyear 2004.* Washington, DC: Bureau of Justice Statistics.

Hesketh, N. (2001). Prison health care: Opening the debate, *British Journal of Nursing, 10*, 1234.

Howse, K. (2003). *Growing old in prison.* London: Prison Reform Trust.

Hutchinson, C. (1998). Health care for prisoners: Humane—and the law. *Infections in Medicine, 15*, 160–161.

Jails and Prisons Task Force. (1976). *Standard for health services in correctional institutions.* Washington, DC: American Public Health Association.

Knapp, J., & Elder, K. B. (1998). Assessing prison personnels' knowledge of the aging process. *Journal of the Oklahoma Criminal Justice Research Consortium, 4*, 1997/1998. Retrieved July 15, 2005 from http://www.doc.state.ok.us/DOC/OCJRC/OCJRC 97–98/1997_research.htm.

Lamb-Mechanik, D., & Nelson, J. (2000). *Prison health care survey: An analysis of factors influencing per capita costs.* National Institute of Corrections Information Center. Retrieved December 17, 2005 from http:www.nicic.org/pubs/2000/015999/PDF

Linder, J., Enders, S., Craig, E., Richardson, J., & Meyers, F. (2002). Hospice care for the incarcerated in the United States: An introduction. *Journal of Palliative Medicine, 5*, 549–552.

Lindquist, C. H., & Lindquist, C. A. (1999). Health behind bars: Utilization and evaluation of medical care among jail inmates. *Journal of Community Health, 24,* 285–303.

Lipson, S. (1990). Aging inmate: The challenge for corrections. In *Long term confinement and the aging inmate population.* Washington, DC: Federal Bureau of Prisons.

Mara, C. (2004). Chronic illness, disability, and long-term care in the prison setting. In P. R. Katz, M. D. Mezey, & M. B. Knapp, (Eds.), *Vulnerable populations in the long-term care continuum* (pp. 39–56) New York: Springer Publishing Co.

Mara, C. (2002). Expansion of long-term care in the prison system: An aging inmate population poses policy and programmatic questions. *Journal of Aging and Social Policy, 14,* 43–61.

McDonald, D., Hassol, A., & Carlson, K. (1999, April). Can telemedicine reduce spending and improve prisoner health care? *National Institute of Justice Journal,* 20–25.

McMahon, P. (2003). Aging inmates present prison crisis. *USA Today.* Retrieved August 10, 2003 from http://www.usatoday.com/news/nation/2003-08-10-prison-inside-usat_x.htm

Mezey, M., Dubler, N. N., Mitty, E., & Brody, A. A. (2002). What impact do setting and transitions have on the quality of life at the end of life and the quality of the dying process? *Gerontologist, 42,* 54–67.

Moore, E. O. (1989). Prison environments and their impact on older citizens. *Journal of Offender Counseling, Services, and Rehabilitation, 13,* 175–191.

Morton, J. (1992). An administrative overview of the older inmate. U.S. Department of Justice. Washington, DC: National Institute of Corrections.

National Center on Institutions and Alternatives. (1998). *Imprisoning elderly offenders: Public safety or maximum security nursing homes?* Executive Summary, Alexandria, VA: NCIA.

National Commission on Correctional Health Care. (2003). *Standards for health services.* Retrieved May 24, 2005 at http://www.ncchc.org/

National Correctional Industries Association. (1996). *Real war on crime.* New York: Harper Collins.

National Institute of Corrections. (2001). Provision of mental health care in prisons. Washington, DC: National Institute of Corrections, February, 2001. Retrieved December 17, 2005 from http://www.nicic.org/pubs/2001/016724.pdf

National Prison Hospice Association. (2005). *What is hospice?* Retrieved October 20, 2005 from www.npha.org

Newton, E., & Kendig, N. (2004). Correctional health care systems and collaboration with academic medicine, *Journal of the American Medical Association, 292,* 501–503.

Norman, A., & Parish, A. (1999). Prison health care: Work environment and the nursing role. *British Journal of Nursing, 8,* 653–656.

Older Offenders Initiative Work Group. (1997). *Older offenders: The Ohio initiative.* Columbus, OH: Ohio Department of Rehabilitation and Correction.

Paris, J. E. (1998). Care of the impaired and disabled. In M. Puisis (Ed.), *Clinical practice in correctional medicine* (326–331). St. Louis: Mosby.

Raimer, B. G., & Stobo, J. D. (2004). Health care delivery in the Texas prison system. *Journal of the American Medical Association, 292*, 485–48.

Riviere, R., & Young, V. (2004). Aging behind bars: Health care for older female inmates. *Journal of Women Aging, 16*(1–2), 55–69.

Robert, D. (2004). Understanding health care utilization in custody: Situation of Canadian penitentiaries. *Journal of Correctional Health Care, 10*, 239–256.

Selye, H. (1978). *The stress of life.* New York: McGraw-Hill.

Smyer, T. Gragert, M., & LaMere, S. (1997). Stay safe! Stay Healthy! Surviving old age in prison. *Journal of Psychosocial Nursing and Mental Health Services, 35*, 10–17.

Stana, R. (2000). *Testimony by Richard Stana. Federal prisons: Containing health care costs for and increasing inmate population.* The Subcommittee on Criminal Justice Oversight, Committee on Judiciary. Washington, DC: US Senate General Government Division (GEO).

Stanford University. (2002). *Understanding prison health care.* Retrieved May 24, 2005 www.movementbuilding.org/prisonhealth/index.html

Stanford University. (1994). *Elderly prisoners to pose major problems in Three Strikes law.* Retrieved February 7, 2005 www.stanford.edu/dept/news/pr/94/941102Arc4063.html

Stein, T. (2000). *The medicine show: Video treatments offer more opportunities to nurses, inmates.* Retrieved February 10, 2006 from http://www.nurseweek.com/features/00-04/correct.html.

Stevens, R. (1993). When your clients are in jail. *Nursing Forum, 28*(4), 5–8.

U.S. Department of Justice. (2001). *Mental health treatment in state prisons, 2000.* Retrieved February 7, 2005 from http://ojp.usdoj.gov/bjs/pub/pdf/mhtsp00/pdf

U.S. Department of Justice. (1998). *Hospice and palliative care in prisons: Special issues in corrections.* Washington, DC: National Institute of Corrections.

U.S. Department of Justice. (1997). *Medical problems of inmates, 1997. Special Report.* Washington, DC: Bureau of Justice Statistics. Retrieved February 10, 2006 from http://www.ojp.usdoj.gov/bjs/abstract/mpi97.htm

Volunteers of America GRACE Project. (2001). *Incarceration of the terminally ill: Current practices in the United States.* Alexandria, VA: Volunteers of America.

Volunteers of America GRACE Project. (2004). *End-of-life care in corrections:* Alexandria, VA: Volunteers of America.

Vaughn, M., & Carroll, L. (1998). Separate and unequal: Prison versus free-world medical care. *Justice Quarterly, 15*(1), 3–40.

Wahidin, A. (2004). *Older women in the criminal justice system: Running out of time.* Philadephia: Jessica Kingsley.

Watson, R., Stimpson, A., & Hostick, T. (2004). Prison health care: A review of the literature. *International Journal of Nursing Studies, 41*, 119–128.

Whitehead, D. (2006). The health promotion prison (HPP) and its imperative for nursing. *International Journal of Nursing Studies, 43*, 123–131.

Word, R. (2004). *Elderly inmates swell nation's prisons.* Associated Press. Retrieved February 7, 2005 www.angelfire.com/f13/starke/elderlyswell.html

PART III

Homeless Older Adults

Health Issues of Homeless Older Adults

D. C. Martins and M. A. Sullivan

Older adults who are homeless have been called an invisible population, ignored by service providers and policymakers (Cohen, 1999). Few sights are more tragic than that of the older homeless man or woman, huddled in a doorway or sleeping on a heating grate, or wandering on freezing city streets in winter carrying all of his or her belongings, often wasting away from a host of illnesses. It is indeed hard to imagine a more marginalized and vulnerable group of people with less political power than older homeless adults. As the homeless problem in the United States continues to grow unabated, the number of older homeless people will increase dramatically as the baby boomers begin to turn 60 (Cohen, 1999) and their options for reintegration into society dwindle.

Homelessness in later life is a topic that has been largely neglected in the gerontology literature. Research into the causes of homelessness in older adults and the needs of this vulnerable population are scarce. Both research and public policy on homelessness have focused primarily on younger homeless people and, in particular, on the increasing numbers of families with children. This chapter will define older-adult homelessness, discuss the prevalence of older adults who are homeless, and identify risk factors for becoming homeless. Physical and mental health issues common to older adults who are homeless will also be described.

DEFINING HOMELESSNESS

The definition of who is actually homeless is hotly debated. This is related to the disagreements between policy makers and homeless advocates about who should be defined as homeless. Not surprisingly, there is little agreement on this basic issue. Numbers are extremely important because they affect the willingness of government agencies to fund programs for the homeless. Some define homelessness strictly in terms of the guidelines provided by the Stewart B. McKinney Act (1994), that is, "literal homelessness," which restricts the definition of homelessness to persons who stay in shelters or public spaces. This definition excludes persons in institutions with no known address, persons living in single-room occupancy hotels, persons who live in inadequate housing, with no plumbing or heating, for example, or persons doubled up with unwilling relatives or friends. Disagreement also exists as to at what age "older homelessness" begins, but recently researchers and service providers have agreed that "older homeless" should be defined as age 50 and older (Cohen, 1999; Crane, 1999; Stergiopoulos & Herrmann, 2003). Researchers have argued that such a definition is appropriate because at age 50, homeless persons have physical illnesses and disabilities resembling those in the general population who are 10–20 years older. (Cohen & Sokolovsky, 1989; Gelberg, Linn, & Mayer-Oaks, 1990). In this chapter, the older homeless will be defined as age 50 and older.

PREVALENCE OF HOMELESSNESS AMONG OLDER ADULTS

As a result of methodological and financial constraints, estimating the number of older adults who are homeless is especially challenging. Surveys designed to evaluate the numbers of older homeless persons typically use data provided by health clinics, shelters and soup kitchens (Burt, Aron, Lee, & Valente, 2001). Numbers reveal a wide range of estimates, between 2.5–27.7% of the total homeless population (Cohen, 1999). Many older homeless adults comprise what is called the "hidden homeless." This category includes older adults who stay with friends or those who are temporarily housed in prisons and hospitals. Another factor is that many older homeless are reluctant to use services for the homeless (Crane & Warnes, 2001). Older homeless adults may not be reached through the network of services designed to care for their needs because of fears of robbery or assault from younger clients or negative attitudes of providers (Martins, 2003).

In most studies, older adults are under-represented among the homeless compared with the general population (Stergiopoulos & Herrmann,

2003). This may be attributed to the higher mortality rates of older homeless persons (Barrow, Herman, Cordova, & Struening, 1999; Cheung & Hwang, 2004; Hwang, Orav, O'Connell, Lebow, & Brennan, 1997), or to the safety net of social security benefits, which begin at the age of 65. Older homeless adults tend to be young elderly, with few over the age of 75 (Crane, 1999). The absolute numbers of older adults who are homeless are increasing (Cohen, 1999; Tully & Jacobson, 1994). With the doubling of the population of those aged 50 and older expected during the next three decades, the number of older homeless adults is anticipated to increase from the current level of 60,000–400,000 to 120,000–800,000, (Cohen, 1999). The current aging population has more risk factors for homelessness; thus, these numbers represent a conservative estimate. The risk for homelessness is substantially greater for those aged 50–65 than for those aged 65 and older (Cohen, 1999). This is related to social service programs that will provide housing to the older adults who are aged 65 and more.

The causes of homelessness among older adults are multifactorial (Bottomly, Bissonette, & Snekvik, 2001; Cohen & Sokolovsky, 1989; Crane & Warnes, 2001; Snow & Anderson, 1993; Stergiopoulos & Herrmann, 2003). Several researchers have proposed that homelessness results from the interaction of individual personal traits and societal forces (Cohen, 1999; Susser, Moore, & Link, 1993). Cohen (1999) provides a model useful in understanding homelessness among older adults. The model suggests that individual background risk factors from early life and later life, as well as sociodemographic risk factors, interact with macro-level structural forces to make a vulnerable person become homeless. Once homeless, a person may become enculturated to a shelter-dependent life, which leads to prolonged homelessness (Cohen, 1999) (see Figure 5.1).

The risk factors of homelessness among persons aged 50 and older are multiple. The factors include being male, African American, having low income, low job skills, difficult childhoods, chemical abuse, mental illness, cognitive deficits, chronic health problems, abuse, limited social network, and history of being single, divorced, or never married (Cohen, 1999).

SOCIODEMOGRAPHIC RISK FACTORS

Homelessness can best be understood if viewed as the interplay between sociodemographic individual risk factors and macro-level structural processes, such as the labor and housing market. Gender is an important risk factor. In the general population, women aged 50 and older outnumber men. In the aging homeless population, however, the number of men

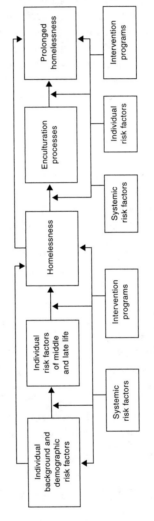

FIGURE 5.1 A model of homeless and aging. From Cohen, 1999. Reprinted with permission.

generally far exceeds that of women. Although numbers vary based on geographic location, most studies of older homeless adults have found that older men outnumber older women at least by 4:1 (Cohen, 1999). Men are at greater risk of becoming homeless in early and middle adulthood through repeated episodes of homelessness, whereas women tend to become homeless after the age of 50. Because of entitlement programs that are oriented toward women and children as well as other cultural factors, women seem to be able to avoid becoming homeless earlier in life. Women become vulnerable to homelessness at midlife because of physical abuse, separation, divorce, onset of psychiatric illness, or widowhood (Crane & Warnes, 2001). A higher probability of poverty combined with the growing shortage of affordable housing places older women at risk of homelessness. Some researchers argue that older women in the United States are now more vulnerable than older men to becoming homeless, a trend that will continue as the baby boom generation ages (Hobbs & Damon, 1996; Kisor & Kendal-Wilson, 2002).

Race

Studies conducted in large metropolitan areas in the United States have shown that among homeless persons aged over 50, the majority are Caucasian (Cohen, 1999); however, Blacks make up the majority of younger homeless people. The majority of the "new" generation of older homeless is predicted to be Black because of their higher levels of poverty and individual risk factors. Latinos historically have been underrepresented among homeless people inspite of their high poverty levels. It has been suggested that Latinos may experience less housing and job discrimination than Blacks and that they are more likely to incorporate additional family members into a single household. Studies of new Latino immigrants to the United States found reduced risk factors for homelessness related to tight family bonds and community protection (Vega et al., 1998). Latinos also have lower levels of personal risk factors, such as psychiatric or substance abuse disorders, rendering them less vulnerable than their White and Black cohorts among the very poor. As Latinos become acculturated, however, the risks for homelessness may become similar to other populations (Vega, 1998).

Poverty and Lack of Housing

Poverty is overwhelmingly associated with homelessness; the causes of homelessness are best understood by examining the causes of poverty (Susser et al., 1993). Most older homeless adults come from poor backgrounds and tend to have spent their lives at or near the poverty level.

During their lifetimes, the majority worked as semiskilled or unskilled laborers. The two components most cited that have contributed to the rise in homelessness among older adults are lack of income and lack of affordable housing. Gentrification and governmental indifference in U.S. cities has decimated the numbers of affordable housing units. In a comparison of rates of homelessness among persons aged 50 and older, New York had rates 22 times greater than London, a city of comparable demographic size (Cohen & Crane, 1996). This is directly attributable to greater numbers of public and extremely low-cost housing units in London.

Support for poor U.S. citizens is inadequate. In the United States, only persons who are 65 and over are provided health coverage and Social Security benefits. Homeless adults aged 50–64 fall under the safety net, and are especially vulnerable to homelessness. Cohen (1999) identifies structural and personal risk factors which lead to homelessness. This includes diminished availability of affordable housing, decreased income support and entitlement programs, decreased low-skilled jobs, decreased housing for adults who are disabled, and lack of outreach programs.

Disruptive Childhood and Life Experiences

In addition to backgrounds of poverty, childhood background and family experiences may be critical in explaining homelessness in late life. Studies have found a consistent relationship between increased risk of homelessness and disruptive family events in childhood (Cohen, 1999, Crane 1999, Susser et al., 1993). Crane (1999), in her studies of homeless older adults in London and Northern England, stated that different events and illnesses from earlier life stages may trigger and contribute to homelessness in old age. These are considered antecedents and include childhood experiences, such as abuse and foster care, early adulthood mental illness and drinking, midlife marital breakdown or death of last parent, and later life death of spouse, marital breakdown, difficulty with retirement, discharge from armed services, and mental illness (Crane, 1999) (see Table 5.1).

Substance Abuse/Addictions

As many as one half to three fourths of homeless persons have diagnoses of alcohol or other drug dependences (Wenzel, Ebener, Koegel, & Gelberg, 1996). Homeless substance abusers seem to have needs and characteristics different from those of substance abusers who have more stable housing situations. For example, compared with the domiciled counterparts, homeless substance abusers have been found to have greater severity and chronicity of alcoholism, greater social and economic

TABLE 5.1   Antecedents of Homelessness in Older Adults

Stage in life	Antecedent event
Childhood/Adolescence	Disturbed homes/broken homes Involvement in foster care Runaway/throwaway child Time in shelter
Early Adulthood	Discharge from military service Mental illness Problems with alcohol use Itinerant working life
Midlife	Death or deteriorating health of last surviving parent Separation or divorce Loss of work Mental illness Problems with alcohol use
Later Life	Separation or divorce Death of spouse Discharge from military service Retirement and loss of work accommodations Retirement and loneliness Inability to manage finances Mental illness

Adapted from Crane (1999).

disadvantages, greater psychological distress, and more pervasive medical problems (Stahler & Cohen, 1995). Homeless persons are often provided inferior treatment services, compounded by their substance abuse. Their involvement in the service system is often episodic, of short duration, and punctuated with relapses.

Mental Illness

Deinstitutionalization is often associated with a high rate of mental illness within the homeless population (Backrach, 1992; Lamb, 1992). The streets have become the newest dumping ground for discharged mental health patients (Hopper, 1988). On any given night it is estimated that approximately one third of the single homeless adults suffer from the added burden of severe mental illnesses. Severe mental illness includes persistent mental or emotional disorders including, but not limited to schizophrenia, schizoaffective disorders, mood disorders such as depression, and severe personality disorders (Walker, 1998). Herman, Susser, and Struening (1994) found in their study of 1,849 homeless adults that those subjects who report current severe depressive symptoms are more likely to have had childhood out-of-home care, such as foster, group, or institutional care. Daily hassles, social supports, and coping skills are essential ingredients in determining depressive symptoms with the homeless (Belcher & DiBlasio, 1990; LaGory, Ritchey, & Mullis, 1991). Unresolved grief has also been associated with the downward social mobility of the homeless. The cause of such social collapse is thought to be an experience of relationship loss (Hughs & Fleming, 1991).

Mental illness significantly interferes with a person's ability to carry out primary aspects of daily life, such as self-care, household management, interpersonal relationships, and work or school (Federal Task Force on Homelessness and Severe Mental Illness, 1992). It is estimated that at least 20% of the homeless population has been treated for mental illness (Mason, Jenson, & Boland, 1992). In an ethnographic study, Desjarlais (1994) found that mentally ill homeless people struggle through their daily encounters. Fragmentation of service delivery was recognized as a serious impediment for homeless mentally ill people (Rosenheck et al., 1998). The homeless mentally ill also had high rates of criminal victimization; they are victims of crimes that increase their social adjustment problems (Lam & Rosenheck, 1998).

HEALTH PROBLEMS OF OLDER HOMELESS ADULTS

Homelessness itself causes illness. Older homeless adults must cope with lack of shelter, severe poverty, exposure to the elements, crime, lack of medical care, and social marginalization. Deleterious health consequences result from chronic exposure to the stressors of homelessness. Homelessness brings with it an overall deterioration of physical health, especially for older adults who have the most urgent needs for health care. Homeless older adults have higher rates of physical morbidity and mortality than their cohorts in the general population (Bottomly, 2001; Crane, 1999; Stergiopoulos & Herrmann, 2003). The lifestyles of older homeless adults complicate health promotion practices and health protection. The health problems of older homeless adults are exacerbated by age, severe living conditions, poor nutrition, lack of proper sleeping arrangements, lack of health care, and extreme stress from living on the streets. In comparison with the general population aged 50 and older, homeless older adults are significantly more likely to have a chronic disease, functional disabilities, high blood pressure, elevated creatinine levels, and elevated cholesterol (Cohen, 1999; Gelberg et al., 1990).

Homeless adults age prematurely on the streets. The health and functional problems of homeless people aged more than 50 years resemble those in the general population of adults who are 65 and older (Cohen, 1999). For older homeless adults, the risks to health increase with the time they remain without adequate housing (Bottomly, 2001). The older adult on the street is disadvantaged at multiple levels. Homelessness itself is a survival level of existence that is brutalizing, exhausting, and dehumanizing. The effort of securing basic survival needs, such as food, a safe place to sleep, and somewhere to perform personal hygiene, leaves little time or energy to seek necessary medical care or to comply with treatment plans. The homeless older adult lacks social support from family and friends at a time of life when most people can expect to draw on a safety net of resources and relationships.

PHYSICAL HEALTH PROBLEMS

Older homeless adults experience higher rates of every type of physical illness than their cohorts in the housed population (Bottomly, 2001; Crane, 1999). They are also more likely than the general population to be hospitalized for a preventable condition. Older homeless adults have at least three major chronic health problems with the most common diagnoses being hypertension, alcohol abuse, and psychiatric problems (Rich, Rich, & Mullins, 1995). Major medical problems frequently reported among older homeless adults include dental problems, glaucoma, asthma, bronchitis and pneumonia, chronic obstructive pulmonary disease, hypertension, arthritis, circulatory problems, anemia, diabetes, gastrointestinal problems, and sensory impairment (Stergiopoulos & Herrmann, 2003). Health problems also stem directly from homelessness. Homelessness increases the older homeless person's exposure to infectious and communicable diseases, to accidents, criminal assaults, skin disorders, parasite infestations, malnutrition, peripheral vascular disease, leg ulcers, and cellulitis (Crane, 1999; Gelberg et al., 1990; Stergiopoulos & Hermann, 2003, Wright, 1990). Health problems that are more prevalent with older homeless adults than with domiciled older adults include hypothermia, dehydration, urinary incontinence, sleep deprivation, infectious diseases, musculoskeletal, food and leg ailments, and accidents and assaults. The homeless also have untreated chronic illnesses, both physical and mental.

Hypothermia

Older adults have impaired thermoregulatory mechanisms and are less able to adjust to extremes of environmental temperatures (Kane, Ouslander, & Abrass, 2004). Age-related changes involved in temperature dysregulation include declines in thermoregulatory mechanism, perception of temperature changes, efficiency in adjusting to change of temperature, resting peripheral blood flow, shivering, muscle mass, fat stores, and metabolic rate (Leuckenotte, 2000). Hypothermia is an extremely common problem seen in the older homeless population. Owing to strict regulations, many older homeless adults must vacate night-time shelters very early in the morning and linger out on the streets until shelters re-open in the evening, thereby prolonging exposure to cold stress. For older homeless adults, the risks to physical health are greatest when living on the street.

As stated earlier, older homeless adults may avoid public shelters because of fears of being assaulted or robbed, or because staff may be abusive and insensitive to their needs. They may often prefer to sleep outdoors in cold, damp conditions, in abandoned cars and derelict housing, in old factories, in cemeteries, in parks, doorways, subways, and the likes. Some older homeless persons who sleep outdoors create beds from cardboard, newspaper, and sleeping bags. Others have no bedding at all, and lack appropriate clothing. Those who sleep outside are at risk of hypothermia and frostbite, which can develop into gangrene and eventually lead to amputation. Hypothermia and frostbite are hazards of life on the streets and have been shown to be risk factors for early death in homeless people (O'Connell, 2004). In addition to prolonged exposure to cold stress, older homeless adults have many comorbid conditions, which contribute to the high risk for hypothermia. Psychiatric illness, alcoholism, smoking, cardiac disease, peripheral vascular disease, malnutrition, and metabolic disorders such as hypothyroidism and hypoglycemia, contribute to an increased risk for hypothermia.

Dehydration

Thirst regulation is affected as the body ages, making dehydration a primary risk among older adults. The older homeless adult is particularly vulnerable, due to lack of food and access to nonalcoholic fluids, as well as excessive alcohol consumption. Most older homeless adults seen at homeless healthcare clinics suffer from some degree of dehydration (Bottomly, 2001). Dehydration is a risk factor for falls and hospitalizations in older homeless adults.

Urinary Incontinence

Both older homeless men and women suffer from all types of urinary incontinence: stress, urge, functional, and mixed. Functional incontinence is the most common form seen among older homeless adults (Bottomly,

2001). This is caused by the lack of available or accessible public bathrooms, cognitive impairments, and multiple layers of clothing. Problems associated with incontinence include skin breakdown from wet clothing and lack of access to care for basic hygiene needs.

Sleep Deprivation

Sleep deprivation ranks as one of the most prevalent complaints among older homeless people. In normal aging, periods of deep sleep are decreased, with increased periods of wakefulness. Homeless adults staying at night-time shelters may have difficulty in sleeping. Shelters are noisy and beds are very close together. Fear of assault is always present and fatigue is constant. Sleep deprivation compromises the immune system, further exposing the homeless older adult to a host of illnesses.

Infectious Diseases

Age-related changes in the immune system coupled with the environmental hazards of homelessness greatly increase the rates of infectious disease among older homeless adults. The older adult is much more susceptible to diseases, such as tuberculosis (TB), respiratory infections, skin infestations, and gastroenteritis. The often over-crowded and unsanitary conditions of shelters promote the transmission of infectious and communicable diseases (Wright, Rubin, & Devine, 1998). The incidence of tuberculosis is steadily increasing among the homeless, who may be unable to comply with treatment and who often find themselves in the close quarters of a shelter. TB is also underdiagnosed among older adults and is undergoing resurgence (Rich et al., 1995). In large shelters, the space between beds and necessary ventilation systems are far less than recommended for the prevention of air-borne infections (Robertson & Greenblatt, 1992). Positive skin test rate for TB increases progressively with the length of time people spend in shelters (Brickner, Scanlan, & Conanan, 1986). Older homeless people are more susceptible to tuberculosis infections, and to lesions becoming re-activated because of general ill health, poor diet, poor adherence to treatment, and because early detection and treatment is rare in the homeless population (Crane, 1999). For some homeless adults, TB infections are drug-resistant because of failures to comply with treatment or they have been infected with resistant strains of the organisms by contact with others who were not treated appropriately (Crane, 1999). TB treatment regimens may require taking medication over a period of nine months or more. Compliance with these treatment regimens proves difficult, if not impossible, for homeless older people, because of their daily challenge of finding a suitable sleeping arrangement for the night and lack the necessary storage space for medications. Surveys in large metropolitan areas in the United States have shown the rate of positive skin tests to be as high as one in three of homeless persons. (Gelberg, 2000). Some estimates have placed the rate of TB among the homeless in the United States to be 25–100 times more than that in the adult population as a whole (Wright, 1989).

Upper respiratory disorders of varying degrees of severity are endemic to homelessness. Minor upper respiratory complaints represent 40% of acute medical complaints of people who are homeless (O'Connell, 1991; Raoult, Foucault, & Brouqui, 2001). Death from respiratory diseases is reported to be seven times higher in the homeless than in the general population (Raoult et al., 2001). It is estimated that 90% of shelters users smoke (www.streetlevel.ca/newsArticlesStats/homeless_health_facts.htm). Crowded shelters and soup kitchens provide ideal circumstances for the spread of respiratory infections. Respiratory illnesses such as colds, flu, sore throat, bronchitis, and pneumonia, are common among older homeless adults. Recuperation from these illnesses is difficult given their poor living conditions and poor nutritional status. Older homeless adults are also highly susceptible to gastroenteritis, due to unsanitary living conditions, poor hygiene, and poor diets. Many older street homeless people avoid soup kitchens and day centers, preferring to eat discarded food from trash bins, because they fear intimidation and violence from younger homeless people (Crane, 1999).

Scabies and lice infestations are the major parasitic disorders of homeless people. Close contact in crowded shelters, lack of laundry facilities, sharing clothing and bedding, and poor hygiene permit easy passage of these parasites. These infestations cause severe pruritus and can cause significant secondary disorders, such as impetigo and internal abscesses. The louse-transmitted bacterium, *Bartonella quintana*, has recently been found to cause clinical conditions in the homeless, such as urban trench fever, bacillary angiomatosis, endocarditis, and chronic afebrile bacteremia (Raoult et al., 2001).

Musculoskeletal Ailments

Osteoarthritis, osteoporosis, fractures and foot deformities are commonly seen in the older homeless population. Because of lack of access to health care, these disorders become much more acute in the older homeless person, resulting in severe pain and loss of functioning. Falls are a major cause of morbidity in the older adult population (Kane et al., 2004). The environmental hazards of daily life on the streets predispose older homeless adults to falls. Age-related factors, which contribute to instability, such as muscle weakness, decreases in proprioception, and sensory changes interact with the environmental hazards of homelessness. Untreated medical and neuropsychiatric conditions, dehydration, medications, malnutrition, accidents, and poor-fitting shoes and clothing are potential contributors to falls.

Foot and Lower Leg Problems

Some shelters impose limits on the numbers of nights one may stay, and/or operate on a first-come, first-serve basis. Older adults who may be suffering from a host of chronic illnesses must vacate the shelter early in the morning regardless of the weather or how they feel, carrying with them all of their belongings. Often the only mode of transportation for them is their feet. The older adult who is homeless often walks miles each day to food kitchens, churches, or other places for sanctuary until the evening shelter opens again. In some cities, it is illegal to sit in downtown areas with belongings that occupy more than 3 feet. In other cities, common activities of homeless persons, such as sleeping in parks are criminal activities (Cohen, Sokolovsky, & Crane, 2001). Older adults who are homeless are often persecuted by police, and told to "move along" if they sit in malls, libraries, cafes, or bus stations.

Of all the health problems associated with homelessness, foot and lower leg problems are among the most common. Thirty percent of older adults who are homeless report foot or lower leg problems (Brickner et al., 1986; Raoult et al., 2001). Prolonged walking and standing in poor-fitting shoes causes blisters and corns; cold and moisture and lack of good foot hygiene promote primary foot lesions, athletes' foot (*tinea pedis*), and nail fungus (*onychomycosis*). Overgrown toenails promote the development of lesions, which contribute to the formation of ulcers. These infections may result in cellulitis, osteomelitis, and gangrene leading to amputation of the limb (Raoult et al.). Tetanus may also occur.

Peripheral vascular disease (PVD) is another very common condition reported in homeless older adults (Brickner et al, 1986). Heavy use of alcohol and tobacco, as well as the high prevalence of hypertension and diabetes mellitus in older adults who are homeless are causes and exacerbating factors in the development of peripheral arterial disease (Caton, 1990). The problems of peripheral arterial disease are compounded in homeless older adults by their lifestyle, which could include exposure to a subfreezing environment, poorly fitting or badly worn shoes, poor foot hygiene, and delay in seeking medical assistance should injury of frostbite occur. Complications resulting from PVD, such as gangrene and amputation, are higher among homeless adults than in the general population (Caton, 1999).

Venous disease of the lower extremities in homeless people is more common than arterial disease. The older adult is at increased risk to developing lower leg venous dysfunction because they are frequently unable to lie supine at night, and because of prolonged standing and walking during the day. Many homeless older adults must spend nights sleeping in a sitting position, semiupright and flexed at the waist, on park benches or in cramped spaces. The most prevalent form of peripheral vascular diseases among the homeless is the chronic venous stasis ulcer (Brickner et al., 1986). For the older homeless adult, once the ulcer has formed, the likelihood of infection is increased due to the environmental hazards of homelessness.

Accidents and Assaults

Trauma is one of the leading causes of death and disability among homeless persons (Brickner & Scharer, 1985). The homeless suffer an alarmingly high incidence of repeat trauma and hospitalization. They are 50 times more likely than the housed population to be fatally assaulted (Bottomly, 2001). Older adults live under constant threat of assault. They are easy targets for robbery and live in a constant state of danger. Lack of a safe refuge and impaired functional capacity due to malnutrition, alcoholism, or sensory impairment render older homeless adults extremely vulnerable to assaults. Surveys from large US cities found that half of older homeless persons had been robbed and nearly one third had been physically assaulted during the prior year (Cohen & Sokolovsky, 1989). Two thirds of all homeless women have a history of physical and sexual abuse, and one in three women report that an abusive relationship led directly to homelessness (Cohen, 1999). In Detroit, in one year, 30% of older homeless women reported they had been raped (Cohen, 1999). Trauma interacts with poverty, inadequate housing, physical and mental illnessess to produce and perpetuate homelessness in older homeless adults.

CHRONIC DISEASES AMONG HOMELESS OLDER ADULTS

Diabetes Mellitus

The most common uncontrolled medical condition among people who are homeless is diabetes mellitus (Bottomly, 2001). Chronic disease management, while difficult for anyone, poses special problems for older adults who are homeless. Homeless people have to eat whatever is available, and meals are irregular, often only one or two per day, with limited or no dietary choices. Most food in shelters and soup kitchens is high in starch, sugar, and fat. To avoid hypoglycemia, an individual must eat three meals plus two snacks per day, a very difficult task for a homeless older adult. Glucometers for self-monitoring are difficult to obtain, particularly for the uninsured. Glucometers are often stolen in shelters. Test strips are expensive and hard to come by. Consistent administration of insulin is hampered by limited access to refrigeration. The cost of oral hyperglycemic medications is high, which restricts their availability for indigent populations. The older homeless adult often lacks health insurance, which limits access to specialty referrals to opthalmology, nephrology, endocrinology, and podiatry. Treatment for diabetes mellitus in older homeless adults is further complicated by cognitive deficits, depression, and alcoholism.

Cardiovascular Diseases: Hypertension, Hyperlipidemia, and Heart Failure

Cardiovascular diseases are highly prevalent among people experiencing homelessness (Burt, 1999; Gelberg et al., 1990; Hwang, 2001; Kinchen & Wright, 1991; Kleinman, Freeman, Perlman, & Gelberg, 1997; Szerlip & Szerlip, 2002; White, Tulskey, Dawson, Zolopa, & Moss, 1997; Wright, 1990). The most commonly seen disorders in the homeless population are hypertension, hyperlipidemia, and heart failure (Brammer et al., 2004). Homeless older adults are significantly more likely to have hypertension than their cohorts in the housed population. The rate of hypertension exceeds that reported for the general population by a factor of two (Wright, 1990).

Elevated serum cholesterol also has been found to be more prevalent among homeless adults than in the general adult population. Studies have shown the rates to be 55% in adults over the age of 50 in the homeless population (Gelberg et al., 1990). By comparison only 25% of all U.S. adults over the age of 50 have high serum cholesterol (National Health & Nutrition Examination Survey, NHANES III [Center of Disease Control (CDC), 2003]).

Homeless adults bear a higher risk for heart disease, although they are chronologically younger than the general adult population (Brammer et al., 2004). Heart failure is frequently seen among middle-aged homeless adults, secondary to alcohol use disorders and to chronic, uncontrolled hypertension and hyperlipidemia. Heart disease is a leading cause of death in middle-aged homeless persons aged 45–64 years (Hwang, 2000). Seventy percent of homeless people smoke compared with 25% of the general U.S. population (Sachs-Ericsson, et al., 1999). Practitioners serving homeless adults report that treatment of heart disease often involves earlier hospitalization than their cohorts in the housed population because of difficulty controlling sodium and fat intake and obtaining bedrest (Fleischman & Farnham, 1992). Older homeless adults have extreme difficulty adhering to treatment plans. Multidose regimens may be confusing for those who are cognitively impaired. Inadequate water intake and lack of access to bathroom facilities complicate the use of diuretics. Living in shelters requires that homeless people carry all medications with them due to lack of storage space. As a result, medications are frequently lost, stolen, or crumble in pockets.

Mental Health Disorders

SUBSTANCE ABUSE

The most prevalent psychiatric disorders found in homeless populations are substance use disorders (DeMallie, North, & Smith, 1997). Half of all homeless people have had a diagnosable substance abuse disorder at some point in their lives (Koegel, Burnam, & Baumohl, 1996). Alcoholism has long been identified as a dominant characteristic of homeless people. Problems with alcohol are six to seven times more prevalent among homeless persons than in the general population (Hwang, 2001). Recent surveys have shown lifetime rates of alcohol use disorders in 71% of men and in 63% of women (Robertson, Zlotnick, & Westerfelt, 1997). In older homeless adults, the reported prevalence of alcohol abuse is about three or four times higher among older men than among older women, and both older homeless men and women have higher abuse rates than their same-age peers in the general population (Cohen, 1999). Older homeless people who drink heavily tend to be in poorer physical and mental health overall (Cohen & Sokolovsky, 1989). Studies involving older homeless persons suggest that problem-drinking and alcohol consumption tend to decrease with advancing age. This may be due to high mortality related to alcoholism in older homeless adults. Surveys report that higher rates for alcohol abuse occur in homeless persons in the age group of 30–64, with prevalence rates at about 30%; in those aged 65 and older, only 18% are reported to be problem drinkers. Older adults who drink heavily have higher rates of depression (Crane & Warnes, 2001). Faced with the hopelessness and desperation of homelessness, older adults will continue to drink even though they may know they have serious health problems such as cirrhosis of the liver, renal failure and peripheral neuropathy (Crane, 1999). They are likely to neglect self-care and are subject to falls, seizures, incontinence, and general poor health. As people age on the street, they tend to become solitary drinkers (Cohen & Sokolovsky, 1989).

Illegal drug use is rare among older homeless adults (Cohen, 1999) and may be a generational phenomena. Drug abuse is much higher among the homeless baby boomer generation. Older homeless people, compared to younger homeless people, are less likely to have psychotic symptoms, drink alcohol frequently, or use illegal drugs (Gelberg et al., 1990). Drug use disorders are much more prevalent in younger compared to older homeless people (DeMallie et al., 1997). After the age of 50, drug use among homeless people drops off sharply. This trend may change, however, as the baby boomer generation ages.

MAJOR MENTAL DISORDERS

A good deal of research has been conducted on the psychiatric and addictive disorders of homeless people. The best estimates now indicate about 22% of homeless men and 29% of homeless women suffer from diagnosable psychiatric disorders (Cohen, 1999). Mental illness is certainly one of the most challenging issues encountered in older homeless adults, yet very little research exists about psychiatric disorders in the current older homeless population. Mental illness in old age is an important contributory factor to homelessness, particularly among those who lack cohesive support networks. Once homeless, mental health problems impair the older adult's capacity to seek and accept help. Studies involving homeless adults have shown a correlation between gender, age, and mental illness. Although studies indicate low levels of mental illness among older homeless populations, levels among older women seem to increase with age (Cohen). Individual studies have shown that mental illness is higher among older homeless women than among older homeless men. Research has found that older homeless men tend to have more depression, whereas older women tend to have more psychosis (Crane, 1998).

Homelessness is a downward spiral characterized by deep feelings of helplessness, hopelessness, loss of self-esteem, and self-neglect. The longer people remain homeless, the greater the likelihood that they will become resigned to their circumstances, and slip into a despondent and apathetic state. Individual studies in large metropolitan areas of the US have shown that one-half to three-quarters of older homeless people are depressed and demoralized (Cohen, 1989; Crane, 1998).

COGNITIVE IMPAIRMENT

Levels of cognitive impairment in older homeless range from 10–25%. About 5% of older homeless people have severe cognitive impairment, which is comparable to rates in the general population. In a study by Bubrick, Hodder, and Teesson (2003) 10% of the homeless showed evidence of cognitive impairment as assessed by the Mini Mental State Examination. Subjects with cognitive impairment were significantly older than those without impairment.

SUMMARY

Older adults who are homeless have largely been neglected in the literature on homelessness and gerontology. Researchers and public policy have primarily focused on younger homeless people, especially women and children. Although older homeless adults have been shown to represent only a small proportion of the overall homeless population, their numbers are growing. As the baby boomer generation ages, these numbers will increase dramatically, as will the numbers of at-risk persons. Homelessness results because of the interplay between individual vulnerabilities and the larger structural forces of society. Lack of adequate income and affordable housing place older adults at significant risk of homelessness. Homeless adults are much more likely to suffer from a host of chronic illnesses than their cohorts in the housed population. Homelessness itself causes illness. Superimposed on the normal aging process and chronic illnesses often associated with aging are the health and environmental hazards of homelessness, leading to extreme vulnerability for morbidity and mortality. Programs must be developed and expanded to respond to the needs of this extremely vulnerable population.

REFERENCES

Backrach, L. (1992). What we know about homelessness among mentally ill persons: An analytical review and commentary. *Hospital and Community Psychiatry, 43*, 453–464.

Barrow, S., Herman, D., Cordova, P., & Struening, E. (1999). Mortality among homeless shelter residents in New York City. *American Journal of Public Health, 89*, 529–534.

Belcher, J., & DiBlasio, F. (1990). The needs of depressed homeless persons: Designing appropriate services. *Community Mental Health Journal, 26*, 255–266.

Bottomley, J. (2001). Health care and homeless older adults. *Topics in Geriatric Rehabilitation, 17*(1), 1–21.

Bottomley, J., Bissonette, A., & Snekvik, V. (2001). The lives of homeless older adults: Please, tell them who I am. *Topics in Geriatric Rehabilitation, 16*(4), 50–64.

Brammer, S., Gee, G., Hale, A., Kopydlowski, M., Post, P., Rabiner, M., et al. (2004). Adapting your practice: Treatment and recommendations for homeless patients with cardiovascular diseases. *Health Care for the*

Homeless Clinicians' Network, National Health Care for the Homeless Council, Inc. Retrieved May 30, 2005. http://www.guidelines.gov/sum-mary/summary.aspx?ss=15&doc_id=4851&nbr=3492

Brickner, P. W., Scanlan, B. C., & Conanan, B. (1986). Homeless persons and health care. *Annals of Internal Medicine, 4,* 405–409.

Brickner, P. W., & Scharer, L. (Eds.). (1985). *Health care of homeless people.* New York: Springer Publishing.

Bubrick, N., Hodder, T., & Teesson, M. (2003). Schizophrenia among homeless people in inner Sydney: Current prevalence and historical trends. *Journal of Mental Heatlh. 12*(1), 51–57.

Burt, M. (1999). Demographics and geography: Estimating needs. In L. B. Fosburg & D. L. Dennis (Eds.), *Practical lessons: The 1998 National Symposium on Homelessness Research, 1*(pp. 1–24). Washington, DC: U.S. Department of Housing and Urban Development and U.S. Department of Health and Human Service.

Burt, M., Aron, L., Lee, E. & Valente, J. (2001). Homeless families with children. *Fact Sheet, no. 7. National Coalition for the Homeless,* June 2001. Retrieved on June 5, 2005 from http://www.nationalhomeless.org/education/families.html

Caton, C. (1990). *Homeless in America.* New York: Oxford University Press.

Center of Disease Control. (2003). *National Health and Nutrition Examination Survey (NHANES-2001-2002).* National Center for Health Statistics. Retrieved 5/30/05 http://www.cdc.gov/nchs/nhanes.htm

Cheung, A., & Hwang, S. (2004). Risk and death among homeless women: A cohort study and review of the literature. *Canadian Medical Association Journal, 170,* 1243–1247.

Cohen, C. (1999). Aging and homelessness. *Gerontologist, 39,* 5–14.

Cohen, C., & Crane, M. (1996). Old and homeless in London and New York City: A cross-national comparison. In D. Bhurga (Ed.), *Homelessness and mental health* (pp. 150–69). London: Cambridge University Press.

Cohen, C., Sokolovsky, J., & Crane, M. (2001). Aging, homelessness and the law. *International Journal of Law and Psychiatry, 24,* 167–181.

Cohen, C. I., & Sokolovsky, J. (1989). *Old men of the Bowery: Strategies for survival among the homeless.* New York: Guilford Press.

Cohen, M. B. (1989). Social work practice with homeless mentally ill people: Engaging the client. *Social Work, 34*(6), 505–509.

Crane, M. (1998). The association between mental illness and homelessness among older people: An exploratory study. *Aging and Mental Health,* 2(3). Retrieved February 21, 2004 from www.ebscohostResearch Databases

Crane, M. (1999). *Understanding older homeless people.* Philadelphia: Open University Press.

Crane, M., & Warnes, A. (2000), Evictions and prolonged homelessness. *Housing Studies, 15,* 757–773.

Crane, M., & Warnes, A. (2001). Older people and homelessness: Prevalence and causes. *Topics in Geriatric Rehabilitation, 16*(4), 1–14.

120   HOMELESS OLDER ADULTS

DeMallie, D., North, C., & Smith, E. (1997). Psychiatric disorders among the homeless: A comparison of older and younger groups. *Gerontological Society of America, 37*(1), 61–66.

Desjarlais, R. (1994). Struggling along: The possibilities for experience among the homeless mentally ill. *American Anthropologist, 96*(4), 16. Retrieved January 16, 2003 from InfoTrac database.

Federal Task Force on Homelessness and Severe Mental Illness. (1992). *Outcasts on Main street.* Washington, DC: National Institute of Mental Health, Department of Health and Human Services.

Fleischman, S., & Farnham, T. (1992). Chronic disease in the homeless. In D. Wood (Ed.), *Delivering health care to homeless persons: The diagnosis and management of medical and mental health conditions.* New York: Springer Publishing.

Gelberg, L. (2000). The behavioral model for vulnerable populations: Application to medical care use and outcomes for homeless people. *Health Services Research, 34*, 1273–1302.

Gelberg, L., Linn, L. S., & Mayer-Oakes, S. A. (1990). Differences in health status between older and younger homeless adults. *Journal of American Geriatrics Society, 38*, 1220–1229.

Herman, D., Susser, E., & Struening, E. (1994). Childhood out of home care and current depressive symptoms among homeless adult. *American Journal of Public Health, 84*(11), 1849–1851.

Hobbs, F., & Damon, B.(1996). *65+ in the United States.* Washington DC: US Bureau of Census. Retrieved on June 5, 2005 from http://www.census.gov/prod/1/pop/p23-190/p23190-f.pdf

Hopper, K. (1988). More than a passing strange: Homelessness and mental illness in New York City. *American Ethnologist, 15*(1), 155–167.

Hughs, C., & Fleming, D. (1991). Grief casualties on skid row. *Omega, 23*, 109–118.

Hwang, S. (2001). Homelessness and health. *Canadian Medical Association Journal, 164*, 229–233.

Hwang, S, Orav, J., O'Connell, J., Lebow, J., & Brennan, T. (1997). Causes of death in homeless adults in Boston. *Annals of Internal Medicine, 126*, 665–628.

Hwang, S. W. (2000). Mortality among men using homeless shelters in Toronto, Ontario. *Journal of the American Medical Association, 283*, 2152–2157.

Kane, R. L., Ouslander, J. G., & Abrass, I. B. (2004). Disorders of temperature regulation. In *Essentials of clinical geriatrics* (pp. 328–331). New York: McGraw-Hill.

Kinchen, K., & Wright, J. D. (1991). Hypertension management in health care for the homeless clinics: Results from a survey. *American Journal of Public Health, 81*, 1163–1165.

Kisor, A., & Kendal-Wilson, L. (2002). Older homeless women: Reframing the stereotype of the bag lady. *Affilia, 17*, 354–370.

Kleinman, L., Freeman, H., Perlman, J., & Gelberg, L. (1997). Homing in on the homeless: Assessing the physical health of homeless adults in Los Angeles County using an original method to obtain physical examination data in a survey. *Health Service Research, 31*, 533–549.

Koegel, P., Burnam, M. A., & Baumohl, J. (1996). The causes of homelessness. In *Homelessness in America*. Washington, DC: Oryx Press. Available from the National Coalition for the Homeless, 2201 P St NW, Washington, DC 20037.

LaGory, M., Ritchey, F., & Mullis, J. (1991). Depression among the homeless. *Journal of Health and Social Behavior, 31*, 87–101.

Lam, J., & Rosenheck, R. (1998). The effect of victimization on clinical outcomes of homeless persons with serious mental illness. *Psychiatric Services, 49*, 678–683.

Lamb, H. R. (1992). Perspectives on effective advocacy for homeless mentally ill persons. *Hospital and Community Psychiatry, 43*, 1209–1212.

Lueckenotte, A. (2000). *Gerontologic nursing* (2nd ed.). St. Louis: Mosby.

Martins, D. C. (2003). *Health care experiences of homeless people*. UMI ProQuest Digital Dissertations Online. UMI Publication Number: AAT 3089752.

Mason, D., Jensen, M., & Boland, D. (1992). Health behaviors and health risks among homeless males in Utah. *Western Journal of Nursing Research, 14*, 775–790.

National Coalition for the Homeless. (1999). *NCH Fact Sheet# 15: Homelessness among elderly persons*. Washington, DC: Author, O'Connell, J. (1991). Nontuberculous respiratory infections among the homeless. *Seminars in Respiratory Infections, 6*, 247–253.

O'Connell, J. (2004). Dying in the shadows: The challenges of providing health care for the homeless. *Canadian Medical Association Journal, 170*, 1251–1252.

Raoult, D., Foucault, C., & Brouqui, P. (2001). Infections in the homeless. *Lancet Infectious Diseases, 1*(2), 77–84.

Rich, D. W., Rich, T. A., & Mullins, L. C. (1995). *Old and Homeless–Double Jeopardy: An Overview of Current Practice and Policies*. Westport, CT: Auburn House.

Robertson, M., & Greenblatt, M. (1992). *Homelessness: A national perspective series. Topics in social psychiatry*. New York: Springer Publishing.

Robertson, M., Zlotnick, & C., Westerfelt, A. (1997). Drug use disorders and treatment contact among homeless adults in Alameda County, California. *American Journal of Public Health, 87*, 221–228.

Rosenheck, R., Morrissey, J., Lam, J., Calloway, M., Johnsen, M., Goldman, H., et al. (1998). Service system integration, access to services, and housing outcomes in a program for homeless persons with severe mental illness. *American Journal of Public Health, 88*, 1610–1615.

Sachs-Ericsson, N., Wise, E., Debrody, C. P., & Paniucki, H. B. (1999). Health problems and service utilization in the homeless. *Journal for the Poor and Underserved, 10*, 443–452.

Snow, D., & Anderson, L. (1993). *Down on their luck: A study of homeless street people*. Berkeley: University of California Press.

Stahler, G., & Cohen, E. (1995). Homelessness and substance abuse in the 1990's [Special issue]. *Contemporary Drug Problems, 22*(2), 169–192.

Stergiopoulos, V., & Herrmann, N. (2003). Old and homeless: A review and survey of older adults who use shelters in an urban setting. *Canadian Journal of Psychiatry, 48*, 374–380.

Stewart McKinney Act. (1994). Definition of homelessness. The Steward B. Mc Kinney Homeless Assistance Act. (U.S.C. 42 § 11302).

Susser, E., Moore, R., & Link, B. (1993). Risk factors for homelessness. *Epidemiologic Reviews, 15*, 546–556.

Szerlip, M., & Szerlip, H. (2002). Identification of cardiovascular risk factors in homeless adults. *American Journal of Medical Sciences, 324*, 243–246.

Tully, C., & Jacobson, S. (1994). The homeless elderly: America's forgotten population. *Journal of Gerontology and Social Work, 23*(3/4), 61–84.

Vega, W., Kolody, B., Aguilar-Gaxiola, S., Alderete, E., Catalano, R., Caraveo-Anduaga, J. (1998). Lifetime prevalence of DSM-III-R psychiatric disorders among rural and urban Mexican Americans in California. *Archives of General Psychiatry, 55*, 771–782.

Walker, C. (1998). Homeless people and mental health. *American Journal of Nursing, 98*(11), 26–32.

Wenzel, S., Ebener, P., Koegel, P., & Gelberg, L. (1996). Drug-abusing homeless clients in California's substance abuse treatment system. *Journal of Psychoactive Drugs, 28*, 147–159.

White, M., Tulskey, J., Dawson, D., Zolopa, A, & Moss, A. (1997). Association between time homeless and perceived health status among the homeless in San Francisco. *Journal of Community Health, 22*, 271–282.

Wright, J. D. (1989). *Address Unknown: Homelessness in Contemporary America.* Hawthorne, New York: Aldine de Gruyter.

Wright, J. D. (1990). Poor people, poor health: The health status of the homeless. *Journal of Social Issues, 46*(4), 49–64.

Wright, J., Rubin, B., & Divine, J. (1998). Beside the golden door: Policy, politics and the homeless. New York: Aldine de Gruyter.

CHAPTER SIX

Health Care Strategies for Homeless Older Adults

D. C. Martins and M. A. Sullivan

The issue of elder homelessness is a serious one that needs to be addressed by all sectors of the community. Elder's needs are often neglected by a climate of eroding government and sporadic social program supports. This chapter will address strategies to assist professionals to care for older adults who are homeless or at risk of becoming homeless and to work with this population effectively. Several approaches will be suggested including preventing elder homelessness, advocating to end elder homelessness and caring for those who are homeless. Diversity within the homeless population presents numerous challenges for service delivery. The development of policies and services for the homeless is complex. Services for the person who is homeless compete for scarce resources along with health and social care, and older homeless peoples' needs vie for attention with the new younger homeless families with children (Crane, 1999). Programs and services of the aging network were not designed to serve the homeless, and specialized programs for elders are few (Cohen, Teresi, Holmes, & Roth, 1988; Doolin, 1986; Hecht & Coyle, 2001; Keigher & Greenblatt, 1992).

There are obstacles that further marginalize homeless older adults and keep them lost and invisible in a society in which poor people have no safe place. It is extremely difficult for homeless people to become reestablished and resettled. There are multiple challenges for professionals including creating a sense of privacy in an open environment, mistrust and conflicts with the shelter and soup kitchen staff, and the agony of maintaining relationships with family members, friends, and lovers, both within and outside the shelters. The professional working to end elder homelessness will be dealing with multiple clients needing service as funding sources and other support declines; the frustrations of dealing with an inefficient public bureaucracy; and the homeless person's struggle to maintain a sense of community in the face of destructive forces, such as ageism, sexism, racism, and mental illness.

INTERVENTIONS AND SERVICE DELIVERY FOR OLDER ADULTS WHO ARE HOMELESS

Three tiers comprise the service delivery system to the homeless population that is now present (Markos & Allen, 2001). The first tier involves the direct care given at emergency shelters, soup kitchens, drop-in centers and detoxification clinics. The goal of the first-tier services is for basic survival and health needs. The second tier is more long-term in nature and includes midstream interventions, such as transitional housing and empowerment of elders. The third tier is permanent and supportive and involves policy changes, changes in professional's perspectives, and permanent housing. The three tiers move from the first tier with "downstream" interventions and an individual, micro focus to the third tier "upstream" or macro focus, to address the interventions needed for older adults who are homeless. The upstream focus was first described by McKinlay (1986) and later Butterfield (1990) to address the political economy of illness. Downstream interventions refer to those activities that health providers perform to maintain the status quo by providing basic survival needs to our clients, whereas upstream interventions are those changes that must be made at the sociostructural level with political activity and policy changes.

Both macro- and micro-level factors need to be considered when examining the causes of homelessness among older adults, as well as strategies and interventions for professionals to assist this population. Macro-level factors include poverty and lack of affordable housing. The micro-level factors include individual vulnerabilities, such as mental illness, substance abuse, and disability. These may undermine an individual's ability to negotiate for jobs, housing, and services from the welfare system (Snow & Anderson, 1993). In this chapter both micro/downstream and macro/upstream level interventions and programs will be discussed.

TIER 1: DOWNSTREAM STRATEGIES

The immediate needs of homeless older adults are related to their emergency- or survival-oriented needs. This includes the need for food, shelter, mental health, physical health, and safety from street living. These needs cannot be addressed via traditional elder service programs. The existing soup kitchens, food pantries, emergency shelters, drug and alcohol programs, homeless medical clinics, and mental health programs exist to respond to the growing numbers of emergency needs. The treatment is generally problem-focused and is ameliorative rather than rehabilitative or long term in nature (Doolin, 1986). The downstream strategies include multipurpose centers, shelter programs, food service programs, health service programs, social service programs, emergency elder shelters, small day programs, large day programs, outreach programs, and establishing homeless/provider relationships.

In one study, homeless older people reported that homelessness could have been prevented if they had received outside assistance at a critical time in their life (Crane & Warnes, 2001). Downstream emergency services during a life crisis may prevent people who are experiencing difficulty when young or middle aged from becoming the future older homeless population (Crane & Warnes, 2001).

Multipurpose Centers

Multipurpose centers offer programs to meet the emergency health needs of the older adult homeless. Multipurpose programs are seen in many cities throughout the United States. The Multipurpose Center is a large, urban program that provides a variety of programs, including medical care, dental services, drop-in center, clothing, laundry facilities, and social services such as job training. In some programs, a hot line is available to respond to issues related to abuse and violence 24 hours a day. These centers are often frightening for older adults who are homeless with different needs from homeless children, families, and younger adults. The centers tend to be fast moving and occupied by many transient homeless adults that may be involved in drugs, alcohol, or violent behavior. The older adults tend to be hesitant to use these centers owing to fears of robbery or abuse. The older homeless people could benefit from special elder programs in the centers with an interdisciplinary staff that focused on the special needs of the older homeless populations.

Shelter Programs

The shelters for the homeless are available predominately for one-night stays. They often open at dinner time, serve a dinner, and have dormitory-style rooms for sleeping. Many shelters are dehumanizing places where the homeless elder is among the most disenfranchised. The elderly street person is often more severely physically and mentally disabled than his or her younger counterpart, needing an extra measure of support to survive. More important, the younger homeless people tend to "squeeze out" and take advantage of the older street people (Doolin, 1986). This is caused by the older homeless person's increased vulnerability due to increases in chronic illnesses and decreases in agility and sensation from the effects of street life. A shelter program organized specifically for older homeless people could increase their safety and focus their service needs.

Food Service Programs

Many food service programs exist within a variety of settings. Some of the programs are privately operated services that function purely as free eating places. These are often sponsored by church groups. Often the food service programs are referred to as *soup kitchens*. The foods offered are usually donated items from local supermarkets, restaurants, or private donations. The extensive nutritional deficiency in daily food intake of homeless older adults is not surprising. Most of the food offered is low-cost and high quantity, and hence is limited in fresh fruits and vegetables, dairy product, and whole-grain foods. Instead, the majority of food is highly refined and relatively high in fats, starches, and sugars. This sometimes leads to food items that may be filling but not always suited for the older adults nutritional needs. *Food pantries* are also established either as part of some soup kitchens or as food pantries only. The food pantries usually have a variety of nonperishable food items available for the older homeless person to select.

Johnson and McCool (2003) suggest several strategies that can improve the food intake of older homeless women. One suggestion is the incorporation of oatmeal into the breakfast offering. Oatmeal not only adds fiber to the diet but may also help in lowering cholesterol. Another suggestion is to add canned tomatoes or tomato juice into products prepared at the soup kitchens because they are an excellent source of vitamins A and C. Lastly, including nonfat dry milk products into the preparation of food adds calcium, Vitamin D, and protein. These strategies in the soup kitchens may improve the long-term health of frequent soup kitchen clients.

Health Service Programs

Poor health is linked closely with homelessness in the older adult population (Bottomley, 2001b). For an older adult who is struggling to pay for housing, a serious illness can lead to homelessness. Although the seniors generally have health coverage through Medicare, many older adults do not receive these benefits, whereas others get only a portion for Medicare coverage (Bottomley, 2001c). This is caused by their lack of social connections with social service programs, mistrust and fear of the system, and the amount of paperwork and follow-up that is needed to initiate coverage. Poverty and lack of health insurance often result in a failure to get medical attention. Scott (2001) argues that in a society where geriatric clients cannot afford health care, pro bono service should be established. This has developed in many communities as free clinics or outreach medical units. One difficulty with the pro bono service is that the older adult clients may have a different health care provider at each encounter because the staff is comprised of volunteers. Access to care is also problematic due to the need for transportation, remembering the appointments, and limited clinic hours.

Health services must be delivered to homeless older adults with unconditional positive regard. First discussed by Carl Rogers, unconditional positive regard is the universal need for positive regard by others. It is unconditional when it has no criteria for acceptance; it is positive when it offers warm acceptance; and it is regard in that the provider recognizes the client's experience as his/her own and that the provider does not possess it. It is with this perspective that care is provided for the client who is homeless (Rogers, 1962).

Coordinated services are more effective than crisis-oriented health care. Outreach health service programs allow for screening and intervention before the client's condition requires hospitalization. Outreach medical units have been used successfully with homeless people in many communities (Dziobek & Martins, 1992). Many of the health care programs for the homeless are funded by the Stewart B. McKinney Homeless Assistance Act of 1994, the first national initiative for the homeless crisis. The Health Care for the Homeless (HCH) program was developed to improve the health of the homeless population by providing primary health care to the homeless. This program was developed by health providers for homeless across the United States. Health and social service workers in HCH programs provide screening and comprehensive care in clinics that are accessible to the homeless population. HCH programs are interdisciplinary, and they offer informational material for providers as well as linkages for outreach, case management, housing, income and transportation (Bottomley, 2001c).

The National Health Care for the Homeless Council (NHCHC) suggests that to meet the health care needs of the homeless adequate Medicare and Medicaid payments for the homeless health care providers must be incorporated, ideally with universal coverage that would guarantee older adults' access to care (Bottomley, 2001c). NHCHC suggests that federal and state Medicare and Medicaid agencies should include linkages with health care providers of the homeless. Gelberg (2000) examined a Health Care for the Homeless Program with such a linkage.

Gelberg's (2000) research examined a designated Health Care for the Homeless Program providing health care with a primary provider as a regular source of care for older homeless adults. The research findings indicated that the program was beneficial. This was seen as a predictor of improved health status for vision impairment, skin, leg, and foot problems.

Jezewski (1995) explored the way nurses may facilitate health care for the homeless person. This study was conducted in a nurse-managed shelter. The findings indicated that the core category needed for health care was "staying connected." There were three aspects of staying connected: links with the homeless person, networks with other providers, and facilitating the homeless person's connections with the health care system.

A connection with health care and social service providers that treats the older person who is homeless with dignity and respect needs to be established. Bottomley, Bissonnette, and Snekvik (2001) present older adults' concerns about what it is like to find themselves homeless. Their findings indicate that some of the homeless older adults avoid contact with the system because "they are chastised; are made to feel inferior; and cannot tolerate the rules, long lines, long waits, crowded shelter, lack of staff, inconsistent advice, loss of independence, and being made to feel as if they have been stripped of status and dignity, and self-esteem" (Bottomley, Bissonette, & Snekvik, 2001, p. 55).

Carter, Green, Green, and Dufour (1994) suggested that *nurse-managed free clinics* might be an effective way to provide heath care to the homeless. The belief is supported by the Health Care for Homeless Clinician's Network supported by the U.S. Department of Health and Human Services. This approach is a downstream or micro approach that would help decrease labeling, disrespect, and "patient dumping" (Berliner, 1988). In a study of patient dumping, Kellermann and Hackman (1988) reviewed the "dumping" or immediate transfer of poor patients from one emergency department to another emergency department. In their study almost all transferred patients (91%) were sent for economic reasons. One out of four was found to be unstable on arrival, based on clinical criteria. Eighty-two patients who were transferred for economic reasons (34%) required emergency hospitalization. Of these three patients died prior to discharge where two had been transferred for primarily economic reasons.

McCormick and Macintosh (2001), in their grounded theory study, explored the health experiences of 11 homeless people living in shelters. They looked at the strategies used by participants to attain, maintain, or regain health. The authors found that active participation of the homeless person helped. They suggested that a fragmented system of help hinders access to heath care services.

Research on the homeless older adults indicates a high prevalence of psychiatric disorders and cognitive impairment. Stergiopoulos and Herrmann (2003) recommend that special geriatric mental health services are needed with this population, including comprehensive evaluation and referral and geriatric psychiatrists as members of an interdisciplinary team to deliver services to homeless elders.

Social Service Programs

Although homeless persons older than age 64 are entitled to Social Security benefits, many do not use the benefits, or the benefits are inadequate to cover the costs. The procedure to register for Social Security benefits is difficult for many, and therefore many older homeless do not access the benefits.

Over half the homeless population is eligible for some type of benefits under the Social Security programs, but less than 10% actually receive the benefits. The reason for this is related to issues with follow-up with this transient population, the amount of detail and time needed to apply for programs, and a lack of address or phone numbers to receive information and requests to complete benefit information packets and case finding (Bottomley et al., 2001; National Law Center on Homelessness and Poverty, 2004). "In 1999, combined Social Security income, food stamps, and medical and housing assistance totaled $5016.00 for a single older adult, which is 84.3% of the poverty level. By themselves, assistance programs may not be sufficient to lift an older individual out of poverty; in fact, in many cases, it is not enough to keep the older adults off the streets" (Bottomley et al., 2001, p. 56). Bottomley (2001b) suggests that social service programs such as Medicare and Medicaid should include explicit language requiring managed care organizations to create linkages with the health care providers for the homeless and that adequate Medicare and Medicare payments be in place for health care providers to the homeless.

Emergency Elder Shelters

Many programs have provided outreach to older homeless adults and some have addressed their special needs. One type of program is the emergency shelter for the frail elderly. Older homeless individuals are recruited from church groups, foster care programs, and community organizations so that the elders can stay in the shelter until more permanent arrangements can be made (Bruckner, 2001). Elder shelters have been established in eight states including Arizona, California, District of Columbia, Florida, Indiana, New York, Oklahoma, and Tennessee [National Clearing House on Abuse in Later Life (NCALL), 2005]. In Tennessee, Catholic Charities have initiated short-term housing for seniors and their families (Samaritan Place, 2005).

Small Day Program for Elders

A small day program serves fewer than 100 elder adults exclusively (Bruckner, 2001; Doolin, 1986). The programs include a nutritious mid-day meal, a safe haven from weather and street violence, and a friendly place to play cards, chat, or read the newspaper. Case management for emergency assistance, job referral, housing assistance, access to primary health care and alcoholism treatment are provided. The Cardinal Medeiros Center in Boston was one of the first-day programs in the city (Wood-Boyle, 2004). The day program started as a lunch site with housing, counseling, and case managers. The elders are then able to return to shelters in the evening until more stable housing can be established.

Large Day Program for Homeless Elders

Cohen, Onserud, and Monaco (1992) describe Project Rescue, a large day program in New York's Bowery neighborhood. Components of this type of program include breakfast, lunch, and snacks. Primary medical care is also included, as well as psychiatric and alcohol rehabilitation. Housing assistance as well as financial and vocational counseling may be included. The first goal of the project was to establish contact and trust with the older homeless adult. Once inside the day program, the staff tried to establish a relationship that would encourage the client to have a needs assessment. Finally, when the client was ready, the professional would offer the services needed, such as programs for mental health, alcoholism, drug abuse, lack of housing, and the accessing income from entitlement programs. A follow-up of 132 clients that used Project Rescue found a reduction in the number of problems. The greatest improvements were found with income and physical health; the least improvements in sobriety and permanent housing (Bruckner, 2001; Cohen et al., 1992).

Outreach Programs

Establishing contact and creating relationships with the homeless older person who cannot or will not access the social service programs is the focus and challenge of outreach (Sullivan-Mintz, 1995). Older adults are among the homeless population especially in need of outreach. Outreach encourages these persons to take advantage of available services and assists them with accessing these resources (Sullivan-Mintz, 1995). Outreach services can be stationary or mobile, depending on the needs of the group. Outreach is provided in the client's own setting and takes place on the streets, shelters, drop-in centers, emergency rooms, psychiatric centers, and soup kitchens (Axelroad & Toff, 1987; Sullivan-Mintz, 1995). Older adults that are homeless are candidates for outreach not only because of their fear of accessing help but also because of their poor physical health and physical frailty. Many older persons are in need of outreach due to poor physical health, poor mental health, and lack of family support (Sullivan-Mintz, 1995).

According to Sullivan-Mintz (1995), the first step in outreach is entering the community to identify and locate the person needing assistance. Observations on the streets, shelters, and soup kitchens must be made to see who is most vulnerable. Sometimes referrals are made from law enforcement, city workers, local citizens, hotel managers, and landlords. Outreach can only be effective if the outreach workers develop trusting relationships with the homeless with unconditional positive regard for each homeless person they encounter.

Establishing Homeless/Provider Relationships

The recognition and respect of human dignity of older adults who are homeless is essential for professionals working with the older adults who are homeless. The staff at one of the Committee to End Elder Homelessness programs (CEEH) suggested that one needs to be open minded, nonjudgmental, flexible, and respectful. Patience also was frequently mentioned as a desirable attribute. A Rogerian perspective using genuine concern and unconditional positive regard would also be beneficial in their encounters with the clients.

The homeless person's view of self calls for special sensitivity on the part of the professional staff. This need is evident from Snow and Anderson (1993) who described the homeless as falling to the bottom of the status system with doubts about self-worth and the meaning of existence. Snow and Anderson (1993) further described the homeless person as being defined as less worthy of attention by members of dominate classes and are subjected to subtle face-to-face deprivation. Goffman's (1959) work sought to understand the meaning that underlies all social interactions. Whenever individuals want the presence of others, they need to assess them, that is, they need to discover facts of the situation. To become visible, Snow and Anderson (1987), in their ethnographic study, suggest that individuals at the bottom of status systems attempt to generate identities that provide them with a measure of self-worth and dignity. Sometimes this is done by great story-telling with much embellishment. Professionals may listen to the great story-telling in the development of the trust relationship. This trust relationship allows the professionals working with the homeless to recognize when the person is ready to take a step toward improvement in quality of life.

Homeless older adults will not utilize services if they feel the treatment is demeaning. Bottomley et al. (2001) report that older adults who are homeless cannot deal with what they refer to as arbitrariness and irrationality of social service systems. "For them, there is not nearly so much craziness among the homeless persons as there is in the systems ostensibly designed to help them" (Bottomley et al., 2001, p. 55). Often the social service system tries to separate out the undeserving from the deserving poor and sees clients as ungrateful and unreasonable. At the same time the social service system is understaffed, and the staff that is present is overworked. In this type of system, the staff does not have the strength to reach out to the homeless, and the homeless population does not have the strength continue to try to get services.

The desirability of a staff skilled in working with older homeless adults was described in an exploratory research project by Gibeau (2001). Gibeau (2001) described several themes in interviews with older adult homeless about what they wanted to experience in the professionals that worked with them. One theme was the ability of the staff member to exhibit a caring attitude toward them. The respondents also suggested that they would like being related to as a person. Other themes were the comprehensiveness and practicality of the professional person's interventions.

TIER 2: MIDSTREAM STRATEGIES

Empowerment of the Older Adult

The professionals working with the homeless population may empower the older adult by recognizing their resourcefulness. McCabe, Macnee and Anderson (2001), in their study of 17 homeless people, found resourcefulness was expressed as experiences of ingenuity and self-pride at being able to negotiate and survive despite being homeless.

Resourcefulness was related to homeless individuals' own behaviors and to assistance from others, especially other homeless people. This included the "attributes of being able to take care of yourself, figuring out how to get needs met, not asking for much from others, and the realization that it takes a lot for a homeless person to ask for help with certain things. Homeless people served as support for one another" (p. 82).

Martins (2003) described the difference between a member of society with higher social standing and a homeless person who exhibits resourcefulness as the difference between behaviors that are socially sanctioned and those that are not. Homeless people exhibit both socially sanctioned strategies and underground resourcefulness strategies. Underground resourcefulness strategies used by marginalized persons or those distanced socially are often considered illegal or unethical by mainstream culture. Their marginalized status frequently forces them to use covert means for survival (Martins, 2003). Underground resourcefulness strategies are strategies used by vulnerable populations to obtain what they need to survive. These strategies are not usually accepted by the dominant society and may include such actions as stealing food or medications, feigning symptoms of illness to get health care, or committing crimes to be housed in a prison (Martins, 2003). Factors that make homeless populations vulnerable include their social status, racial and ethnic status, and economic status. It is these same factors that cause homeless persons to become marginalized or distanced from the dominant social majority (Meleis, 1998). Marginalization, or social distancing, magnifies their risks due to the interrelationships between these social issues. These conditions seem to lead to underground resourcefulness (Martins, 2003).

Critical Social Theory views homeless people as a marginalized and oppressed population (Waitzkin & Britt, 1989). One assumption of Critical Social Theory is that people can change their world, and have the capability to transform organizational situations. The status quo can be changed, and is done though emancipating people. From a critical perspective, there is a need to find alternatives to the existing social conditions of the homeless. It is also understood within this framework that all social knowledge is value-laden, and that all scientific knowledge is a social construction. There is an assumption that reason and critique are inseparable. Application of a critical perspective by health care professionals could provide opportunities to empower the homeless in their survival strategies and to initiate social action to eliminate the structures of oppression (Snow & Mulcahy, 2001). Professionals need to understand the role that power and control play not only in society but also at a personal level in their day-to-day interactions with homeless people. There is a need to examine the professionals' part in creating and supporting larger social structures and systems, their relationships and inequities (Drevdahl, 1995). Professionals must recognize older home-less people as active participants in attempting to solve the problems related to homelessness. An important strategy is the need to focus on strengths for marginalized people and build on these strengths, such as individual strategies as toughness, hope, and tenacity; and socio-structural strategies including begging, developing homeless communities, and scavenging (Martins, 2003).

Montgomery (1994) suggests that there is a need to create a new definition for older homeless people by acknowledging them as heroic people, thus transforming their stigma into respect for what they over-come on a daily basis. There are major ramifications of viewing homeless peoples as overly victimized or rendered helpless by the nature of their oppression (Molina, 2000). This view could inhibit emancipatory efforts through empowerment.

Documenting strengths of homeless people lends credence to those who say that we should be building on strengths rather than focusing on "helping victims overcome their problems" (Banyard, 1995; Baumann, 1993). To focus on the homeless person's problems disempowers them. In-terpersonal strengths and the psychosocial survival strategies used by the homeless in this analysis suggest that health care providers can act as part of the homeless person's support network through humanistic character-istics, such as unconditional positive regard and respect for the homeless. Recognizing their right to decide and contribute to their social services and health care decisions accomplishes this.

Health care professionals' motives in working with socially oppressed populations must be emancipatory in nature. This will include bringing the least powerful into relationships of participation to challenge the dom-inant ideological paradigm. Through this lens of critical perspective, the situation of homelessness can be understood and improved.

Temporary Housing Programs

Temporary accommodations are provided in the form of large hostels, sin-gle occupancy hotels, and temporary housing complexes. Some of these fa-cilities accommodate people with special needs, such as substance abusers or people with mental illness. There is a lack of temporary accommodations with adequate facilities in most cities. Over the past few decades there has been a significant decline in the number of housing units available to low-income persons. With temporary housing some *energy assistance programs* will also be needed. Assistance may be developed with oil companies in the community. This helps to make heat accessible and affordable. The cur-rent escalation of energy costs makes this type of program very beneficial for the older adult at risk of becoming homeless (Bottomley, 2001a).

TIER 3: UPSTREAM STRATEGIES

Professionals also need to advocate for changes at the socioeconomic and structural level that create this social situation. This includes national policies that increase affordable homes, education, and jobs as well as health care, as a right. There is a need for further exploration of strategies used by oppressed populations to survive. Future research must increase efforts to understand both qualitatively and quantitatively the diversity of homeless populations. There needs to be an understanding of how structures of poverty affect diverse groups of individuals. Research should address the balance of social service support and empowerment and be directed toward validation of interventions that foster empowerment of the older homeless person.

POLICY IMPLICATIONS

The United States is one of the few industrialized nations without universal health coverage for all people. At the upstream level, professionals need to advocate for universal health coverage with guaranteed access to health care. Bottomley (2001b) suggests that universal health care coverage would ensure that older adults have comprehensive health care, which would reduce homelessness. This was described in the previous chapter, which presented causes of homelessness in older adults. Many elder homeless have had a history of chronic illness, lack of treatment for substance abuse or mental health issues or premature discharge from health facility that precipitated their homelessness.

Policy options may also include program development that revolves around managed care. Often these programs are based on the medical model with an integration of social and mental health services. There are also senior care policies for projects with case management through outpatient primary care physicians' offices. The most upstream policy option would involve programs that allow target elders to stay in the community in flexible housing arrangements with social, medical, and mental health supports.

PERMANENT SUPPORTIVE HOUSING

The most important intervention for the homeless older adults is permanent low cost housing. Housing is what homeless older adults need first and foremost and is the first form of treatment for older adults with medical problems. The housing needs to be supportive of the multiple physical, mental, and social issues experienced by the older adult who has been homeless.

Rosenheck et al. (1998) found that housing programs need integration and coordination between agencies and service systems for improved access to services, and for improved client housing outcomes. According to the National Coalition for the Homeless (1999), many older adults are poor and in need of housing assistance. The U.S. Housing and Urban Development (HUD) office recognizes the need for addressing the housing and community development needs for the low- and moderate-income population. HUD's goal is to help homeless people obtain appropriate permanent housing and prevent others from becoming homeless (Mullins, 1995).

Identify Early Warning Symptoms for Eviction

Several risk factors have been identified for eviction and prolonged homelessness. Crane and Warnes (2000) interviewed 45 evictees who were sleeping in the street or in temporary shelters. The researchers found that the circumstances preceding eviction were retirement, death of parent, widowhood or separation, increased severity of mental illness, and coping difficulties. This needs to come to the attention of housing providers and welfare agencies. The identification of risk factors increases the possibility of identifying people at risk of becoming homeless, and therefore taking preventive actions. Mechanisms suggested for preventive actions are pooling and linking information about vulnerable people; and second, clarifying and locating the responsibility for the care for the person at risk. The third action includes determination of practical, effective, and affordable prevention procedures. Last is to actively pursue funding for this preventive activity.

According to Gibeau (2001), there is no single level of accountability for addressing elder homelessness in this country. As with many health and social services, the creation of housing, services, and programs for the older homeless adults is supported by a combination for both private and public funding. This needs to include private donations, foundations, corporate grants and bank loans, as well as government programs that provide rent assistance and health services.

Intervention Program Models for Interdisciplinary Professional Practice

It is essential that any interventions and strategies used for ending elder homelessness incorporate all three tiers in their programming. The downstream approaches of outreach work, soup kitchens, food pantries, clothing distribution centers, health care for the homeless programs, and drop-in centers must be connected with midstream approaches such as temporary housing, attitudinal changes of health care workers, and policy changes.

The Dwelling Place

One of the first programs using the three-tier model was the Dwelling Place (2004). It was developed in New York City in 1977 by Sister Nancy, a nurse and a Franciscan Sister of Allegheny, when she recognized that there were no shelters for women. The Dwelling Place is located in the heart of New York City's Hell's Kitchen, and it predominately serves the older women on the streets referred to by the public as "bag ladies." The focus is on the women who live in the streets near the mouth of the Lincoln Tunnel. The sisters who staff The Dwelling Place go out to the streets at night, greet the "bag ladies," offer a blanket and food; and eventually a connection is made. Once trust is established, the elders living on the street may accept help. The journey from the street to the front door of the drop-in center is often a long process. At first the elder may only accept a care package from the door. At a later point, the elder may enter the center and sit to eat. Perhaps with time and patience on the behalf of the sisters doing outreach, the elder may eat, shower, and rest for the night. The Dwelling Place's staff develops relationships, then offer connections to health care services and social service benefits, and finally their ultimate goal is long-term housing (Sr. Gloria, personnel communication, September 2004). Along with serving the older women food in the dining room, the sisters also advocate for the women with the mayor in City Hall in an effort to increase funding and find alternatives to homelessness.

Pathways from Street to Resettlement Model

Pathways from Street to Resettlement is a first-, second- and third-tier program beginning with outreach workers identifying older homeless adults in the streets by establishing trust to allow the older adult to enter a street center for food and shelter. The street center then provides temporary shelter and some rehabilitation. Eventually a resettlement program is established with social service connections and preparation for permanent housing. Finally, permanent supportive housing is established. Crane (1999) calls these "high care homes." The model used by Warnes and Crane (2002) moves from outreach on the streets to identify the older homeless through gaining trust, then referring to drop in centers,

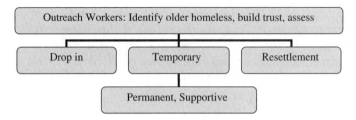

FIGURE 6.1   Pathways from street to resettlement.
Model modified from Crane and Warnes (2002) and Crane (1999).

temporary housing and resettlement programs. Finally, the elder homeless are provided permanent supportive housing (Figure 6.1).

Warnes and Crane (2000) describe Pathways from Street to Resettlement Model, which was described by Cohen and Sokolovsky (1989), Doolin, (1986) and later by Crane (1993) who applied the model in the United Kingdom from 1997 to 1998 (Warnes & Crane, 2000). Their study examined two outcomes of the model: whether users returned to the streets or whether they were resettled in long-term housing. Many of the older homeless people had been sleeping on the street for years, were isolated, had untreated physical and mental illnesses, and were not claiming welfare benefits or accessing services. This led to a proposal to develop an experimental center that would provide multiple services from street outreach to resettlement for people aged 50 years or older. It was modeled on the day centers and outreach work for older homeless people in New York City and Boston.

The primary goal of the project's outreach staff is to persuade street people to enter the drop-in center. Initially, the outreach worker's goal is to develop a trusting relationship with people on the streets. This component is essential in order to connect the homeless person to other services. Warnes and Crane (2000) found 491 older people (448 men and 43 women) sleeping on the streets during the 23 months of the Lancefield Street Project in London. Each month of the 23 month project, the outreach workers discovered at least 10 new people on the streets, sleeping in deserted buildings, parks, and sheds. The outreach team referred 239 homeless people to the Lancefield Street Center and to other hostels. For some older homeless, this step took intensive work and diverse help on the streets. The beginning stages were offerings of food, clothing, and blankets, and then offers of medical treatment and assistance with welfare benefits. As soon as a client showed readiness to accept help it was important to act on that need immediately. Those who were homeless for many years were more resistant to assistance from the outreach workers. The women were found to be the most difficult to help, since many had severe mental illness and seemed less willing to trust the outreach workers (Warnes & Crane, 2000).

Once the outreach team connected with the homeless person on the streets, the older adult would then be referred to the drop-in center, which had sitting rooms, a place to eat, and a bathroom. Laundry facilities were also available in the drop-in center. This center served as a stepping stone from the streets to the hostel for the distrustful and anxious older adults who lived on the streets. A residential hostel was available with stays ranging from less than 30 days to over 9 months. The average length of stay was 101 days (Warnes & Crane, 2000). According to Warnes and Crane (2000), many of the older adults using the residential hotel had physical health problems (55%), and mental health problems (39%) and many (58%) were heavy drinkers. In the United Kingdom, separate supportive housing was created for older adult heavy drinkers. They used daily support staff. For some of the older adults, the opportunity to have their own place to live reduced the amount of drinking (Crane, 1999). The health problems included tuberculosis, liver and renal failure, heart problems, and neurological diseases. Eventually the model works to establish resettlement in long-term accommodations for older adults but more difficulty was experienced with those experiencing alcohol dependency. The researchers suggest that this model could be applied to other entrenched street people who are severely incapacitated by mental health or substance abuse problems (Warnes & Crane, 2000).

ENDING ELDER HOMELESSNESS: THE COMMITTEE TO END ELDER HOMELESSNESS

In 1992, the Committee to End Elder Homelessness (CEEH) was established by Elisabeth Babcock and six other professionals who worked with the elder homeless (CEEH, 2002). The CEEH provides essential services to older adults or those at risk of being homeless. Many CEEH residents require support with activities of daily living, such as dressing, eating, or bathing. The mission of CEEH was to develop a blend of prevention, placement, and housing programs designed to help older adults be placed in homes of their own. The CEEH developed supportive housing in Massachusetts to provide programs within housing facilities that would help older adults remain domiciled. The housing operated by CEEH provides a creative combination of supportive services that assist residents to age with dignity, regardless of their mental health or social needs. The CEEH advocates that supportive housing ends homelessness for people with chronic barriers to health and housing stability.

First, CEEH established the need to document the number of home-less elders. Then, CEEH developed the Case Management Model for giv-ing interdisciplinary care for elder adults at risk of being homeless. The CEEH interdisciplinary team consists of director, nurses, social workers, activities director, and older adult resident personnel. Each older adult is assigned one professional case manager. If the resident has significant mental health issues, the case manager may be a mental health specialist; if the resident has severe medical problems then the case manager may be a nurse (CEEH, 2002).

CEEH Interdisciplinary Case Management Model

The model has four major components: housing, mental health, health, and activity. The *housing* component addresses issues of finances and rent payment. The *mental health* component looks at elders that suffer from mental illness who may also be isolated and have problems with neglect and exacerbations of illnesses. The elders receive counseling, medication education, and socialization programs. The *health* compo-nent addresses elders with multiple health problems that have limita-tions in activities of daily living. They receive assistance from a nurse who monitors their medical condition, schedules appointments and ini-tiates a personal care helper. The model is focused on helping the elders achieve their own goals of independence, satisfaction with *activities* of daily living and health within a community setting (CEEH, 2002).

The ultimate goal of upstream interventions is to eradicate elder homelessness. In addition to permanent affordable supportive housing, there must be programs that advocate for elders at risk of losing their homes. The CEEH (2002) states that supportive housing programs pre-vent elders from having to go to a shelter where they are often vulner-able to victimization and where services are not well-adapted to meet the specific needs of this frail and complex population.

To evaluate the effectiveness of the model, CEEH (2002) completed a resident outcome analysis of the 110 CEEH residents who participated in the study. The majority of the respondents were between the ages of 65–74. Males represented 51.8% of the respondents. Self-reported races were Blacks 51%, White 41%, Hispanic 4%, and others 4%. The most prevalent chronic illnesses in this population were mental illness and de-mentia, followed by hypertension, cardiac, diabetes, COPD, arthritis, asthma, genitourinary problems, and stroke. Assessment of functional status found the population to be very frail and complex; however, they did exhibit stabilization of functional decline. There were statis-tically significant improvements in the functional status of the CEEH residents over time. The description of CEEH participants in the study indicates that the majority of the participants were homeless or institutionalized prior to entering CEEH housing. Results indicate that there were improvements in the areas of physical and emotional functioning, cognition, social integration and well-being when compared to the national norms. The researchers suggest that the CEEH housing model is a unique housing, case management model that delivers consistent and intensive management of holistic needs of the older adult with potential for improving health outcomes. This finding has medical, social, economic and policy implications that could improve the quality of life for the frail older adult (Massachusetts Health Policy Forum, 2002).

Hamel (2002) developed a service learning model with a collaborative partnership between academia and the community within the CEEH program. Graduate students were introduced to formerly homeless older adults to learn about interdisciplinary collaboration, service, and advocacy issues as well as social responsibility. Students from a variety of professional programs received practical experience while providing pro bono service to the older homeless, their caregivers, and the supporting agency. This interdisciplinary approach allowed different disciplines work interdependently to care for the complexities of the older homeless adult in the CEEH programs. An interdisciplinary service learning model was created starting with problem identification and resulting in increased public awareness of the issues, collaboration among professionals, community partnerships, service learning, health promotion programs, research development, increase in funding, and rehabilitation of the elders, the building, and the community (Hamel, 2002).

SUMMARY

Many professionals know that the homeless are often unpopular clients. Many homeless people feel labeled and stigmatized. In his book *Discipline and Punishment*, Foucault (1979) considers the constraints of conformity and sees that the judges of normality are present everywhere. We are a society of the "teacher–judge, the doctor–judge, the educator–judge, and the social-worker–judge...we are entering an age of infinite examination and of compulsory objectification" (Snow, Anderson, & Koegel, 1994, p. 461). Evaluative labels of people are socially constructed and are based on social judgments by the professional. The social worth of individuals is judged when health professionals balance competing demands on their time and other health and social resources. This social judgment is analogous to the concepts of moral evaluation, social evaluation, and labeling. Hallebone (1997) found that homeless people experienced social discomfort and a sense of stigma resulting from their homelessness. The upstream efforts for the older homeless will need to include ideological shifts for many professionals.

Many people have been led to believe that elder homelessness is a tragic but an unavoidable consequence to American individualism (Bissonnette & Hijjazi, 1994). The concept of collective good and social justice is often distant to the ideology of market justice individualism. The answers to older adult homelessness cannot be based totally on the downstream individual responses often used. There needs to be sociopolitical or macro-level changes with social programs that resist the effects of poverty. In a social justice framework, health care access and housing for the older adult is a human right.

The solution to the human and economic dilemma of care for older adults cannot be answered by fragmented programs of shelters, homeless health care programs and drop-in centers. Federal policy is needed that will encourage fair and equitable housing and health care for all older adults (Bottomley, 2001c). To prevent older adults from becoming homeless, we must provide enough low-income housing, income supports, and health care services to sustain independent living. For those older adults who have already lost their homes, a comprehensive outreach health and social services must be made available, as well as special assistance to access existing public assistance programs. Finally, like all people who are homeless or at risk of becoming homeless, older people need an adequate income, affordable housing, and affordable health care in order to stay securely housed (National Coalition for the Homeless, 1999).

REFERENCES

Axelroad, S. E., & Toff, G. E. (1987). *Outreach services for homeless mentally ill people*. Washington, DC: Intergovernmental Health Policy Project.

Banyard, V. (1995). Taking another route: Daily survival narratives from mothers who are homeless. *American Journal of Community Psychology, 23*, 871–891.

Baumann, S. L. (1993). The meaning of being homeless. *Scholarly Inquiry in Nursing Practice, 7*(1), 59–73.

Berliner, B. (1988). Patient dumping—no one wins and we all lose. *American Journal of Public Health, 78*, 1279–1280.

Bissonnette, A., & Hijjazi, K. (1994). Elder homelessness: A community perspective. *Nursing Clinics of North America, 29*, 409–416.

Bottomley, J. (2001a). Energy assistance programs: Keeping older adults housed and warm. *Topics in Geriatric Rehabilitation, 17*(1), 71–81.

Bottomley, J. (2001b). Health care and homeless older adults. *Topics in Geriatric Rehabilitation, 17*(1), 1–21.

Bottomley, J. (2001c). Politics of health care and the needs of the older adult: The social context of changes in the delivery system. *Topics in Geriatric Rehabilitation, 16*(4), 28–44.

Bottomley, J., Bissonette, A., & Snekvik, V. (2001). The lives of homeless older adults: Please, tell them who I am. *Topics in Geriatric Rehabilitation, 16*(4), 50–64.

Bruckner, J. (2001). Walking a mile in their shoes: Sociocultural considerations in elder homelessness. *Topics in Geriatric Rehabilitation, 16*(4), 15–27.

Butterfield, P. G. (1990). Thinking upstream: Nurturing a conceptual understanding of the societal context of health behavior. *Advances in Nursing Science, 12*, 1–8.

Carter, K., Green, R., Green, L., & Dufour, L. (1994). Health needs of homeless clients accessing nursing care at a free clinic. *Journal of Community Health Nursing, 11*(3), 139–147.

Cohen, C., Onserud, H., & Monaco, C. (1992). Project rescue: Serving the homeless and marginally housed elderly. *Gerontologist, 32*(4), 466–471.

Cohen, C. I., & Sokolovsky, J. (1989). *Old men of the Bowery: Strategies for survival among the homeless.* New York: Guilford Press.

Cohen, C., Teresi, J., Holmes, D., & Roth, D. (1988). Survival strategies of older homeless men. *Gerontologist, 28*(1), 58–65.

Committee to End Elder Homelessness (CEEH). (2004). *The Committee to End Elder Homelessness Annual Report.* Boston, MA. Retrieved September 9, 2004 from www.ceeh.org

Crane, M. (1993). *Elderly people sleeping on the streets in inner London: An exploratory study.* London: Age Concern Institute of Gerontology, King's College.

Crane, M. (1999). *Understanding older homeless people.* Philadelphia: Open University Press.

Crane, M., & Warnes, A. (2000). Evictions and prolonged homelessness. *Housing Studies, 15*, 757–773.

Crane, M., & Warnes, A. (2001). Older people and homelessness: Prevalence and causes. *Topics in Geriatric Rehabilitation, 16*(4), 1–14.

Crane, M., & Warnes, A. (2002). *Resettling older homeless people.* Sheffield, United Kingdom: Sheffield Institute for Studies on Ageing.

Doolin, J. (1986). Planning for the special needs of the homeless elderly. *Gerontologist, 26*(3), 229–231.

Drevdahl, D. (1995). Coming to voice: The power of emancipatory community intervention. *Advances in Nursing Science, 18*(2), 13–24.

Dwelling Place. (2004). *Dwelling Place of New York.* retrieved September 30, 2004 from http://www.catholiccharitiesny.org/empoweringgroups

Dziobek, L., & Martins, D. (1992). Outreach to the homeless. *New England Public Health Association Conference Proceedings.* Falmouth, MA.

Foucault, M. (1979). *Discipline and punishment.* New York: Vintage.

Gelberg, L. (2000). The behavioral model for vulnerable populations: Application to medical care use and outcomes for homeless people. *Health Services
Research, 34*, 1273–1302.

Gibeau, J. (2001). Home free: An evolving journey in eradicating elder homelessness. *Topics in Geriatric Rehabilitation, 17*(1), 22–52.

Goffman, E. (1959). The presentation of self in everyday life. Chicago: University of Chicago Press.

Hallebone, E. (1997). Homelessness and marginality in Australia: Young and
old people excluded from independence. In M. J. Huth & T. Wright (Eds.),
International critical perspectives on homelessness (pp. 71–103). Westport,
CT: Praeger.

Hamel, P. (2002). Interdisciplinary perspectives, service learning, and advocacy:
A nontraditional approach to geriatric rehabilitation. *Topics in Geriatric
Rehabilitation, 17*(1), 53–70.

Hecht, L., & Coyle, B. (2001). Elderly homeless. *American Behavioral Scientist,
45*(1), 66–79.

Jezewski, M. (1995). Staying connected: The core of facilitating health care for
homeless persons. *Public Health Nursing, 12*, 203–210.

Johnson, L., & McCool, A. (2003). Dietary intake and nutritional status of
older homeless women: A pilot study. *Journal of Nutrition for the Elderly,
23*(1), 1–21.

Keigher, S., & Greenblatt, S. (1992). Housing emergencies and the etiology of
homelessness among the urban elderly. *Gerontologist, 32*, 457–465.

Kellermann, A., & Hackman, B. (1988). Emergency department patient
'dumping': An analysis of interhospital transfers to the Regional Medical
Center at Memphis, Tennessee. *American Journal of Public Health, 78*,
1287–1292.

Markos, P., & Allen, D. (2001). A model of primary healthcare service delivery for individuals who are homeless. *Guidance and Counseling,
16*(4), 127.

Martins, D. C. (2003). *Health care experiences of homeless people*. UMI
ProQuest Digital Dissertations Online. UMI Publication Number: AAT
3089752.

Massachusetts Health Policy Forum. (2002). *Keeping elders home: New lessons
learned about supporting frail elders in our communities*. Issue Brief (No. 17):
The Massachusetts Health Policy Forum.

McCabe, S., Macnee, C., & Anderson, M. K. (2001). Homeless patients' experience of satisfaction with care. *Archives of Psychiatric Nursing, 15*(2),
78–85.

McCormick, D., & Macintosh, J. (2001). Research with homeless people uncov-
ers model of health. *Western Journal of Nursing Research, 23*(7). Retrieved
June 11, 2002 from www.citation.asp

McKinlay, J. (1986). A case for refocusing upstream-the political economy of
illness. In P. Conrad & R. Kern (Eds.). *The sociology of health and illness: Critical perspectives*, New York: St. Martin Press. (Original work
published 1975).

McKinney Act. (1994). *Definition of Homelessness.* The Steward B. McKinney Homeless Assistance Act (U.S.C. 42 § 11302).

Melies, A. (1998). Revisions in knowledge development: A passion for substance. *Scholarly Inquiry for Practice: An International Journal, 12*(1), 87–94.

Molina, E. (2000). Informal non-kin networks among homeless Latino and African American men. *American Behavioral Scientist, 43*(4), 663–686.

Montgomery, C. (1994). Swimming upstream: The strengths of women who survive homelessness. *Advances in Nursing Science, 16*(3), 34–45.

Mullins, L. (1995). Housing policy. In D. Rich, T. Rich, & L. Mullins. *Old and homeless–Double jeopardy: An overview of current practice and policies* . Westport, CT: Auburn House.

National Clearing House on Abuse in Later Life (NCALL). *Elder Abuse.* (2005). Retrieved June 6, 2005 from http://www.ncall.us/docs%5CElder_Shelters.pdf

National Coalition for the Homeless. (1999). *NCH Fact Sheet# 15: Homelessness among elderly persons.* Washington, DC:Author.

National Law Center on Homelessness and Poverty. (2000). *Homelessness and poverty in America.* Retrieved March 21, 2006 at http://www.hlchp.org/content/pubs/homeless%20 persons%20m%20america.pdf

Rogers, C. (1962). The interpersonal relationship: The core of guidance Harvard. *Educational Review, 32,* 416–429.

Rosenheck, R., Morrissey, J., Lam, J., Calloway, M., Johnsen, M., Goldman, H., et al. (1998). Service system integration, access to services, and housing outcomes in a program for homeless persons with severe mental illness. *American Journal of Public Health, 88*(11), 1610–1615.

Samaritan Place. (2005). *Samaritan Place: An Independent Living Community, Knoxville, TN.* Retrieved June 6, 2005 from www.samaritanplace.com/Elder_Shelters.html-9k

Scott, R. (2001). Pro bono health service delivery to the indigent: Legal and ethical issues. *Topics in Geriatric Rehabilitation, 16*(4), 45–49.

Snow, D., & Anderson, L. (1987). Identity work among the homeless: The verbal construction and arousal of personal identities. *American Journal of Sociology, 92*(6), 1136–1171.

Snow, D., & Anderson, L. (1993). *Down On Their Luck: A Study of Homeless Street People.* Berkeley: University of California Press.

Snow, D., & Mulcahy, M. (2001). Space, politics, and the survival strategies of the homeless. *American Behavioral Scientist, 45*(1), 149–169.

Snow, D., Anderson, L., & Koegel, P. (1994). Distorting tendencies in research on the homeless. *American Behavioral Scientist, 37*(4), 461–476.

Stergiopoulos, V., & Herrmann, N. (2003). Old and homeless: A review and survey of older adults who use shelters in an urban setting. *The Canadian Journal of Psychiatry, 48,* 374–380.

Sullivan-Mintz, J. (1995). Outreach and empowerment. In D. W. Rich, T. Rich, & L. Mulling (Eds.), *Old and homeles–Double-jeopardy: An overview of current practices and policies* (pp. 79–89). Westport, CT: Auburn House.

Waitzkin, H., & Britt, T. (1989). A critical theory of medical discourse: How patients and health professionals deal with social problems. *International Journal of Health Services, 19*, 577–597.

Warnes, A., & Crane, M. (2000). The achievements of multiservice project for older homeless people. *Gerontologist, 40*, 618–626.

Wood-Boyle, D. (2004, May 6). Rising elder homeless ranks tests shelters. *Dorchester Reporter.*

PART IV

Lesbian, Gay, Bisexual, and Transgender Older Adults

Health Issues of Lesbian, Gay, Bisexual, and Transgender Older Adults

P. Burbank and G. Burkholder

The population of lesbian, gay, bisexual, and transgender (LGBT) older adults is among the most invisible of all Americans. Stigma, bias, and fear of discrimination against LGBT people in general can cause many, especially older adults, to hide their identity and become invisible. Hiding one's identity is emotionally costly, whereas fear of discrimination results in LGBT elders limiting visits to health care providers, selectively choosing social activities, and experiencing denial of partner rights in health care and disenfranchised grief. There is also a lack of awareness of these issues by health care providers and the public in general. All of these factors contribute to the increased risk of health problems and vulnerability of the older LGBT population.

Kinsey and colleagues reported in their seminal studies (Kinsey, Pomeroy, & Martin, 1948; Kinsey, Pomeroy, Martin, & Gebhard, 1952) estimates of approximately 10% of the population who do not identify as exclusively heterosexual. A more recent population-based study (Michael, Gagnon, Laumann, & Kolata, 1994) provided estimates of the percentages of males and females who identify themselves as homosexual as approximately 3% and 1%, respectively. Thus, with a total population of almost 35 million older adults (U.S. Census, 2005) and using the low and high estimates, it can be expected that anywhere from

350,000 to 3.5 million older adults are gay, lesbian, or bisexual. This higher estimate is consistent with other reports (e.g., Davidson, 2001). Because of the stigma and discrimination associated with being homosexual or transgender, these figures are probably underestimated rather than over-estimated.

The number of transgender individuals is more difficult to identify. Using Gender Identity Disorder as the marker of prevalence (American Psychiatric Association, 1994), approximately 1 in 30,000 males and 100,000 females would be classified as transgender. Other estimates of prevalence are higher, however, (e.g., see Seil, 2004) in countries where transgender is more accepted. In the United States, 25,000 have undergone sexual reassignment surgery with another 60,000 considering themselves as candidates for the surgery (Goldberg, 1996). It should be noted that transgender people are of all sexual orientations (Green, 2000).

Very little is actually known about older gay, lesbian, bisexual, and transgender adults. It has been noted that adults who participate in studies tend to be more comfortable with their sexual orientation (Meyer, 2001; Reid, 1995); thus, it is difficult to obtain information on the health issues of a larger group of older adults who may be "closeted" or are otherwise not comfortable with their sexual orientation. This runs the risk of creating biased results that may misrepresent the information about and the actual risks associated with being lesbian, gay, bisexual, or transgender and being older (Meyer, 2001).

The purpose of this chapter is to describe the lesbian, gay, bisexual, and transgender population and their health issues. This task is made more difficult by the dearth of literature on LGBT public health issues (Boehmer, 2002) and even less on issues facing LGBT elders. First, definitions are provided to give the reader a contemporary understanding of how those who have sexual and gender orientations outside the mainstream are identified. Next, a description of stigma and bias against this population provides insight into health care issues. Lastly, demographics describe these populations along with a summary of physical, psychosocial, and spiritual health and health care issues facing LGBT adults.

DEFINITIONS OF TERMS

Sexual orientation is defined as "the basis of one's sexual desires and attractions" (Peterkin & Risdon, 2003, p. 6). The nature of understanding of sexual orientation has changed over time, and these changes have reflected the societal constructions around what is/was considered to be "normal" behavior. At the turn of the century, the term "invert" referred to one who was physically of one sex but whose "mind" was of the opposite sex (Freud, 1905/2000). This gendered notion of inversion (later referred to as *homosexuality*) became increasingly identified as a medical disorder, particularly as the social order became increasingly less tolerant of deviations from accepted gender and sex roles. Treatment for homosexuality included a number of medical procedures such as aversion therapy, which included electric shock treatments intended to condition heterosexual thoughts and desires (Haldeman, 1994). Many older LGBT adults came of age during a time when the term "homosexual" in its medical form was the standard for identifying same-sex desire and thus still refer to themselves and think of themselves as such (Rawls, 2004).

In 1969, the Stonewall Rebellion in New York City ushered in the Gay Rights movement in America. Public and scientific understanding of homosexuality began to change as lesbian and gay individuals began to publicly affirm their homosexuality. An outcome of this was the removal of homosexuality as a mental disorder from the *DSM II* (American Psychiatric Association, 1968), and in 1973 (Hooker, 1993). It was also during this time that the term *homosexual* was replaced by the designations *gay* and *lesbian* as a protest against the medical connotations associated with the term *homosexuality*. Interestingly, given that the initiation of the gay rights movement was the direct result of transgender activists (Duberman, 1994); transgender and bisexual individuals had a more difficult time gaining acceptance into both the mainstream scientific research as well as the gay and lesbian community.

Sexual orientation is no longer defined solely by behavior (Peterkin & Risdon, 2003). Michael et al. (1994), in their population-based survey of sexual practices, asked questions that characterized multiple dimensions of sexual orientation including same sex desire (the person's erotic attraction), behavior (how the person acts sexually), and self-identification (the sociopolitical identification of sexual orientation). Results of this survey suggested that how sexual orientation is defined (and thus how prevalence is determined) depends on how the question is asked, and that identification as gay or lesbian does not necessarily imply behavior.

Transgender is a term that embraces all forms of biological sex and gender variances (Denny, 2004). This includes, for example, crossdressing (heterosexual and otherwise), transsexual lives, and intersexed conditions. The distinction between sex and gender are critical to understanding differences among groups under the transgender umbrella. *Sex* is generally reserved as the term to describe the biological/physical characteristics of an individual, whereas *gender* describes the ways that society prescribes roles appropriate to those of a specific sex. *Gender orientation* then, is different from sexual orientation, and entails one's sense of self as male or female which may be different from one's biological sex.

Intersex refers to individuals who exhibit physical characteristics that can be ascribed to both sexes and conditions in which individuals are born with both male and female organs (Fausto-Sterling, 2000).

Fausto-Sterling (2000) estimates that 1.7% of infants are born as inter-sexuals, not an insignificant number. Transsexuals, on the other hand, are those individuals whose *gender* orientation is in opposition to their biological sex; they often report feeling "trapped" in the wrong physical body or an "incongruity between mind and body" (Brown & Rounsley, 1996. p.7). Transsexuals choose to live their lives in a variety of ways ranging from assuming the characteristics of the opposite sex in dress and mannerism only to complete sexual reassignment via surgery.

In current society, then, distinctions between sex and gender are less clear and individuals have choices regarding their assumed gender identity. In addition, there are cultural variations in dealing with transgender people with transgender acceptance varying as a function of time and situation (Feinberg, 1997). In current American culture, gender polarization dominates (Bem, 1995) and those whose gender identity goes against the cultural norm tend to be marginalized individually, socially, and politically.

STIGMA AND BIAS

The numbers of LGBT older adults are not insignificant. This LGBT population of older adults today came of age in an era when homosexuality and violation of gender norms were subsumed under the medical model as deviant (Faderman, 1998; Feinberg, 1997; Katz, 1996). Most adults face similar issues in aging such as increasing numbers of losses, ageism, and transition out of the work role and into retirement. A key difference, however, is that LGBT individuals live in a culture that is still largely nonaccepting of people whose affections, identities, and behaviors fall outside of the mainstream.

The term "homophobia" generally refers to negative attitudes toward lesbian and gay men. "Heterosexism" has been defined as an "ideological system that denies, denigrates, and stigmatizes any non-heterosexual form of behavior, identity, relationship, or community" (Dean et al., 2000). Transphobia, or fear, hatred, or revulsion of anyone who transgresses traditional gender roles and expectations, may be even more pervasive than homophobia. Fear of and ignorance about trans-genderism perhaps, stems from firmly rooted beliefs that there are two and only two genders (men and women) (Finnegan & McNally, 2002). Internalized transphobia may also cause the transgender person to see themselves as wrong, bad, sick, or at fault (Brown & Rounsley, 1996).

A 1999 poll found that the majority of Americans continue to view homosexuality as morally wrong (Ungvarski & Grossman, 1999). Such views may translate into homophobia and acts of discrimination against

LGBT individuals. The experience of "coming out" into a homophobic, transphobic culture is one that has a number of physical, mental, and psychological consequences throughout the life span. O'Hanlan, Cajab, Schatz, Lock, and Nemrow (1997) suggest that homophobia is linked to all aspects of health and health care and poses a major public health risk for LGBT people. In order to increase their social power and decrease homophobia, LGBT elders who were once "out" may go back in the closet and pass as heterosexual, becoming "invisible."

Issues of discrimination cross cultural boundaries. Black, Latino, and Asian LGBT people struggle with religious issues, family concerns, racism, homophobia, discrimination, and development of a homosexual identity, thus resulting in the management of multiple identities (Adams & Kimmel, 1997; Gonzalez & Espin, 1996; Lopez & Traung, 1998). To understand the enthno-racial experiences of same-sex sexuality within the lesbian and gay community, one must consider the degree of tolerance each ethnic community has toward such behavior (Zamora-Hernandez & Patterson, 1996).

Older lesbian and bisexual women have "triple minority status" (due to age, gender, and sexual orientation; Deevey, 1990, p. 35). Older lesbian women of color add yet another minority status. Elders in LGBT community must also confront the bias of ageism just as their heterosexual counterparts (McKee, 1999). Within the LGBT community, however, there has been a general lack of outreach to elders and few programs designed specifically to honor their contributions. Organizers against ageism are taking steps to mobilize the LGBT community to take action to remedy this ageism (Cahill, South, & Spade, 2000).

Discrimination and barriers to health care for LGBT people of all ages have been documented (e.g., Cahill et al., 2001; Peterson, 1996). The assumption of heterosexuality and stereotyping of LGBT people may silence them about health concerns (Schatz & O'Hanlan, 1994). This cohort of LGBT elders has been referred to as "preliberation" to highlight their particular socio-historical reality (Brotman, Ryan, & Cormier, 2003). Those who grew up in the era before gay liberation often experience great stigma and shame associated with their sexual orientation (Kaufman & Raphael, 1996). The need to stay hidden to prevent discrimination has remained a prominent coping strategy for many older LGBT adults (Cook-Daniels, 1997; Harrison & Silenzio, 1996; Rosenfeld, 1999).

Internalized Homophobia

Internalized homophobia occurs when negative feelings (or even self-hatred) toward one's self result from growing up in a heterosexist environment that devalues and denigrates nonheterosexuals (Rostosky & Riggle, 2002). Based on this definition, it is expected that most, if not all, individuals who identify as gay, lesbian or bisexual will experience at least some degree of internalized homophobia. In order for development of a positive homosexual or bisexual identity to occur, one must recognize the impact of internalized homophobia and work to eradicate it (Cass, 1979, 1984; Fox, 2002; Troiden, 1989). Internalized homophobia has been found to be associated with substance abuse (e.g., Amadio & Chung, 2004; Bobbe, 2002), mental health issues such as suicide and depression (Igartua, Gill, & Montoro, 2003; Szymanski, Chung, & Balsam, 2001) and higher levels of distress associated with cancer (McGregor et al., 2001). Friend (1991) suggested that positive aging in gay and lesbian adults is associated with positive identity development that tends to be associated with lower levels of internalized homophobia (Rowen & Malcolm, 2002).

DEMOGRAPHIC PROFILE

Just as the older adult population in general is very heterogeneous, older LGBT people are also extremely diverse. Additionally, although researchers have attempted to sample the LGBT population more accurately, sampling bias continues to exist and caution must be used in interpreting the results.

The demographic profile of the older LGBT population differs from the heterosexual profile in several ways including education, income, percent in committed relationships, living alone, and having children (see Table 7.1). Although there is a dearth of research on the experiences of gay, lesbian, bisexual and transgender individuals who are members of racial minority groups (Brotman et al., 2003), there is evidence that samples of GLB people are as racially diverse as heterosexual samples (Cahill et al., 2000).

In the discussions below, lesbians and bisexual women have been grouped together and gay men grouped with bisexual men, with differences noted. It is important to recognize that, although bisexuality is a distinct sexual orientation (Fox, 2002; McVinney, 2001), the paucity of literature on bisexuals is a direct reflection on the lack of understanding of this orientation among public health researchers. Health issues of older transgender adults are also discussed.

Studies, including data from the General Social Survey (GSS) and National Health and Social Life Survey (NHSLS), generally indicate that gays and lesbians are better educated than their heterosexual counterparts. Evidence suggests that this is not a result of sample selection

TABLE 7.1. Profile of Gay Men, Lesbians, and Heterosexuals Age 65 and Over (%)

	Gay men	Lesbians	Heterosexuals
Bachelors degree and above	74[*]	66[*]	15.4[§]
Partnered (GL) or married (hetero)	36[*]–46[**]	51[*]–79[**]	75 men 43 women[†]
Live alone	66[*]	52[*]	21 women 6.9 men[†]
Formerly married	33[**]	42[**]	NA
Have children	15[*]	30[*]	20[††]

[*]Cantor, Brennan, and Shippy (2004).
[**]Herdt, Beeler, and Rawls (1997).
[†]Gist and Hetzel (2004).
[††]SAGE (2001).
[§]Federal Interagency Forum on Aging-Related Statistics (2004).

bias (Black, Gates, Sanders, & Taylor, 1998). The widespread belief that gay men and lesbians are more affluent than the general population is a myth, however. Bailey's (1998) study of 40 metropolitan areas with gay and lesbian concentrations showed a slightly negative correlation between homosexuality and income. Several studies have shown that gay men earn less than their heterosexual counterparts (Bailey, 1998; Klawitter & Flatt, 1998), with one study reporting that gay men earned as much as 27% less than heterosexual men (Badgett, 1995). Lesbians seem to earn slightly more than heterosexual women (Black et al., 1999); however, Klawitter and Flatt (1998) found no differences from heterosexual women when other factors were considered. Poverty and wage discrimination are widespread among transgender people of all ages according to anecdotal evidence (Cahill et al., 2000).

A higher percentage of older lesbians and fewer older gay men are partnered than their heterosexual counterparts. Additionally, more lesbians than gay men report being in a committed relationship (Cantor, Brennan, & Shippy, 2004; Herdt, Beeler, & Rawls, 1997). The differences in rates of being partnered or married for gay men, lesbians, and heterosexuals may reflect differences in life spans of males and females.

Evidence suggests that LGBT seniors are nearly twice as likely as heterosexual seniors to live alone (Cahill et al., 2000). It should be noted, however, that the stereotype of the lonely old gay man or lesbian is a myth and has not been supported. Research evidence has not shown differences in prevalence of loneliness between older gays and lesbians and older heterosexuals (Berger, 1982).

Social support networks of LGBT seniors include family and close friends. The majority of older LGBT individuals do not seem to be estranged from their families of origin as some have suggested (Grossman, D'Augelli, & Hershberger, 2000). Cantor et al. (2004) report that 90% of older gay and lesbian respondents with living parents were close or very close to them with 59% having close siblings and 84% of those with children having close relationships with them. Friendship networks are especially important to gays and lesbians of all ages. In one study, over 90% of respondents had an average of six friends in their network (Cantor et al., 2004). Friends become families of choice or "fictive kin" for many older LGBT people (Barranti & Cohen, 2000; Brotman et al., 2003; Weinstock, 2004). Close friends were cited as the most frequent sources of support among older LGBT adults (90%), followed by their partners (44%; Grossman, D'Augelli, & Hershberger, 2000).

Loss of functional status and chronic illness sometimes necessitates the need for caregivers in old age. In a recent study of LGBT older adults, when asked who would take care of them if they needed care, 27% said they did not know, 59% indicated their partner, 34.5% stated a friend, and 8.8% indicated a child would care for them. Friends were identified most often by 78.4% as helping them get through a personal crisis, whereas 60.8% listed their partner, and 5.5% did not know who would help them (Burbank & Manning, 2005). These numbers underscore the necessity for high-quality, LGBT-friendly health care.

Exit polling data suggest that more openly lesbian, gay, and bisexual seniors live in urban areas than rural or suburban areas (Bailey, 1998). Another study found that most lived in single-family dwellings (48.8%) or condominiums (13.8%) with 31.3% in apartments (Quam & Whitford, 1992). Sixty-one percent owned their own homes with 38.8% renting. When LGBT elders concerns were surveyed, the need for LGBT affirming housing emerged as an important concern (Burbank & Manning, 2005).

PHYSICAL HEALTH ISSUES

Older Lesbian/Bisexual Women

Lesbians do not seem to be at higher risk for particular health problems simply because of their sexual orientation, but rather because of differential risk factors more prevalent among lesbians (Solarz, 1999).

Although heterosexual and nonheterosexual women appear to have similar incidences of chronic diseases, lesbians seem to have higher rates of important risk factors such as smoking, obesity, and alcohol use. Further discussion of smoking and alcohol use can be found in the section on substance abuse, which follows.

One study of health behaviors of lesbians found that 34.2% of lesbians (mean age 40) reported no physical activity in the past month compared with 31.4% of a comparable sample of heterosexual women. More heterosexual women (86.3%) than lesbians (63.2%) reported having no regular vigorous activity, however. More lesbians were overweight with higher body mass indices (BMI) than heterosexual women (Aaron, Markovic, Danielson, Honnold, Janosky, & Schmidt, 2001). Other studies also reported this same finding of increased BMI among lesbians (Case et al., 2004; Roberts, Dibble, Nussey, & Casey, 2003). Yancey, Cochran, Corliss, and Mays (2003) reported 45.1% of their sample of lesbians and bisexual women exercised three or more times per week with a mean BMI of 27. Other risk factors more prevalent in lesbians are nulliparity (never having given birth), less use of oral contraceptives, and fewer screening examinations of all kinds (Denenburg, 1995; Haynes, 1995).

Studies have, in general, supported the hypothesis that lesbian and bisexual women are at higher risk for breast cancer (Dibble, Roberts, & Nussey, 2004); however, to date, no conclusive data confirm higher rates among lesbians. Another study did not find an increase in self-reported breast cancer in lesbian and bisexual women; however, those women were more likely to exhibit risk factors such as smoking, higher consumption of alcohol, nulliparity, and obesity associated with breast cancer (Cochran et al., 2001). Additionally, research suggests a higher risk among lesbian women for ovarian cancer (likely due to fewer pregnancies and lower use of birth control pills; Dibble, Roberts, Robertson, & Paul, 2002). Given that lung cancer is the number one cause of cancer death in women, and that numerous studies suggest that lesbian and bisexual women are more likely to smoke, it appears that these women may be at differential risk for this form of cancer.

Cardiovascular disease is the number one killer of women in North America, including lesbians (Ulstad, 1999). Based on current data, the actual risk of coronary artery disease is unknown among lesbians (Solarz, 1999). Although they have increased rates of smoking and higher BMI than heterosexual women, they also used fewer oral contraceptives that may have reduced their risk (Peterkin & Risdon, 2003). Some sources do indicate that they are at higher risk because of increased smoking and body weight, however (Case et al., 2004).

In summary, although conclusive research evidence is not available, it seems that lesbian and bisexual women have more risk factors related to reproductive cancers and lung cancer than heterosexual women. Cardiovascular disease is also a problem among this group of women, as with women in general. It is not clear how lesbian and bisexual women may differ on risk factors because, in most empirical studies, lesbian and bisexual women are grouped together and compared with heterosexual women.

Older Gay/Bisexual Men

Gay and bisexual men are at higher risk of cardiovascular disease and some cancers, as are lesbian and bisexual women, for many of the same reasons. Gay (but not bisexual) men were more likely to smoke than their heterosexual counterparts (Ryan, Wortley, Easton, Pederson, & Greenwood, 2001; Tang et al., 2004), increasing their risk for lung cancer (Peterkin & Risdon, 2003). Very few studies have examined cancer risk among gay or bisexual men. Daling et al. (1987) and Koblin et al. (1996) found an increase in risk of anal cancer among gay men. Koblin et al. (1996) also documented increased risk of nonHodgkins lymphoma and Hodgkins disease among gay men. What is interesting for gay and bisexual men (as well as for lesbian and bisexual women) is that the rates of smoking among adolescents in this population continue to be higher than for their heterosexual counterparts (e.g., D'Augelli, 2004; Rosario, Schrimshaw, & Hunter, 2004), indicating that it is likely that the increase in risk for cardiovascular disease and cancer will continue.

Gay and bisexual males, more than nonheterosexual males, are at risk of human immunodeficiency virus (HIV) and other sexually transmitted diseases (STD) such as hepatitis. HIV places gay and bisexual men at higher risk for Kaposi's sarcoma (Koblin et al., 1996). It appears that older gay men have more difficulty changing to safer sex practices and may not use condoms with every sexual encounter (Linsk, 1997). Issues related to HIV and AIDS among older adults are addressed in detail in other chapters and are not covered in more detail here.

Older Transgender Adults

Much less is known about health issues related to transgender adults, and research on older transgender adults is rare (Berreth, 2003). Substance abuse rates among transgender individuals are probably much higher than the norm (Leslie, Perina, & Mequeda, 2001). Additionally, rates of HIV are significant. Leslie et al. (2001) reported that 35% of male-to-female transgender individuals in one study tested positive for HIV. There also appears to be significant risk of physical violence and harassment toward transgender individuals. In a recent study, Lombardi,

Wilchins, Priesing, and Malouf (2001) found that about 25% of the respondents reported violence against them, whereas over 50% reported either physical violence or harassment.

Little is known about the long-term effects of hormone use and of surgeries associated with sexual reassignment. Hansbury (2004) reported a first-person account of the extreme physical side-effects of initial testosterone injections, and Berreth (2003), in her review of the literature, indicated that some evidence exists linking hormone injections to increased risk of a number of diseases (including cardiovascular), thus increasing risk to this population. Additionally, sexual reassignment surgeries have great impact on the physical body, and little is known about the increased health risks for the transgender individual who is post-operative. After sexual reassignment has taken place, health concerns associated with the previous sex remain (for example, males who undergo reassignment to females still need to have prostate exams; Berreth, 2003).

PSYCHOSOCIAL AND SPIRITUAL HEALTH ISSUES

This section addresses general psychosocial issues common among LGBT older adults including adjustment, substance abuse, violence and sexual assault, and spiritual issues. Issues specific to lesbians, gays, and transgender older adults are addressed in separate sections.

Adjustment

The stereotypical view presents older gay and lesbian people as lonely, depressed, and alienated with extreme internalized homophobia. An opposing view described in the research literature are those gay and lesbian older adults who are well-adjusted, vibrant, and adapting well to the aging process. They have responded to heterosexism by reconstructing a positive and affirmative sense of self. These two opposing views of older gays and lesbians can be thought of as representing two ends of a continuum. In the center of the continuum is a group called "passing" older lesbian and gay people who marginally accept some aspects of homosexuality but who have some internalized homophobia and still believe heterosexuality is optimal (Friend, 1991). Even considering the hostile historical period in which they were raised, the research literature suggests that the majority of older gays and lesbians are at the well-adjusted end of the continuum with high levels of self-acceptance with being lesbian or gay (Brown et al., 1997; Ehrenberg, 1996; Friend, 1991). In fact, positive experiences and healthy adjustment to age seem to be the norm for gay men (Wahler & Gabbay, 1997) and lesbians (Gabbay & Wahler, 2002).

A common issue associated with aging is loneliness. The risk for loneliness may be higher among gay, lesbian, bisexual, and transgender elders because many, particularly gay men, may have no children. In a study of gay, lesbian, and bisexual adults over 60 years, Grossman et al. (2000) found that about a quarter of their sample reported lacking companionship and that about 13% felt isolated. Those who were living with partners reported fewer feelings of loneliness than those who were not. Reid (1995) noted in his review of the literature on older gay and lesbian adults that social networks can be important to counteract the negative attitudes toward homosexuality by society.

The finding that older gays and lesbians may be better able to cope with aging than their heterosexual counterparts has been explained by their past experiences at coping with homophobia and discrimination. This may reflect a sampling bias, however, as those who are depressed and lonely may not participate in studies (Ehrenberg, 1996).

The term "crisis competence" refers to a person's ability to successfully manage challenges and crises, based on previously developed coping skills. Many older LGBT adults age with a sense of crisis competence that they have developed in response to earlier pain and life crises around homophobia and discrimination and losses of loved ones from the AIDS epidemic (Friend, 1991; Cahill et al., 2000). In addition, lesbians and gays may be more prepared for aging because of the blurring of gender role responsibilities throughout life and mastery of independence (Friend, 1991). This crisis competence perspective has been criticized by Lee (1991) as only applicable to the more affluent segment of the LGBT population, however.

Gay men may experience "accelerated aging" or perceive themselves as being old at an earlier age than their chronological age (Baron & Cramer, 2000). These feelings may occur as early as age 30 (Berger, 1982). Lesbians, on the other hand, seemed to have advantages over heterosexual women in that intimate relationships may not be as strongly based on youthful appearance (Laner, 1979). They also tend to have a wider intergenerational circle of family and friends than gay men (Baron & Cramer, 2000).

Substance Abuse

There seems to be no definitive agreement in the literature on the prevalence of alcohol and drug use among the LGBT population. Some studies report increased use of alcohol and drugs (Skinner & Otis, 1996), whereas others did not find a difference in use compared to the heterosexual population (Bloomfield, 1993; Cochran, Keenan, Schober, & Mays, 2000). McKirnan and Peterson (1989a, 1989b) found that although gay men and lesbians accounted for twice as many reported alcohol problems as heterosexuals, they had similar patterns of heavy drinking. Another study found that gay men were more likely than heterosexual men to either drink heavily or abstain making the overall quantity and frequency of consumption comparable to heterosexual counterparts (Stall & Wiley, 1988). Roberts, Patsdaughter, Grindel, and Tarmina (2004) found an increased rate of alcohol use among older lesbians. There does seem to be agreement that alcohol consumption does not decline with age in the gay and lesbian population as it does among those who are heterosexual (McKirnan & Peterson, 1989a, 1989b; SAMHSA, 1996; Skinner, 1994). One study suggested that, for lesbian women, internalized homophobia was related to tobacco and alcohol use (Amadio & Chung, 2004).

Related to drug use, gay men reported higher overall rates of illicit drug use than lesbians (Skinner & Otis, 1996), but do not seem to have higher rates of dependence or addiction than heterosexual men (Stall & Wiley, 1988). They do report using a greater variety of illicit drugs than heterosexual men, however (Stall & Wiley, 1988; Stall, Greenwood, Acree, Paul, & Coates, 1999). The National Household Survey on Drug Abuse report found that lesbians were more likely than heterosexual women to have been diagnosed with drug dependency (SAMHSA, 1996). Little information is available on drug use, specifically among older gays and lesbians.

Numerous studies document higher rates of smoking among both gay men and lesbians than among heterosexual men and women (Sanchez, Meacher, & Beil, 2005; Solarz, 1999; Stall et al., 1999; Tang et al., 2004). Another study did not report this finding for lesbians over 50 years of age, however (Gruskin, Hart, Gordon, & Ackerson, 2001). Evidence on the prevalence of lesbian smoking seems to indicate that more lesbians smoke than gay men (Bradford, Ryan, & Rothblum, 1994; Skinner & Otis, 1996). Fewer lesbians than gay men were heavy smokers, however (Solarz, 1999). Lesbians who smoke may be at higher risk of health problems also because of their higher average body mass index and their more infrequent visits to health care providers (White & Dull, 1997).

Substance abuse problems are also prevalent in the transgender population. Alcohol abuse rates ranged from 27.1% (Valentine, 1998) to 33% (Xavier, 2000). In Clements' study (1999) of 392 male to female transgender people, lifetime noninjected drug use prevalence was: 90% used marijuana; 66%, cocaine; 48%, crack; and 24%, heroin. Because of the difficulties associated with loss of jobs and reduced social support networks often faced by transgender people, they may turn to the sex industry for financial survival (Marcel, 1998), which puts them at an even higher risk for substance abuse.

Violence and Sexual Assault

Domestic violence is an issue in the gay, lesbian, bisexual, and transgender community, and researchers have begun to give more attention to this issue. Evidence suggests that it occurs at approximately the same rate as in heterosexual relationships with about one in every four relationships experiencing some form of abuse (Dolan-Soto & Kaplan, 2005; Elliot, 1996). Researchers have suggested that it is important to understand that victimization in these relationships is real and must be recognized (Lettelier, 1996). Studies reporting physical violence in lesbian relationships have found that 22–46% of all lesbians have been abused by a same-sex partner (Coleman, 1990; Gay and Lesbian Community Action Council, 1987 as cited in Elliot, 1996; Kelly & Warshafsky, 1987 as cited in Elliott, 1996). In one report, incidences of domestic violence peaked among 30–44-year-olds and declined sharply with age, reaching a low among LGBT adults who are 65 years of age. Reports of domestic violence increased slightly again with age after 65 years of age (Dolan-Soto & Kaplan, 2005). This requires further study, however, as these increased numbers may reflect caregiver abuse.

There is a general unwillingness to report violent incidents because of fear of discrimination in the legal system and reluctance to fuel homophobic reactions to such reports (Elliott, 1996; Peterkin & Risdon, 2003). An examination of the domestic violence laws in all 50 states reveals that battered lesbians and gay men are often less protected than heterosexuals or not protected at all (12 states; Fray-Witzer, 1999). Abuse in same-sex relationships may differ from heterosexual domestic abuse in the power of the abuser with either one or both partners being the abuser, a lack of social support from families or friends, and lack of professional support from police, doctors, or clergy. Access to shelters that are gay- or lesbian-affirmative is limited in most communities (Peterkin & Risdon, 2003).

Violence against transgender people is said to have reached epidemic proportions (National Coalition for LGBT Health, 2004). The experience of victimization of some form is probably universal among transgender people as a direct result of their transgender identity or presentation (Dean et al., 2000). Distrust of police and the justice system, along with fears of secondary victimization (in the judicial system), result in underreporting of crimes committed against transgender people. Older transgender people are also at risk of being victimized in the health care system when they may be dependent and unable to care for themselves.

Older Lesbian/Bisexual Women

Research on mental health issues of older lesbians paints a picture of a relatively well-adjusted group of older women. Kehoe (1986) reported that the typical lesbian over 65 years is a survivor who copes with aging in a satisfactory manner. Older lesbians expressed fears related to loss of physical or mental capabilities and income (Almvig, 1982). One study found only 4% of older lesbians indicated current problems with depression and 1% with anxiety (Bradford et al., 1994). Grossman et al., (2001) found the majority of older lesbians to be psychologically well-adjusted with good self-esteem. In another study, however, 25% reported being lonely and 10% had at some point in their lives been depressed about their sexual orientation and had suicidal thoughts (Barker, 2004). There is general agreement that, although midlife lesbians comprise the most "out" group of lesbians to date (Adelman, 2000), many older lesbians continue to be closeted (Bradford et al., 1994; Quam, 1997).

Losses are an inherent part of the lives of all older adults and older lesbians are no different. What is different is that often the most significant and difficult loss, the loss of a life partner, is not recognized, validated, or valued. The heterosexual widow who loses a spouse usually receives open and caring support from a wide circle of friends and family. Depending on the degree of disclosure and acceptance of the older lesbian's (or gay man's) relationship the remaining partner may be left to grieve alone. This has been discussed as "disenfranchised grief" by Doka (1989) and may complicate the mourning process. Because in most states same-sex couples cannot legally marry, they are excluded from rights of spouses. This may have a serious impact in health care settings, on health care decision-making, and in estate settlement after the death a partner.

Older Gay/Bisexual Men

The experiences of gay and bisexual older men are multifaceted. Kertzner, Meyer, and Dolezal (2004) found that gay and bisexual men were more likely to report more depressive symptoms, lower scores on self-acceptance, a lower purpose in life, and were less likely to be in relationships than were heterosexual men. Rawls (2004) reported similar results related to symptoms of depression. He reported that about 40% of the men in their 60's reported high levels of disclosure of sexual orientation, and only about 28% of those in their 70's high disclosure; this supports the notion that older men are less likely to have disclosed sexual orientation to others. What was interesting in this study is that degree of disclosure was related to depression only in those 50–59 years of age; for those over 60 years, the relationship was nonexistent.

Although the same discussion of loss among lesbians applies to gay men, this generation of older gays has lived through multiple losses of many friends from AIDS. The concept of global loss has been used to describe the experience of the multiple losses due to AIDS in the gay community. Global loss affects all aspects of life and identity, and is experienced as a loss of community, with no safe haven (Marion, 1996). Four symptoms of pervasive loss may be especially pronounced: psychological fatigue, depression, survivor guilt, and shame (Marion, 1996). This global loss experience is carried with the gay man into old age and may increase their vulnerability to the psychological effects of subsequent losses.

It is commonly understood that marital status in older age is related to positive health outcomes. Hostetler (2004) found that more than half of the sample of gay men ($M = 52$ years) indicated being somewhat or very concerned about being isolated and growing older in general. Their perception and positive acceptance of being single by choice predicted well-being, however, thus challenging the stereotype of the "old and lonely" homosexual. Butler (2004) reached a similar conclusion as a result of her review of the literature on older GLBT elders. Although they are more likely to be living alone and without children than their heterosexual counterparts, these elders are generally not reporting the experience of being lonely. In fact, Berger and Kelly (2001) suggested, from results of their studies, that the unique problems faced by older gay men include discrimination, uninformed health professionals, and legal issues (wills, domestic partnerships, etc.).

Older Transgender Adults

One important issue that needs to be explored among transgender individuals is the effect of their changing lives on family connections in which family ties may have been severed due to the stress of the transition (Berreth, 2003). Midence and Hargreaves (1997), in their review of the correlates of psychopathology in those undergoing sexual reassignment found that, in general, poor social support and negative family reactions predicted post-surgery psychopathology. It was also noted that the rates of suicide attempts, completed suicides, depression, and substance use were high (Dean et al., 2000).

Spiritual Issues

Spirituality is very important to older gays and lesbians. In one study of older lesbians, many credited their spirituality with providing them with the strength they needed to face challenges of life (Clunis, Fredriksen-Goldsen, Freeman, & Nystrom, 2005). Some religions, however, attack same-sex identities. In another study, over 90% of older gays and lesbians surveyed in a recent study reported being raised with a religions affiliation, although 65.5% currently had no religious affiliation. The majority indicated that spirituality was very important, however (Burbank & Manning, 2005). Religious homophobia can cause LGBT people to stop going to church because they feel guilty or because of the hostile treatment they have received (Finnegan & McNally, 2002).

HEALTH CARE ISSUES

As people age, the risk for disease increases and thus the need for more frequent access to health care; for LGBT individuals, other factors can complicate the aging process. These factors include issues related to disclosure (or lack thereof) of sexual orientation, potential lack of social support by families, and sensitivity by health care providers (Brotman et al., 2003; Butler, 2004; Dean et al., 2000). In addition, health care providers in general lack information on gay and lesbian health-related matters (Peterkin & Risdon, 2003). This is not surprising, given the lack of general awareness of LGBT people in general, of issues affecting the lives of LGBT individuals, and that members of this population, particularly older adults, tend to be ignored in public health research (Boehmer, 2002).

Gay men and lesbians tend to visit doctors less often than heterosexual women (Harrison & Silenzio, 1996) and lesbians postpone treatment longer than heterosexual women (Carroll, 1999). This is presumably due, at least in part, to a health care system perceived to be homophobic (Klitzman & Greenberg, 2002; Owen, 1996; Peterkin & Risdon, 2003). One study found that 72% of lesbian respondents reported negative treatment in health care experiences (Stevens & Hall, 1988). Lesbians also receive less frequent gynecological care than heterosexual women (Robertson & Schacter, 1981), putting them at higher risk for mortality and morbidity from gynecological cancers. This may also be attributed to a lack of education about their need for examinations. There is some evidence to suggest that lesbian women are increasingly using primary care services, however (Roberts et al., 2004). Rankow and Tessaro (1998) found that women whose providers were more sensitive to lesbian issues were more likely to report regular screening.

SUMMARY

Lesbian, gay, bisexual and transgender older adults are an invisible population in the United States. This invisibility has multiple causes, including a general lack of awareness by the public (including health care professionals), general denial of the reality of same-sex and transgender identities, widespread homophobia, and elders who feel it necessary to hide their LGBT identity. Research with this population is made especially difficult by a reluctance of its members to self-identify; this necessitates the cautious interpretation of what limited research findings are available. These elders live in a society in which stigma, homophobia, transphobia, and discrimination are realities that impact health status and well-being as well as influence the development of a healthy psychosocial identity.

A general lack of information on LGBT health-related matters and discrimination among health care providers causes barriers to health care for LGBT people of all ages. Although more research on the older LGBT population is greatly needed, a greater awareness on the part of health care providers that this population exists and has special health needs is imperative. Ongoing research and education is necessary to improve the health of this vulnerable group of older adults.

REFERENCES

Aaron, D. J., Markovic, N., Danielson, M. E., Honnold, J. A., Janosky, J. E., & Schmidt, N. J. (2001). Behavioral risk factors for disease and preventive health practices among lesbians. *American Journal of Public Health, 91,* 972–975.

Adams, C. L., & Kimmel, D. C. (1997). Exploring the lives of older African American gay men. In B. Greene (Ed.), *Ethnic and cultural diversity among lesbians and gay men: Psychological perspectives on lesbians and gay men* (3rd ed.). Thousand Oaks, CA: Sage.

Adelman, M. (Ed.). (2000). *Midlife lesbian relationships: Friends, lovers, children, and parents.* Binghamton, NY: Harrington Park Press.

Adin, E. K. (2004, Spring). Where's the old dyke's home? City planners leave older lesbians out in the cold. *Women & Environments* pp.10–11.

Almvig, C. (1982). *The invisible minority: Aging and lesbianism.* Syracuse, NY: Utica College of Syracuse.

Amadio, D. M., & Chung, Y. B. (2004). Internalized homophobia and substance use among lesbian, gay, and bisexual persons. *Journal of Gay & Lesbian Social Services: Issues in Practice, Policy & Research, 17*(1), 83–101.

American Psychiatric Association. (1968). *Diagnostic and statistical manual of mental disorders* (2nd ed.). Washington, DC: Author.

American Psychiatric Association. (1994). *Diagnostic and statistical manual of mental disorders* (4th ed.). Washington, DC: Author.

Badgett, M. V. L. (1995). The wage effects of sexual orientation discrimination. *Industrial and Labor Relations Review, 48,* 737.

Bailey, R.W. (1998). *Gay politics, urban politics: Identity and economics in the urban setting.* New York: Columbia University Press.

Barker, J. C. (2004). Lesbian aging: An agenda for social research. In G. Herdt & B. deVries (Eds.). *Gay and lesbian aging* (pp. 29–72). New York: Springer Publishing.

Baron, A., & Cramer, D. W. (2000). Potential counseling concerns of aging lesbian, gay, and bisexual clients. In R. M. Perez, K. A. DeBord, & K. A. Bieschke (Eds.), *Handbook of counseling and psychotherapy with lesbian, gay and bisexual clients* (pp. 207–224). Washington, DC: American Psychological Association.

Barranti, C., & Cohen, H. (2000). Lesbian and gay elders: An invisible minority. In R. Schneider, N. Kropt, & A. Kisor (Eds.), *Gerontological social work: Knowledge, service settings, and special populations* (2nd ed., pp. 343–367). Belmont, CA: Wadsworth/Thompson Learning.

Bem, S. (1995). Dismantling gender polarization and compulsory heterosexuality. Should we turn the volume down or up? *Journal of Sex Research, 32*(4), 329–334.

Berger, R. M. (1982). The unseen minority: Older gays and lesbians. *Social Work, 27,* 236–242.

Berger, R. M. (1984). Realities of gay and lesbian aging. *Social Work, 29*(1), 57–76.

Berger, R. M., & Kelly, J. J. (2001). What are older gay men like? An impossible question? *Journal of Gay & Lesbian Social Services, 13*(4), 55–64.

Berreth, M. (2003). Nursing care of transgendered older adults: Implications from the literature. *Journal of Gerontological Nursing, 29*(7), 44–49.

Block, S. (2004, May 17). Gay couples enter golden years with more risk. *USA Today.*

Bobbe, J. (2002). Treatment with lesbian alcoholics: Healing shame and internalized homophobia for ongoing sobriety. *Health & Social Work, 27,* 218–222.

Boehmer, U. (2002). Twenty years of public health research: Inclusion of lesbian, gay, bisexual, and transgender populations. *American Journal of Public Health, 92,* 1125–1130.

Black, D., Gates, G., Sanders, S., & Taylor, L. (1999). *Demographics of the gay and lesbian population in the United States: Evidence from available systematic data sources.* Center for Policy Research Working Papers 12, Center for Policy Research, Maxwell School, Syracuse University. Retrieved July 25, 2005 from http://ideas.repec.org/p/max/cprwps/12.html

Bloomfield, K. A. (1993). A comparison of alcohol consumption between lesbian and heterosexual women in an urban population. *Drug and Alcohol Dependence, 33,* 257–269.

Bradford, J. B., Ryan, C., & Rothblum, E. (1994). National lesbian health care survey: Implications for mental health care. *Journal of Consulting and Clinical Psychology, 62,* 228–242.

Brotman, S., Ryan, B., & Cormier, R. (2003). The health and social service needs of gay and lesbian elders and their families in Canada. *Gerontologist, 43,* 192–202.

Brown, M. L., & Rounsley, C. A. (1996). *True selves: Understanding transexualism— For families, fiends, coworkers, and helping professionals.* San Francisco: Jossey-Bass.

Brown, L. B., Sarosy, S. G., Cook, T. C., & Quarto, J. G. (1997). *Gay men and aging*. New York: Garland.

Burbank, P. M., & Manning, C. (2005). *Meet the older neighbors: Report of the SAGE/ RI survey of lesbian, gay, bisexual and transgender older adults in Rhode Island*. Providence, RI: SAGE/RI.

Butler, S. (2004). Gay, lesbian, bisexual, and transgender (GLBT) elders: The challenges and resilience of this marginalized group. *Journal of Human Behavior in the Social Environment, 9*(4), 25–44.

Cahill, S., South, K., & Spade, J. (2000). *Outing age: Public policy issues affecting gay, lesbian, bisexual, and transgender elders*. New York: The National Gay and Lesbian Task Force Policy Institute.

Cantor, M. H., Brennan, M., & Shippy, R. A. (2004). *Caregiving among older lesbian, gay, bisexual, and transgender New Yorkers*. New York: National Gay and Lesbian Task Force Policy Institute.

Carroll, N. (1999). Optimal gynecologic and obstetric care for lesbians. *Obstetrics and Gynecology, 93*, 611–613.

Case, P., Austin, B., Hunter, D. J., Manson, J. E., Malspeis, S., Willett, W. C., et al. (2004). Sexual orientation, health risk factors, and physical functioning in the Nurses' Health Study II. *Journal of Women's Health, 13*(9), 1033–1047.

Cass, V. (1979). Homosexual identity formation: A theoretical model. *Journal of Homosexuality, 4*, 219–235.

Cass, V. (1984). Homosexual identity formation: Testing a theoretical model. *Journal of Sex Research, 20*, 143–167.

Clements, K. (1999). *The Transgender Community Health Project: Descriptive results*. San Francisco: San Francisco Department of Public Health.

Clunis, D. M., Fredriksen-Goldsen, K. I., Freeman, P. A., & Nystrom, N. (2005). *The lives of lesbian elders*. New York: Haworth.

Cochran, S. D., Keenan, C., Schober, C., & Mays, V. M. (2000). Estimates of alcohol use and clinical treatment needs among homosexually active men and women in the U. S. population. *Journal of Consulting and Clinical Psychology, 68*, 1062–1071.

Cochran, S. D., Mays, V. M., Bowen, D., Gage, S., Bybee, D., Roberts, S. J., et al. (2001). Cancer-related risk indicators and preventive screening behaviors among lesbian and bisexual women. *American Journal of Public Health, 91*, 591–597.

Coleman, V. E. (1990). *Violence between lesbian couples: A between groups comparison*. Unpublished doctoral dissertation. University Microfilms International.

Cook-Daniels, L. (1997). Lesbian, gay male, bisexual, and trangendered elders: Elder abuse and neglect issues. *Journal of Elder Abuse and Neglect, 9*(2), 35–50.

Daling, J. R., Weiss, N. S., Hislop, G., Maden, C., Coates, R. J., Sherman, K. J., et al. (1987). Sexual practices, sexually transmitted diseases, and the incidence of anal cancer. *New England Journal of Medicine, 317*, 973–977.

Davidson, D. (2001). *Issues facing elderly gay men and lesbians.* Retrieved September 11, 2004, from www.keln.org/bibs/davidson.html

D'Augelli, A. R. (2004). High tobacco use among lesbian, gay, and bisexual youth: Mounting evidence about a hidden population's health risk behavior. *Archives of Pediatric Medicine, 158,* 309–310.

Dean, L., Meyer, I. H., Robinson, K., Sell, R. L., Sember, R., Silenzio, V. M. B., et al. (2000). *Lesbian, Gay, Bisexual, and Transgender Health: Findings and Concerns. Journal of the Gay and Lesbian Medical Association, 4*(3), 102–151

Deevey, S. (1990). Older lesbian women: An invisible minority. *Journal of Gerontological Nursing, 16*(5), 35–37.

Denenberg, R. (1995). Report on lesbian health. *Womens Health Issues, 5*(2), 81–91.

Denny, D. (2004). Changing models of transexualism. In U. Leli & J. Drescher (Eds.), *Transgender subjectivities: A clinician's guide* (pp. 25–40). New York: Haworth Press.

Dibble, S. L., Roberts, S. A., & Nussey, B. (2004). Comparing breast cancer risk between lesbians and their heterosexual sisters. *Women's Health Issues, 14*(2), 60–68.

Dibble, S. L., Roberts, S. A., Robertson, P. A., & Paul, S. M. (2002). Risk factors for ovarian cancer: Lesbian and heterosexual women. *Oncology Nursing Forum, 29*(1), E1–E7.

Doka, K. (1989). *Disenfranchised grief: Recognizing hidden sorrow.* Lexington, MA: Lexington Books.

Dolan-Soto, D. R., & Kaplan, S. (2005). *New York lesbian, gay, transgender and bisexual domestic violence report 2003/2004.* New York: New York City Gay and Lesbian Anti-Violence Project. Retrieved from www.avp.org on July 24, 2005.

Duberman, M. (1994). *Stonewall.* New York: Plume

Ehrenberg, M. (1996). Aging and mental health: Issues in the gay and lesbian community. In C. J. Alexander (Ed.), *Gay and lesbian mental health: A sourcebook for practitioners* (pp. 189–209). Binghamton, NY: Haworth.

Elliott, P. (Ed.). (1996). *Confronting lesbian battering.* St. Paul, MN: Minnesota Coalition for Battered Women.

Faderman, L. (1998). *Surpassing the love of men: Romantic friendship and love between women from the Renaissance to the present.* New York: Perennial.

Fausto-Sterling, A. (2000). *Sexing the body: Gender politics and the construction of sexuality.* New York: Basic Books.

Feinberg, L. (1997). *Transgender warriors: Making history from Joan of Arc to Dennis Rodman.* Boston: Beacon.

Finnegan, D. G., & McNally, E. B. (2002). *Counseling lesbian, gay, bisexual, and transgender substance abusers.* New York: Haworth.

Fisk, A. D., & Rogers, W. A. (2002). Psychology and aging: Enhancing the lives of an aging population. *Current Directions in Psychological Science, 11*(3), 107–110.

Fox, R. C. (2002). Bisexual identities. In L. D. Garnetts & D. C. Kimmel (Eds.), *Psychological perspectives on lesbian, gay, and bisexual experiences* (pp. 86–129). New York: Columbia University.

Fray-Witzer, E. (1999). Twice abused: Same-sex domestic violence and the law. In B. Leventhal & S. E. Lundy, (Eds.), *Same-sex domestic violence*. Thousand Oaks, CA: Sage.

Freud, S. (2000). *Three essays on the theory of sexuality*. New York: Basic Books. (Original work published 1905)

Friend, R. A. (1991). Older lesbian and gay people: A theory of successful aging. *Journal of Homosexuality, 20*(3–4), 99–118.

Gabbay, S. G., & Wahler, J. J. (2002). Lesbian aging: Review of a growing literature. *Journal of Gay and Lesbian Social Services, 14*(3), 1–21.

Gist, Y. J. & Hetzel, L. I. (2004). *We the people: Aging in the United States. Census 2000 Special Reports*. U.S. Census Bureau. Retrieved July 22, 2005 from www.census.gov/prod/2004pubs/censr-19.pdf

Goldberg, C. (1996, Sept. 8). Shunning "he" and "she", they fight for respect. *New York Times*, p. A10.

Gonzalez, F. J., & Espin, O. M. (1996). Latino men, Latino women, and homosexuality. In R. P. Cabaj & R. S. Stein (Eds.), *Textbook of homosexuality and mental health*. Washington, DC: American Psychiatric Press.

Green, J. (2000). Introduction to transgender issues. In *Transgender equality: A handbook for activists and policymakers* (p. 7). New York: Policy Institute of the National Gay and Lesbian Task Force and the National Center for Lesbian Rights.

Grossman, A. H., D'Augelli, A. R., & Hershberger, S. L. (2000). Social support networks of lesbian, gay, and bisexual adults 60 years of age and older. *Journal of Gerontology: Psychological Sciences, 55B*, 171–179.

Grossman, A. H., D'Augelli, A., & O'Connell, T. S. (2001). Being lesbian, gay, bisexual, and 60 or older in North America. In D. C. Kimmel & D. L. Martin (Eds.), *Midlife and Aging in Gay America* (pp. 23–40). Binghamton, NY: Harrington Park Press.

Gruskin, E. P., Hart, S., Gordon, N., & Ackerson, L. (2001). Patterns of cigarette smoking and alcohol use among lesbians and bisexual women enrolled in a large health maintenance organization. *American Journal of Public Health, 91*, 976–979.

Haldeman, D. C. (1994). The practice and ethics of sexual orientation conversion therapy. *Journal of Consulting and Clinical Psychology, 62*, 221–227.

Hansbury, G. (2004). Sexual TNT: A transman tells the truth about testosterone. In U. Leli & J. Drescher (Eds.), *Transgender subjectivities: A clinician's guide* (pp. 7–18). New York: Haworth Press.

Harrison, A. E., & Silenzio, V. M. B. (1996). Comprehensive care of lesbian and gay patients and families. *Primary Care: Models of Ambulatory Care, 23*(1), 31–46.

Haynes, A. (1995). Cancer among special populations: Women, ethnic minorities, and the poor. *Environmental Health Perspectives, 103*, 319–320.

Herdt, G., Beeler, J., & Rawls, T. W. (1997). Life course diversity among older lesbians and gay ment: A study in Chicago. *Journal of Gay, Lesbian, and Bisexual Identity*, 2, 231–247.

Hooker, E. (1993). Reflections of a 40-year exploration: A scientific view on homosexuality. *American Psychologist*, 48, 450–453.

Hostetler, A. J. (2004). Old, gay and alone? The ecology of well-being among middle-aged and older single gay men. In G. Herdt & B. deVries (Eds.), *Gay and lesbian aging: Research and future directions* (pp. 143–176). New York: Springer Publishing.

Igartua, K. J., Gill, K., & Montoro, R. (2003). Internalized homophobia: A factor in depression, anxiety, and suicide in the gay and lesbian population. *Canadian Journal of Community Mental Health*, 22(2), 15–30.

Kaufman, G., & Raphael, L. (1996). *Coming out of shame: Transforming gay and lesbian lives*. New York: Doubleday.

Katz, J. (1996). *The invention of heterosexuality*. East Rutherford, NJ: Plume.

Kehoe, M. (1986). A portrait of the older lesbian. *Journal of Homosexuality*, 12, 157–161.

Kelly, E. E., & Warshafsky, L. (1987, July). *Partner abuse in gay male and lesbian couple*. Paper presented at the Third National Conference for Family Violence Researchers, Durham, NH.

Kertzner, R., Meyer, I., & Dolezal, C. (2004). Psychological well-being in midlife and older gay men. In G. Herdt & B. de Vries (Eds.), *Gay and lesbian aging: Research and future directions* (pp. 97–115). New York: Springer Publishing.

Kinsey, A., Pomeroy, W. B., & Martin, C. E. (1948). *Sexual behavior in the human male*. Bloomington, IN: Indiana University.

Kinsey, A., Pomeroy, W. B., Martin, C. E., & Gebhard, P. H. (1952). *Sexual behavior in the human female*. Bloomington, IN: Indiana University.

Klawitter, M. M., & Flatt, V. (1998). The effects of state and local antidiscrimination policies of sexual orientation. *Journal of Policy Analysis and Management*, 17, 674–675.

Klitzman, R. L., & Greenberg, J. D. (2002). Patterns of communication between gay and lesbian patients and their health care providers. *Journal of Homosexuality*, 42(4), 65–75.

Koblin, B. A., Hessol, N. A., Zauber, A. G., Taylor, P. E., Buchbinder, S. P., Katz, M. H., et al. (1996). Increased incidence of cancer among homosexual men, New York City and San Francisco, 1978–1990. *American Journal of Epidemiology*, 144, 916–923.

Laner, M. R. (1979). Growing older female: Heterosexual and homosexual. *Journal of Homosexuality*, 4, 267–275.

Lee, J. A. (Ed.). (1991). Forward. *Journal of Homosexuality*, 20(3/4), xiii–xix.

Leslie, D. R., Perina, B. A., & Maqueda, M. C. (2001). Clinical issues with transgender individuals. In *A providers introduction to substance abuse treatment for lesbian, gay, bisexual, and transgender individuals* (pp. 91–97). Rockville, MD: U.S. Department of Heath and Human Services.

Lettelier, P. (1996). Twin epidemics: Domestic violence and HIV infection among gay and bisexual men. *Journal of Gay and Lesbian Social Services, 4*(1), 69–82.

Linsk, N. L. (1997). Experience of old gay and bisexual men living with HIV/AIDS. *Journal of Gay, Lesbian, and Bisexual Identity, 2,* 285–308.

Lombardi, E. L., Wilchins, R. A., Priesing, D., & Malouf, D. (2001). Gender violence: Transgender experiences with violence and discrimination. *Journal of Homosexuality, 42*(1), 89–101.

Lopez, R. A., & Traung, L. B. (1998). Social supports among Vietnamese American gay men. *Journal of Gay and Lesbian Social Services, 7*(3), 29–50.

Marcel, A. D. (1998). *Determining barriers to treatment for transsexuals and transgenders in substance abuse programs.* Boston: Transgender Education Network, Justice Resource Institute Health.

Marion, M. (1996). Living in an era of multiple loss and trauma: Understanding global loss in the gay community. In C. J. Alexander (Ed.), *Gay and lesbian mental health: A sourcebook for practitioners* (pp. 61–94). New York: Haworth Press.

McGregor, B. A., Carver, C. S., Antoni, M. H., Weiss, S., Yount, S. E., & Ironson, G. (2001). Distress and internalized homophobia among lesbian women treated for early stage breast cancer. *Psychology of Women Quarterly, 25*(1), 1–9.

McKee, V. (1999). Seniors survey identifies double discrimination for senior lesbians. *Herizons, 13*(1), 9–12.

McKirnan, D. J., & Peterson, P. I. (1989a). Psychosocial and social factors in alcohol and drug abuse: Epidemiology and population characteristics. *Addictive Behaviors, 14,* 545–553.

McKirnan, D. J., & Peterson, P. I. (1989b). Psychosocial and social factors in alcohol and drug abuse: An analysis of a homosexual community. *Addictive Behaviors, 14,* 555–563.

McVinney, D. (2001). Clinical issues with bisexuals. *A providers introduction to substance abuse treatment for lesbian, gay, bisexual, and transgender individuals* (pp. 87–90). Rockville, MD: U.S. Department of Heath and Human Services.

Meyer, I. H. (2001). Why lesbian, gay, bisexual, and transgender public health? *American Journal of Public Health, 91*(6), 856–859.

Michael, R. T., Gagnon, J. H., Laumann, E. O., & Kolata, G. (1994). *Sex in America: A definitive survey.* Boston: Little, Brown.

Midence, K., & Hargreaves, I. (1997). Psychosocial adjustment in male to female transsexuals: A review of the research evidence. *Journal of Psychology, 131,* 602–614.

National Coalition for LGBT Heath. (2004). *An overview of U.S. trans health priorities.* Retrieved July 1, 2005 from www.nctequality.org/HealthPriorities.pdf

O'Hanlan, K., Cajab, R. B., Schatz, B., Lock, J., & Nemrow, P. (1997). A review of the medical consequences of homophobia with suggestions for resolution. *Journal of the Gay and Lesbian Medical Association, 1*(1), 25–40.

Owen, W. F. (1996). Gay men and bisexual men and medical care. In R. P. Cajab & T. S. Stein (Eds.), *Textbook of homosexuality and mental health* (pp. 673–685). Washington, DC: American Psychiatric Press.

Peterkin, A., & Risdon, C. (2003). *Caring for lesbian and gay people: A clinical guide.* Toronto: University of Toronto.

Peterson, K. J. (1996). *Health care for lesbians and gay men: Confronting homophobia and heterosexism.* New York: Haworth Press.

Quam, J. K. (Ed.). (1997). *Social services for senior gay men and lesbians.* Binghamton, NY: Harrington Park Press.

Quam, J. K., & Whitford, G. S. (1992). Adaptation and age-related expectations of older gay and lesbian adults. *Gerontologist, 32,* 367–374.

Rankow, E. J., & Tessaro, I. (1998). Cervical cancer risk and Papanicolaou screening in a sample of lesbian and bisexual women. *Journal of Family Practice, 47,* 139–143.

Rawls, T. W. (2004). Disclosure and depression among older gay and homosexual men: Findings from the Urban Men's Health Study. In G. Herdt & B. de Vries (Eds.), *Gay and lesbian aging: Research and future directions* (pp. 97–115). New York: Springer Publishing.

Reid, J. C. (1995). Development in late life: Older lesbian and gay lives. In A. R. D'Augelli & C. J. Patterson (Eds.), *Lesbian, gay, and bisexual identities over the lifespan: Psychological perspectives* (pp. 215–242). New York: Oxford University.

Roberts, S. A., Dibble, S. L., Nussey, B., & Casey, K. (2003). Cardiovascular disease risk in lesbian women. *Women's Health Issues, 13,* 167–174.

Roberts, S. J., Patsdaughter, C. A., Grindel, C. G., & Tarmina, M. S. (2004). Health related behaviors and cancer screening of lesbians: Results of the Boston Lesbian Health Project II. *Women & Health, 39*(4), 41–55.

Robertson, P., & Schacter, J. (1981). Failure to identify venereal disease in a lesbian population. *Sexually Transmitted Diseases, 8*(20), 75–76.

Rosario, M., Schrimshaw, E. W., & Hunter, J. (2004). Predictors of substance use over time among gay, lesbian, and bisexual youths: An examination of three hypotheses. *Addictive Behaviors, 29,* 1623–1671.

Rosenfeld, D. (1999). Identity work among lesbian and gay elderly. *Journal of Aging Studies, 13,* 121–145.

Rostosky, S. S., & Riggle, E. D. B. (2002). "Out" at work: The relation of actor and partner workplace policy and internalized homophobia to disclosure status. *Journal of Counseling Psychology, 49,* 411–419.

Rowen, C. J., & Malcolm, J. P. (2002). Correlates of internalized homophobia and homosexual identity formation in a sample of gay men. *Journal of Homosexuality, 43*(2), 77–92.

Ryan, H., Wortley, P. M., Easton, A., Pederson, L., & Greenwood, G. (2001). Smoking among lesbians, gays, and bisexuals: A review of the literature. *American Journal of Preventive Medicine, 21*(2), 141–149.

Sanchez, J. P., Meacher, P., & Beil, R. (2005). Cigarette smoking and lesbian and bisexual women in the Bronx. *Journal of Community Health, 30*(1), 23–47.

Schatz, B., & O'Hanlan, K. (1994). *Anti-gay discrimination in medicine: Results of a national survey of lesbian, gay and bisexual physicians.* San Francisco: American Association of Physicians for Human Rights.

Seil, D. (2004). The diagnosis and treatment of transgendered patients. In U. Leli & J. Drescher (Eds.), *Transgender subjectivities: A clinician's guide* (pp. 99–116). New York: Haworth Press.

Skinner, W. F. (1994). The prevalence and predictors of illicit and licit drug use among lesbians and gay men. *American Journal of Public Health, 84,* 1307–110.

Skinner, W. F., & Otis, M. D. (1996). Drug and alcohol use among lesbian and gay people in a southern U. S. sample: Epidemiological, comparative, and methodological findings from the Trilogy Project. *Journal of Homosexuality, 30*(3), 59–92.

Solarz, A. L. (Ed.). (1999). *Lesbian health: Current assessment and directions for the future.* (pp. 70–105). Washington, DC: National Academy Press, Institute of Medicine.

Stall, R. D., Greenwood, G. L., Acree, M., Paul, A., & Coates, T. J. (1999). Cigarette smoking among gay and bisexual men. *American Journal of Public Health, 89,* 1875–1878.

Stall, R. D., & Wiley, J. (1988). A comparison of alcohol and drug use patterns of homosexual and heterosexual men. *The San Francisco Men's Health Study, 22*(1/2), 63–73.

Stevens, P. E., & Hall, J. M. (1988). Stigma, health beliefs, and experiences with health care in women. *Image: Journal of Nursing Scholarship, 20,* 69–73.

Substance Abuse Mental Health Services Administration (SAMHSA). (1996). *National household survey on drug abuse: Main findings of 1996.* Rockville, MD: SAMHSA.

Szymanski, D. M., Chung, Y. B., & Balsam, K. F. (2001). Psychosocial correlates of internalized homophobia in lesbians. *Measurement & Evaluation in Counseling & Development, 34*(1), 27–39.

Tang, H., Greenwood, G. L., Cowling, D. W., Lloyd, J. C., Roeseler, A. G., & Bal, D. G. (2004). Cigarette smoking among lesbians, gays, and bisexuals: How serious a problem? (United States). *Cancer Causes and Control, 15,* 797–803.

Troiden, R. R. (1989). The formation of homosexual identities. *Journal of Homosexuality, 12*(2), 39–51.

Ulstad, V. K. (1999). Coronary health issues for lesbians. *Journal of Gay and Lesbian Medical Association, 3*(2), 59–67.

Ungvarski, P. J., & Grossman, A. H. (1999). Health problems of gay and bisexual men. *Nursing Clinics of North America, 34,* 313–331.

United States Census. (2005). National population estimates-characteristics. Retrieved May 15, 2005 from: http://www.census.gov/popest/national/asrh/NC-EST2003-as.html

Valentine, D. (1998). *Gender Identity Project: Report on Intake Statistics, 1989–April 1997.* New York: Lesbian and Gay Community Services Center.

Wahler, J., & Gabbay, S. G. (1997). Gay male aging: A review of the literature, *Journal of Gay and Lesbian Social Services, 6*(3), 8–12.

Weinstock, J. (2004). Lesbian friendships at and beyond midlife: Patterns and possibilities for the 21st century. In G. Herdt & B. DeVries (Eds.). *Gay and lesbian aging: Research and future directions* (pp. 177–210). New York: Springer Publishing.

White, J. C., & Dull, V. T. (1997). Health risk factors and health seeking behavior in lesbians. *Journal of Women's Health, 6*(1), 103–112.

Xavier, J. M. (2000). *The Washington DC transgender needs assessment survey: Final report for phase two.* Washington, DC: Administration for HIV/AIDS, Department of Health of the District of Columbia Government.

Yancey, A. K., Cochran, S. D., Corliss, H. L., & Mays, V. M. (2003). Correlates of overweight and obesity among lesbian and bisexual women. *Preventive Medicine, 36,* 676–683.

Zamora-Hernandez, C. E., & Patterson, D. G. (1996). Homosexually active Latino men: Issues for social work practice. *Journal of Gay and Lesbian Social Services, 5*(2/3), 69–91.

CHAPTER EIGHT

Health Care Strategies for Lesbian, Gay, Bisexual, and Transgender Older Adults

P. Burbank, G. Burkholder, and P. Fournier

Most health care agencies, along with the majority of the public in the United States, operate under the assumption that everyone is heterosexual. Because of widespread negative attitudes and homophobia among the public, health care providers, and other health care professionals, lesbian, gay, bisexual, and transgender (LGBT) people are frequently subject to discrimination in health care encounters (Dean et al., 2000). They may receive substandard care or choose not to disclose important health information they fear might lead to stigmatization (Bradford & Ryan, 1988; Schatz & O'Hanlan, 1994).

For LGBT older adults, heterosexism, homophobia, and ageism are part of the fabric of life. Many are marginalized in multiple ways. About three quarters of this group are women and many experience sexism, and racism is not uncommon among those identifying with communities of color. By becoming or remaining closeted, lesbian, gay, and bisexual elders can remove one of the major categories of bias, although not without risks to their mental health. Most of these older adults grew up during an era in which homosexuality was considered an adverse medical condition, and some may have directly experienced any one of a number of aversive techniques to change sexual orientation (Haldeman, 1994). Despite an increase in the acceptance of homosexuality over the past two decades (Herek, 1999, cited in Dean et al., 2000), fear of stigma and discrimination continues to impact the daily lives of LGBT individuals. Dean et al. (2000), in their review of the current state of health of lesbian, gay, bisexual, and transgender individuals, suggest that stigma continues to be a major factor in health care provision to LGBT adults.

When considering how to address the needs of LGBT elders, one must take into account a reality resulting from a number of internal and external factors, including (a) sexual identity development; (b) internalized homophobia; (c) homophobia that is experienced from friends, family, and health care practitioners; (d) institutionalized prejudice in the form of ageism, sexism, and heterosexism; and (e) and societal (i.e., legal) structures that perpetuate the legitimacy of cultural heterosexism.

As described in the previous chapter, little is known about older gay, lesbian, bisexual, and transgender adults. It has been noted that adults who participate in studies tend to be more comfortable with their sexual orientation (Dean et al., 2000; Meyer, 2001; Reid, 1995); thus, the health issues of a larger group of adults who may be "closeted" or are otherwise not comfortable with their sexual orientation are unknown. This runs the risk of creating biased results that may misrepresent the actual risks associated with being lesbian, gay, bisexual, or transgender and being older (Meyer, 2001). This also means that it is difficult to know how to provide services or what strategies may be useful in dealing with these older adults.

Older LGBT people experience many of the same health problems as heterosexual older adults; however, there are additional risk factors associated with an LGBT identity. As discussed in the previous chapter, LGBT adults have increased risks for some cancers and cardiovascular disease. Gay men are at higher risk for HIV/AIDS and sexually transmitted diseases. Smoking, alcohol and drug abuse, and domestic violence are also issues for this population. Although LGBT older adults are generally a well-adjusted and resilient group, mental health issues may include problems with self-concept from internalized homophobia, depression, and disenfranchised grief. LGBT elders have expressed concerns about their health and health care in general, about who would care for them if they were unable to care for themselves, and about housing and finances. Older LGBT adults are also less likely to have screening exams and to use health care resources because of fear of discrimination and homophobia.

Although specific treatment of individual health problems such as cancer is the same for seniors regardless of sexual orientation, health care professionals and agencies must be open and affirming to the lives of LGBT people in ways that encourage them to seek out appropriate screening and health care. Regular screening is necessary for cancer detection and early treatment. If LGBT seniors are reluctant to access health care, this screening can be delayed, even to the point of threatening their survival. The main issue in improving care to older LGBT adults, then, is not interventions to address specific health issues, but rather strategies to provide LGBT affirming health care directed at health providers and the larger health care system in general. This must happen before LGBT elders feel comfortable utilizing health care and are able to receive informed, quality care that honors their differences and respects them as human beings.

This chapter will cover specific strategies directed at caring for LGBT elders such as communication techniques and assessment guidelines. Next, it will address education about LGBT issues and attitude change among health care providers and students. The goal of cultural competence in provision of care to the older LGBT population will be discussed. Organizational changes for improving care to the LGBT community along with policy and legal issues will also be described. Lastly, this chapter provides examples of current actions that are being taken by the LGBT community and its allies to ensure access to affirming health care. Suggestions for future strategies to further this work are also discussed.

STRATEGIES FOR CARING FOR LGBT ELDERS

Communicating with LGBT Elders

Quam (1997) wrote about her experiences while educating a group of social workers who worked with elders in long-term care. These social workers had an average of 15–20 years of experience and were open to diversity. She asked them how many gay and lesbian patients they had worked with during their professional careers. "After a period of silence, one of the social workers said 'I remember a man—I think was gay . . . he never exactly came out to me . . . but then I never really asked him about it'" (Quam, 1997, p. xv). This is a common experience in heterosexist environments in which health care providers generally assume everyone is heterosexual and do not ask questions to refute that assumption. Such responses, although typical, seem to reflect a "Don't ask, don't tell" approach to patient interaction that has the effect of reinforcing silence and invisibilty. Providers may assume that everyone, including the older person, is more comfortable not discussing issues of sex or sexual orientation, or they may think that it does not matter because sexual orientation is not central to the health care issue being addressed. Indeed, the person's nondisclosure to health care professionals may contribute to this. One study found that this nondisclosure to be much more pronounced among lesbians than among gay men (Klitzman & Greenberg, 2002). The discomfort that health professionals may feel discussing and dealing with issues of sexual orientation, coupled with the older LGBT person's need to remain invisible to protect themselves from discrimination (or from their own discomfort around dealing with the issue) reinforces a vicious cycle of oppression (Brotman, Ryan, & Cormier, 2003).

Further complicating open communication with LGBT elders is the issue of labeling and language used to describe themselves and their experiences. For instance, older women who would be considered lesbians by current definition may not describe themselves as such. They rarely use the terms "lesbian," "dyke," "queer," or "homosexual" (Simkin, 1998). Lesbians and gay men usually indicate that they are single or divorced on marital status and may state they live with a close friend, housemate, or even a sister if asked. Brotman et al. (2003) quote from a focus group narrative describing one lesbian couple in which "one of the partners changed her last name to her partner's last name so that they would be taken for sisters, to be put in the same room" (p. 197). Older gays and lesbians may acknowledge loving relationships with another of the same sex, but still not identify with the lesbian or gay community. These elders may be deeply offended when others, even younger gays or lesbians, apply labels to them (Deevey, 1990). For these reasons, communication with elders about their sexual orientation must be done with caution and sensitivity. It is suggested that providers listen carefully to how patients describe their living situation and/or partner status. The provider should then follow the patients' leads and use words that are consistent with the ways patients describe themselves.

Assessment Guidelines

The first place in the health care system where an older LGBT person may encounter difficulty is in the health care provider's office completing the intake form. The question about marital status usually lists four options (single, married, divorced or separated, and widowed). There is no option to identify a same-sex long-term partnership, nor is there is a way to describe any of the myriad of living situations describing the same-sex couple. Some suggested ways of changing assessment forms to more accurately reflect LGBT realities are to ask open-ended questions such as, "Who is most important to you? Who lives with you?" If the response is that they live alone, then a follow-up question might be "have you always lived alone?" This will give clues as to whether they may be experiencing a recent loss of a partner.

The Gay and Lesbian Medical Association (GLMA) has developed guidelines for creating a safe clinical environment for lesbian, gay, bisexual, transgender, and intersex patients. (See Table 8.1 for the Web resource.) This guideline includes sample recommended questions for LGBT-sensitive intake forms. This sample form is comprehensive for LGBT people of all ages and may be revised to be more specific for older patients needs. It includes questions about HIV and sexually transmitted infections that are also relevant for older LGBT adults. The Transgender Aging Network (TAN) also provides a resource for assisting organizations that serve the LGBT community with suggestions to make programs more transgender friendly (Cook-Daniels, 2001).

TABLE 8.1   Internet Resources for Lesbian, Gay, Bisexual, and Transgender Elders

Subject	Web address and description
Drug Use and Abuse	http://www.health.org/referrals/resguides.aspx? InvNum=MS489#Organizations Center for Substance Abuse Prevention, SAMHSA; provides alcohol and drug abuse information, resources, and list of organizations serving LGBT people.
Drug Abuse and Recovery for Lesbians	http://www.soberdykes.org/welcome.html Information resources as well as lesbian 12 step support mailing list, newsletter, and list of gay and lesbian AA meetings.
SAGE (Senior Action in a Gay Environment)	http://www.sageusa.org/ Oldest and largest organization devoted to meeting the needs of aging GLBT persons; SAGE New York City provides many direct services and resources to GLBT seniors, education, training for health providers, and advocacy.
Gay and Lesbian Medical Association	www.glma.org National organization committed to ensuring equality in health care for LGBT individuals and health care professionals through professional education, public policy work, patient education and referrals, and the promotion of research; hosts annual conference; publishes the *Journal of the Gay and Lesbian Medical Association*; many links and resources; provides guidelines for Caring for LGBT patients at http://www.glma.org/medical/clinical/lgbti_clinical_guidelines.pdf

(Continued)

TABLE 8.1   (*Continued*)

Subject	Web address and description
Association of Gay and Lesbian Community Centers	http://www.lgbtcenters.org/ The National Association of LGBT Community Centers (NALGBTCC) supports and enhances LGBT community centers; provides list of community centers; technical assistance, training, and networking opportunities; distribution of nationally-coordinated program materials; assistance in forming new centers; and linkages to other national organizations, foundations, and government.
Healthy People 2010 (Companion Document for LGBT Health)	http://www.glma.org/policy/hp2010/index.shtml Focuses on approximately 120 objectives and 12 focus areas from the recently published *Healthy People 2010* document, the federal blueprint for public health for the next ten years; examines these areas and lists specific recommendations regarding improved access, preventative medicine, and cultural competency; Makes recommendations in the following areas: quality health services, mental health, public health infrastructure, HIV, immunization and infectious diseases, tobacco, injury and violence prevention, and substance abuse; includes a comprehensive LGBT health resource list.
National Gay and Lesbian Task Force	http://www.thetaskforce.org/ The first national (LGBT) civil rights and advocacy organization founded in 1973; works to build the political strength of the LGBT community by training state and local activists and leaders, working to strengthen the infrastructure of state and local allies, and organizing broad-based campaigns to build public support for complete equality for LGBT people. Policy Institute, provides research and policy analysis to support the struggle for complete equality; links to several publications including those on elder issues; hosts annual "Creating Change" conference.
National Coalition for Lesbian, Gay, Bisexual, and Transgender Health	http://www.lgbthealth.net/ Committed to improving the health and well-being of LGBT individuals and communities through public education, coalition building and advocacy that focuses on research, policy, education and training.

TABLE 8.1   (*Continued*)

Subject	Web address and description
Mental Health Service Organization in San Francisco	http://www.newleafservices.org/index.htm Provides professional mental health, substance abuse, and social support services to LGBT people of all ages; Outreach to Elders program offers information and referrals, support services, friendly visits for the homebound, educational and cultural activities, holiday events, group outings, and women's and men's social/recreational activities and groups and geriatric mental health services including in-home, senior-specific counseling services and medication management.
Rainbow Train	http://www.rainbowtrain.org/links.html Rainbow Train works to ensure that LGBT cultural competency training becomes a part of the overall training of health care and service providers; training increases the awareness of service providers about the diversity of sexual orientations and gender identities among their senior clients; helps providers to better identify and meet clients' needs by providing care without judgments or assumptions.
Lesbian and Gay Aging Issues Network (LGAIN)	http://www.asaging.org/networks/LGAIN/about.cfm Works to raise awareness about the LGBT elders and about the unique barriers they encounter in gaining access to housing, healthcare, long-term care and other needed services; fosters professional development, multidisciplinary research and dialogue on LGBT issues in the field of aging through publications, conferences, and cosponsored events.
Transgender information resources	http://www.tgguide.com/ TG Guide provides the Transgender community with quality resources, publishing a comprehensive site of services and information, accurately representing the Transgendered community, in a positive manner; one of the largest collections of informative texts on the web.
National Transgender Advocacy Coalition (NTAC)	http://www.ntac.org/ Activist organization founded in 1999; a federal-level lobbyist and supporter of state-level lobbying; works proactively to reform societal attitudes and the law to achieve equal rights for the transgendered and other gender diverse individuals.

(Continued)

TABLE 8.1 (*Continued*)

Subject	Web address and description
Transgender Law and Policy Institute (TLPI)	http://www.transgenderlaw.org/ Advocacy organization brings experts and advocates together to work on law and policy initiatives designed to advance transgender equality; tracks current developments in legal and public policy issues affecting transgender people and their families, and writes summaries of these trends for activists, policymakers, and the media; provides legal, medical, and social science resources to attorneys and others advocating on behalf of transgender individuals; makes freely available litigation, legislative, and education advocacy materials for use by other advocates for transgender people.
Lambda Legal Defense	http://www.lambdalegal.org/cgi-bin/iowa/index.html National organization committed to achieving full recognition of the civil rights of lesbians, gay men, bisexuals, transgender people and those with HIV through impact litigation, education, and public policy work; pursues litigation in all parts of the country, in every area of the law that affects LGBT; website provides many informative links.
Transgender Aging Network (TAN)	http://www.forge-forward.org/tan/index.php Works to improve the lives of current and future trans/SOFFA (significant others, friends, family and allies) elders by promoting communication, providing information and enhancing the work of researchers, service providers, educators, advocates, elders and others who are interested in trans/SOFFA aging issues; advocates for policy changes in public and private institutions, services, organizations, and programs; provides communication channels through which trans/SOFFA elders can give and receive support and information.
Gay, Lesbian and Straight Education Network	http://www.glsen.org/cgi-bin/iowa/home.html A website for educators not geared toward older adults, but many good curricular resources that could be adapted; strives to assure that each member of every school community is valued and respected regardless of sexual orientation or gender identity/expression.

TABLE 8.1   (*Continued*)

Subject	Web address and description,
Gay, Lesbian and Straight Teachers Network	http://www.qrd.org/qrd/www/orgs/glstn/ Also for schools, goal is to create an environment at school in which every member of the school community is valued and respected, regardless of sexual orientation; offers many resources to do this applicable to any agency.
Parents and Friends of Lesbians and Gays	http://www.pflag.org/ Promotes the health and well-being of LGBT persons, families and friends through support to cope with an adverse society; educational programs to improve the general populations understanding of LGBT people; and advocacy, to end discrimination and to secure equal civil rights; provides opportunity for dialogue about sexual orientation and gender identity, and acts to create a society that is healthy and respectful of human diversity.
Lambda Antiviolence Project	http://www.lambda.org/avp_gen.htm#avp Provides victim services to survivors of hate crimes, domestic violence, sexual assault, and other crimes including crime prevention and education, a 24-hour bilingual (English–Spanish) national hotline, peer-to-peer support groups, and accompaniment to and advocacy with police, the courts, and other service providers; lists resources for victims and general information on violence among the LGBT population.
Society for Psychological Study of Lesbian, Gay and Bisexual Issues, Division of American Psychological Association (APA)	http://www.apa.org/divisions/div44/ Founded in 1985 to represent sexual orientation issues within and beyond the APA; has over 1500 members in all 50 states, DC and eleven foreign countries; strives to advance the contribution of psychological research in understanding lesbian, gay, and bisexual issues, to promote the education of psychologists and the general public and to inform psychologists, and the general public, about relevant research, educational, and service activities; website has guidelines for psychotherapy practice with LGBT people; Task Force on Aging link has extensive annotated LGBT Aging Bibliography.

(Continued)

TABLE 8.1 (*Continued*)

Subject	Web address and description
Association for Gay Lesbian and Bisexual Issues in Counseling	http://www.aglbic.org/ A division of the American Counseling Association, promotes greater understanding of GLBT issues among members of the counseling profession and related helping occupations; works to improve standards and delivery of counseling services; fosters interest in counseling-related charitable, scientific, and educational programs; works to secure equality of treatment, advancement, qualifications, and status of GLBT members of the counseling profession and related helping occupations; publishes *The Journal of GLBT Issues in Counseling.*
The Mautner Project	http://www.mautnerproject.org Improves the health of lesbians and their families through advocacy, education, research, and direct client services including support groups; provides "Removing the Barriers," a cultural competency training curriculum designed to assist medical and social service providers in providing quality care for women who partner with women.

Adapted from Peterkin and Risdon (2003).

Physical Environment

Creating a welcoming environment for LGBT patients should begin in the waiting room. Posters depicting older gay and lesbian adults and indicating that this is a facility that welcomes LGBT patients can be hung on the wall. An example of such a poster used by SAGE-RI to distribute to health care facilities is shown in Figure 8.1. Written materials listing community resources for LGBT elders (along with other special patient groups) can also be made available for patients to read. An additional benefit of including such reading material is that other heterosexual patients may increase their awareness about the needs of LGBT older adults as well.

Resources for Care of LGBT Elders

Approaches to specific problems of LGBT elders are presented here first, followed by a description of several multipurpose organizations that provide multiple resources to meet many needs of this population.

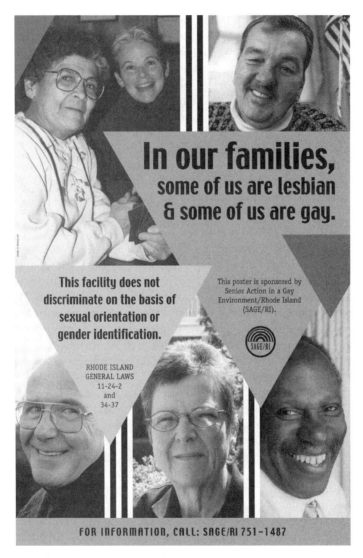

FIGURE 8.1 SAGE poster for health care agencies.
Reprinted with permission. Michael Guy, designer.

SUBSTANCE ABUSE

Research suggests that lesbian, gay, bisexual, and transgender individuals are at higher risk for substance abuse issues than are their majority counterparts (e.g., Roberts, Patsdaughter, Grindel, & Tarmina, 2004; Sanchez, Meacher, & Beil, 2005; Skinner & Otis, 1996; Tang, Greenwood, Cowling,

Lloyd, Roeseler, & Bal, 2004). Thus, early substance abuse prevention programs are important, particularly within these communities. In 2001, the U.S. Department of Health and Human Services (USDHHS) Substance Abuse and Mental Health Services Administration (SAMHSA) published a comprehensive manual for providers to educate them on substance abuse treatment for LGBT individuals. Their Web site (see Table 8.1) contains information on drug use and abuse specifically related to the gay, lesbian, bisexual, and transgender communities. This site provides a clearing house of informative resources that includes Web sites, books, and the names of organizations across the United States. Other web sources are included in Table 8.1. Informative books for counselors of LGBT substance abusers are readily available (e.g., Finnegan & McNally, 2002).

VIOLENCE AND PARTNER ABUSE

Violence is a reality for many LGBT individuals. Many experience this violence as a result of acts of homophobia. The National Coalition for LGBT Health lists violence and murder prevention as their top priority in their Overview of United States Trans Health Priorities (2004). It is also of note that transgender people tend to experience higher rates of violence in general. The Lambda GLBT Community Services Antiviolence Project provides information and support to LGBT victims of violence of all kinds. They also publish a hate crime fact sheet and have a Hate Crime Network for reporting hate crimes. City-wide efforts such as The New York City Gay and Lesbian Anti-Violence Project (www.avp.org) also provide resources to help stop violence of all kinds in the LGBT community.

Domestic violence is another important issue in the gay, lesbian, bisexual and transgender community that has only recently begun to attract more attention from researchers. Evidence suggests that it occurs in same sex relationships at approximately the same rate as in heterosexual relationships (Elliot, 1996). To reduce violence associated with domestic abuse, one primary goal is to educate health care providers in the importance of these issues in the LGBT community. *Same-Sex Domestic Violence: Strategies for Change* (Lundy & Leventhal, 1999) contains information on building community and organizing coalitions around same-sex domestic violence issues. This book also discusses legal issues associated with same-sex domestic violence. *Violence in Gay & Lesbian Domestic Partnerships* (Renzetti & Miley, 1996) is a useful resource for understanding the impact of same-sex domestic violence, issues around service provision, and also discusses issues unique to relationships involving people of color. The Survivor Project (2005) is devoted to the domestic and sexual abuse experienced by transgender individuals (see Table 8.1 for Web addresses).

MENTAL HEALTH

Major mental health problems among LGBT older adults arise from issues of lifetime discrimination, internalized homophobia, and maintaining invisibility. A study in Canada using focus groups with gay and lesbian elders reported on several themes that emerged from the discussions. One theme described repeatedly was the profound marginalization experienced by older gays and lesbians in all aspects of social and political life (Brotman et al., 2003). To address this problem, interventions at two levels are needed. The first involves mental health interventions with older LGBT individuals to help them cope with the psychological effects of this discrimination. The second involves strategies aimed at the policy level designed to change the social and health care environments to make them more inclusive and affirmative of LGBT people. Interventions at the individual level will be discussed here. System-level strategies will be addressed later in the chapter in education, policy, and legal issues sections.

Internalized homophobia can be a difficult concept for those caring for older LGBT adults to comprehend, as it requires being able to identify with the experience of a person who has had to mature in an environment that (in some cases actively) discourages sexual orientations other than heterosexual. It may be helpful for the counselor or therapist to be able to assess this in clients and to open the topic for discussion. Ross and Rosser (1996) developed a comprehensive, reliable, and valid scale for the assessment of internalized homophobia among gay men. This scale consists of four subscales: Public Identification as Gay, Perception of Stigma Associated with Being Gay, Social Comfort with Gay Men, and Moral and Religious Acceptability of Being Gay. Another scale, The Lesbian Internalized Homophobia Scale, contains five subscales that address various aspects of internalized homophobia. These are: Connection with a Lesbian Community, Public Identification as Lesbian, Personal Feelings About Being a Lesbian, Moral and Religious Attitudes Toward Being a Lesbian, and Attitudes Toward Other Lesbians (Szymanski, Chung, & Balsam, 2001). Scales such as these may be useful in helping older gay, bisexual, and lesbian elders to assess attitudes toward their own same-sex attractions and the extent to which those feelings are negatively internalized. Given the relationship between higher levels of internalized homophobia and poorer mental, physical, and psychological health outcomes, understanding how this impacts the lives of LGBT older adults is essential (Amadio & Chung, 2004). In addition, practitioners might benefit from the development of written material that describes, in simple terms, what internalized homophobia is, how to recognize it, and how to cope with its effects.

There are some organizations and resources that address the mental health needs of LGBT elders. For example, Senior Action in a Gay Environment (SAGE) in New York City offers many services targeting mental health issues among older LGBT adults. It is important to note that SAGE has chapters in several major cities across the United States. New Leaf (2005), an organization based in San Francisco, offers one of the largest counseling services directed toward LGBT elders. Several other metropolitan areas also offer mental health services to this community of elders. Books available on the subject, including *Affirmative Psychotherapy and Counseling for Lesbians and Gay Men* (Chernin & Johnson, 2002) and *Gay and Lesbian Mental Health: A Sourcebook for Practitioners* (Alexander, 1996), may be helpful resources for the counselor who wishes to learn more about specific counseling strategies for LGBT clients. A comprehensive outline that can be used to start a group for "maturing gay men" covers topics such as self-esteem, body image, sexuality, and relationships and can be found in Quam, 1997, p. 73).

Housing and Long-Term Care

Although many states have clauses that prohibit discrimination based on sexual orientation, most states do not extend this nondiscrimination to public housing (Kaplan, 2002). This is of concern to elders who are considering moving into retirement communities, senior housing, or who may be facing the reality of long-term care. Retirement communities for LGBT people started in Florida in the late 1990s and are growing in numbers and popularity (Jacobs, 2003). The first affordable housing for LGBT elders is being built in Hollywood, California by the nonprofit group Gay Lesbian Elder Housing Corp. There will be 104 apartments and a community center (Marech, 2005). Some new concepts such as stay at home-assisted living that serves the lesbian and gay elder community are also being developed (Rainbow Gardens, 2005).

In long-term care, the facility becomes the person's home at a time when they are most vulnerable. Given the increased vulnerability of LGBT elders, LGBT-affirmative care is essential. With the number of elder LGBT adults and thus the potential for long-term care needs increasing, LGBT elders raised in a culture of distrust around the medical profession may resist the use of services provided by those systems (Kaplan, 2002). Kaplan noted that homophobic attitudes by service providers working in long-term care facilities were common. Issues may arise because of service providers' discomfort with outward expressions of affection by patients. Brotman et al. (2003) describes a situation where "One woman told me that she would just like to know that if she ever has to go into a facility, that she can hold hands with her partner in the TV room"

(p. 197). Transgender people may be especially fearful of long-term care, as fear of abuse from staff is a very real concern (SAMSHA, 2005). Education and sensitivity training of long-term care staff are needed to ensure quality care of LGBT seniors in this setting.

Multipurpose Community Resources

The oldest direct service agency serving the LGBT elder community is SAGE, founded in 1977. SAGE, New York provides many services including weekly discussion groups, case management and individual advocacy, counseling, SAGE Positive (services for HIV positive LGBT people over the age of 50), an Older Lesbian Project that provides social services, and a Friendly Visitor Program. They have a drop-in center, and sponsor a wide range of educational and social activities to appeal to a wide range of interests.

Reid noted in his review of the literature on older gay and lesbian adults that social networks can be important to counter the negative attitudes toward homosexuality by society. Although SAGE started in New York, other SAGE organizations (SAGE-Net) have been established in 12 other locations and states in the United States, Canada, and Germany.

New Leaf, in addition to providing mental health services to LGBT people of all ages, has an Elder Outreach program that includes services such as information and referral, support services, Friendly Visitors for homebound elders, educational and cultural activities, holiday events, and men's and women's recreational activities. Several other programs similar to New Leaf offer a wide range of resources and are also available in other metropolitan communities. Local community centers can be located through a search tool in the website of the National Association of Lesbian, Gay, Bisexual, and Transgender Community Centers (NALGBTCC; 2005). The mission of this organization is to support the goals of community centers around the country.

STRATEGIES FOR HEALTH CARE PROVIDERS

Health care providers' responses to caring for LGBT older adults range from acceptance and tolerance to ignorance and hostility. Discrimination on the part of health care professionals and perception of bias by LGBT individuals have been identified as barriers to care, leading to a reduction in care sought and in quality of care obtained (Millman, 1993). To change this environment, providers need to become culturally competent in care of older LGBT adults by learning about and understanding the complexities of the lives of LGBT individuals. This can be achieved through consciousness raising (by service providers) to explore their own attitudes toward LGBT people.

Cultural Competence

Cultural competence is "the ability to provide effective and helpful services to people from varied cultures and communities in a respectful and informed manner" (Finnegan & McNally, 2002, p. 67). Although the term "culture" is most frequently used to refer to beliefs, norms, and material traits of people of different ethnic and racial groups, cultural diversity may also extend to differences of many kinds, including those related to sexual orientation and age. A culturally competent model of health care acknowledges the client's cultural strengths, values, and experiences when giving treatment. Culturally responsive services are characterized by the following:

- Staff sensitivity to the cultural nuances of the client population.
- Staff with backgrounds representing those of the client population.
- Treatment modalities that reflect the cultural values and treatment needs of the client population.
- Adequate representation of the client population in decision-making and policy implementation (Wright, Shelton, Browning, Orduna, & Wong, 2001).

There is much debate over what constitutes "gay culture"; however, there is no question that many LGBT people experience a way of life that is considered a culture (Wright et al., 2001, p. 20). The diversity within the LGBT community is great; thus health care providers must be careful to avoid stereotyping when considering the cultural characteristics of the LGBT population. Health care providers can become culturally competent in caring for LGBT older adults through education and awareness of their own attitudes toward sexual orientation and the behaviors that are associated with those attitudes.

Education on LGBT Issues

EDUCATION FOR HEALTH CARE PROVIDERS

The educational system for health professionals has failed to educate providers regarding the unique needs of the LGBT population (Wallik, Cambre, & Townsend, 1992). In a society that is heterosexist, health care professionals trained under this system would also likely share this perspective. Education concerning and the opportunity to examine their attitudes about sexual orientation and gender must be provided to health professionals in order to improve health care for the LGBT population.

There are several educational resources available to health care professionals and agencies. *The Healthy People 2010* Companion Document for LGBT People (Gay and Lesbian Medical Association and LGBT Health Experts, 2001) provides, at the end, a list of health resources by state. The GLMA (2005b) Guidelines for Creating a Safe Clinical Environment for LGBTI (adds intersexuals) Patients lists provider education and training resources at the end also. The Mautner Project of the National Lesbian Health Organization is a nonprofit organization that provides service and support groups for lesbians with cancer, and education and experiential training for providers who care for them (*Removing the Barriers*). Other training curricula for health care professionals are available from Senior Action in a Gay Environment (SAGE), and Midwest AIDS Prevention Project (training called SCRUBS) (Michigan HIV News, 2002).

The GLMA offers a listing of community health centers established specifically to address health issues for LGBT adults (GLMA, 2005a). Most of these health centers also offer training programs for staff of health care agencies. Organizations such as the Fenway Community Health Center in Boston and Gay City Health Project have specialized in serving the medical needs of members of all ages of the community. The LGBT Aging Project in the Boston area also provides speakers and education and technical assistance to those who wish to become LGBT friendly.

Rainbow Train, based in Seattle, provides training for service providers to improve understanding and awareness of the cultural context of LGBT elders. Lesbian and Gay Aging Information Networks (LGAIN) (2005), a constituent group of the American Society on Aging, provides information on the unique needs of LGBT elders, particularly related to access to health care. Additionally, information on physical and mental health needs of these populations is included. Also included in Table 8.1 are weblinks for the Gay Lesbian, and Straight Education Network (GLSEN) and the Gay, Lesbian, and Straight Teacher's Network (GLSTN). Although these web resources are directed primarily to teachers and organizations in schools, many of the educational materials and resources on heterosexism, homophobia, and general consciousness-raising are useful outside of school settings, including those that provide services for LGBT elders.

Standards of Care for gays and lesbians have also been developed and are available from GLMA (2005b), for GLBT population from GLBT Health Access Project (2005), and for transgender people by the

Harry Benjamin International Gender Dysphoria Association (2001). Kaiser Permanante has developed a provider's handbook on culturally competent care for the LGBT population, available through their National Diversity Council. Peterkin and Risdon (2003) provide guidance designed to improve relationships between LGBT individuals and their health care service providers.

There are a number of resources available on the Web for education around transgender issues. These include *Transgender Guide: Strategies for Care Providers* (2005). This site provides comprehensive information on transgender issues and concerns. Included is a directory of transgender service providers and agencies by state.

EDUCATION OF STUDENTS IN THE HEALTH PROFESSIONS

In 1994, the GLMA surveyed their membership and found that 91% of physician and medical student respondents knew of antigay bias directed at patients, whereas 88% had heard colleagues disparage gay or lesbian patients. Sixty-seven percent had seen colleagues deny or reduce care (Schatz & O'Hanlan, 1994). In 1996, The American Medical Association (AMA) recommended greater educational efforts for medical students and physicians regarding the health needs of gay men and lesbians (Council on Scientific Affairs, AMA, 1996). To determine what family medicine departments in the United States were teaching medical students about gay, lesbian, and bisexual issues, Tesar and Rovi (1998) surveyed 95 programs and found that the mean number of hours spent on LGB issues throughout the 4 years was 2.5 h. About half (50.6%) of the respondents indicated that their programs provided no LGB-related content. These statistics underscore the need for increased medical education on the LGBT people in general, and on LGBT elders specifically who need more frequent health care than younger adults. Robinson and Cohen (1996) provided a framework for medical curriculum reform that addresses knowledge, skills, and attitudes through didactic instruction, simulations of patient encounters using trained actors, and directly supervised encounters with gay, lesbian, and bisexual patients. Peterkin and Risdon (2003) also list strategies for improving training on LGBT issues in medical school and residency programs, including adding grand rounds and small group teaching sessions. Although HIV care is often the springboard for discussion of gay men's issues, the content covered needs to be much more inclusive of lesbian, bisexual, and transgender issues and much broader than just limited to HIV and sexually transmitted diseases. Modifications to the curriculum do not need to be lengthy to be effective. For example, a short, 3-hour seminar was shown to increase preparedness and comfort of internal medicine residents in dealing with health care, psychosocial, and sexual issues of lesbians and gays (McGarry, Clarke, Cyr, & Landau, 2002).

The lack of curricular content on LGBT issues is also evident in nursing programs. A 1989 survey among nursing faculty found that 17% thought lesbianism was a disease, 23% believed it was immoral, 34% felt it was disgusting, 52% claimed it was unnatural, 17% thought lesbians molest children, and 8% believed that lesbians were not fit to be nurses (Randall, 1989). A more recent study in Sweden by Rondahl, Innala, and Carlsson (2004) found that 62% of nurses studied felt positively toward gays and lesbians, however. In this study, practicing nurses expressed the most positive attitudes whereas nursing students were the most negative. Although this may indicate that attitudes are changing, the apparent difference may be associated with differences in cultural acceptance of LGBT experiences.

Social work curricula may be the most progressive regarding inclusion of LGBT content. Newman (1989) pointed out that the curriculum policy statement of the Council on Social Work Education requires that curricula include content related to oppression and to the experiences and needs of people who have been subjected to institutionalized forms of oppression, such as gay men and lesbians. Methods and resources for including content on lesbian and gay issues into social work curricula are also discussed (Newman, 1989).

Consciousness Raising About Attitudes

In health care settings in which providers are committed to providing quality care to all of their clients, it is important for staff to examine their own attitudes toward LGBT people. Educational and training programs, to be complete, must assist participants to be self-reflective as an initial step toward attitude change. Consciousness raising techniques can be useful to do this. The Riddle Scale (Riddle, 1994; cited in Peterkin & Risdon, 2003, see Table 8.2) was developed to help people understand the continuum of attitudes toward gays and lesbians. This scale can be used with staff in health care agencies to assess the institutional culture in which the providers work. Another scale to measure attitudes is the 20-item Likert-scaled Homophobic Scale (Peterkin & Risdon, 2003). Health care providers who find that their beliefs are largely negative may not be ready to provide truly effective care to LGBT elders. It is important for providers to understand their own limitations and to be able to identify other referral sources that are LGBT affirming to supplement the care they are able to provide (Peterkin & Risdon, 2003).

TABLE 8.2   The Riddle (1994) Scale of Homophobia

Negative Levels of Attitude	Positive Levels of Attitude
Repulsion: Homosexuality is a crime against nature. LGB people are sick, immoral, sinful or wicked. Anything is justified to change them.	*Support:* The basic ACLU position. Works to safeguard the rights of lesbians, gays, and bisexuals.
Pity: Heterosexual chauvinism: Heterosexuality is more mature and certainly preferred.	*Admiration:* Acknowledges that being LGB in our society takes strength. Willing to examine their own homophobia and attitudes.
Tolerance: Homosexuality is just a phase of adolescent development that most people outgrow. LGB people are less mature than "straights" and should be treated with protectiveness and indulgence.	*Appreciation:* Values the diversity of people and sees LGB people as an important part of that diversity. Works to combat homophobia in themselves and others.
Acceptance: Still implies there is something to accept. Characterized by statements, e.g., "You're not lesbian to me, you're a person" or "That's fine with me as long as you don't flaunt it."	*Nurturance:* Assumes that LGB persons are indispensable in our society. Views them with genuine affection and are willing to be allies and advocates.

Adapted from Peterkin and Risdon (2003).

Quam (1997, pp. 44–45) suggested a staff development exercise to help participants to examine their own attitudes and create action plans for their agencies. A portion of the exercise involves having participants pair-up with a partner and do the following:

- Participants draw a floor plan of their homes or place they spent the most time in growing up. Then they are to take their partner on a "tour," introducing them to people and animals they might find there, and describing relationships that existed at that time. This should take no more than 5 minutes and partners should take turns.
- Then, participants imagine that they have the label "lesbian" or "gay person" on their shirts or blouses. They are to describe what would have been the response of the people they just introduced.
- Next, they imagine they are walking to school with this label on and describe what would have been the response of their neighbors and their classmates.

- Wearing the label, they imagine they are going to their church or synagogue and describe the responses there.
- Then, they imagine that they have "fast forwarded" into the present and imagining they are walking into their agency or place of employment and describe what the response would be of the personnel and staff there.
- Last, they imagine deleting their label so that they no longer have the label of lesbian or gay person and describe how this feels. They discuss what they have learned about sexual orientation and their own barriers, attitudes, and perceptions about it.

Staff development for providers can promote improved services to the older LGBT population. By examining the attitudes of health care professionals, the door is opened for the change to begin.

POLICY AND LEGAL ISSUES

Health Policy

Because so many LGBT older adults are hidden, their issues and concerns typically are not represented in policy objectives (Dean et al., 2000). These elders "lose the critical potential for empowerment and the ability to participate in the design of services and policies that may improve their access to appropriate health care" (p. 28). Issues of gay, lesbian, bisexual, and transgender individuals tend to be ignored at the policy level, and this oversight is particularly evident for elders within these communities. A review of the *Healthy People 2010* document (the primary document that drives public health research funding and interest and outlines the principle concerns of focus for the decade) found very few references to sexual orientation; none of those were related to LGBT older adults (GLMA, 2001). In response, the GLMA, in conjunction with a variety of experts in LGBT health, composed a document to serve as a companion to the *Healthy People 2010* document (GLMA, 2001). Given that HIV has been the issue in the "spotlight," most programs developed have been HIV-related. This has resulted in a critical need for additional nonHIV-related programming (Meyer, 2001). There are also agencies devoted to addressing the policy concerns of transgender individuals. Information sites on transgender activism designed to change policy include the National Transgender Advocacy Coalition (NTAC, 2005) and the Transgender Law and Policy Institute (TLPI; 2005).

The Policy Institute of the National Gay and Lesbian Task Force (Cahill et al., 2000) outlined policy issues affecting the lives of LGBT elders and made several recommendations. Their major recommendations are:

- Government agencies should amend their mandates to include LGBT elders and actively initiate research on LGBT issues.
- The Older Americans Act should be amended to explicitly include services, training, and research on issues of concern to LGBT seniors.
- LGBT families should be legally recognized to ensure equal access to Social Security benefits by partners and children and to minimize discrimination against LGBT seniors in nursing home and senior housing.
- Social services should be expanded to LGBT elders.
- Nondiscrimination laws should be passed to ensure that LGBT people are not vulnerable to discrimination.
- Mainstream aging organizations must expand their programs to respond to the needs of LGBT older adults.

These recommendations can be accomplished through a combination of policy reform, education, research, and advocacy.

Legal Issues

In 1995, a decree of the Canadian Supreme Court prohibited discrimination on the basis of sexual orientation in all provinces, territories, and the federal government. Then, in 1999, it was further ruled that any provincial law that did not extend equality to same-sex couples was ruled unconstitutional (Brotman, Ryan, & Cormier, 2002). Laws in the United States have not followed Canada's example, however, making nondiscrimination of LGBT people a voluntary rather than a mandatory activity in many states.

The heterosexism in American society is evident when one examines the statistics regarding state laws covering nondiscrimination, relationship status, and marriage. Marriage is an extremely important issue for elder LGBT adults. For married couples, visitation rights and survivor benefits are guaranteed through this institution. LGBT individuals are not necessarily guaranteed the same rights. For example, according to the Human Rights Campaign Fund (2005), only one state allows same-sex couples to be married (four states have no specific laws against this, however); all remaining states have existing laws prohibiting same-sex marriage or have enacted laws quickly in response to the Defense of Marriage legislations adopted at the federal level. There are six states that have laws protecting from discrimination based on sexual orientation and gender orientation; an additional 10 states provide protection based only on sexual orientation.

Same-sex partners can be denied rights granted to married heterosexuals in health care settings also. Unless a gay or lesbian couple has signed legal papers specifying durable power of attorney authorizing mutual medical decision making, blood relatives can override the decision made by the person's partner. The partner may also be barred from visitation privileges in some facilities where only legally recognized spouses or blood relatives can visit (Dean et al., 2000). Although in-depth discussion is beyond the scope of this chapter, health care professionals need to be aware of the wide variation in laws among states and consider the impact of those laws on the lives of their LGBT clients.

SUMMARY

At the heart of the increased vulnerability of the older LGBT population is the stigma and bias associated with sexual orientation, and of gender orientations not consistent with the norm. This stigma and bias has resulted in internal and external homophobia that permeates society in general, including the health care system. Fortunately, the potential exists for taking action on a number of levels (individual, organizational, and at the level of policy) to provide a context in which LGBT elders have the same privileges and rights of other Americans. When this happens, vulnerability decreases. Interventions across levels are necessary for this to occur. Change must take place at the individual level among the LGBT elders themselves; recognizing the effects of internalized homophobia on health care would be an important step toward taking a more proactive stand on mental and physical health care needs. The LGBT community in general must continue to advocate for the health of all LGBT individuals, including those who are older. Health care providers need to assess their own attitudes and beliefs around sexual and gender orientation and actively seek ways to improve awareness (consciousness-raising) of the physical, psychological, and mental health needs of LGBT people. They also need to better understand the impact of heterosexism on the state of health of their LGBT patients. Researchers must continue to provide reliable and valid research that minimizes bias associated with sampling of LGBT older adults. It is also critical to ensure that HIV, although an important health concern, is not driving research on the health status and care of LGBT elders. Services that meet the general physical and mental health needs of the general LGBT population are necessary. Finally, advocacy at the policy level needs to include the voices of LGBT elders. Gains made here will do much to counter the legacy of heterosexism and its effects on the lives of older LGBT adults.

At the same time, change must also take place at the larger system level with emphasis on changing attitudes and changing practice through research, policy change and advocacy. The GLMA (2004) strategic plan 2004–2007 focuses on two priority audiences: health care providers and the general community of policymakers and the press. Their overall goals include:

- Heightened awareness among policymakers, funders, and the community at large about the health disparities of LGBT people and the inclusion of them as "vulnerable" or "priority" populations.
- Increased funding for new evidence-based research relating to LGBT health disparities.
- Inclusion of questions about sexual orientation and gender identity on ongoing population surveys.

Key tactics designed to achieve these goals include summarizing available research that documents health disparities; establishing and disseminating clinical guidelines and standards for culturally competent care; establishing a speaker's bureau that provides expert presence in communities; seeking national media coverage; establishing relationships with key federal, state, and local government agencies; undertaking curricular reform with health professional organizations; and advocating for targeted funding (GLMA, 2004). Similar recommendations have been made in the areas of research, education, and training of health professionals, health care systems and direct services, and funding resources (L.A. Gay and Lesbian Center, 2000). Solarz (1999) identified gaps in research and priorities for future research along with several recommendations for improving the knowledge base on lesbian health. These recommendations will not be implemented without committed people to move them forward.

Controversy remains about the rights of LGBT people in American society; however, this does not justify the provision of substandard care to LGBT elders. Health professionals are ethically obligated to provide quality service to all people without discrimination. The first and critical step toward nondiscrimination is an openness to education on the issue of health needs of LGBT elders and exploration of attitudes toward this population. Once the issue of affirming health care for LGBT elders is addressed at the individual level, the door is opened to other more expansive interventions at the system level. Through reduced discrimination and improved quality of care, the LGBT elder population can become less vulnerable and experience healthy aging.

REFERENCES

Alexander, C. J. (Ed.). (1996). *Gay and lesbian mental health: A sourcebook for practitioners.* Binghamton, NY: Haworth Press.

Amadio, D. M., & Chung, Y. B. (2004). Internalized homophobia and substance use among lesbian, gay, and bisexual persons. *Journal of Gay & Lesbian Social Services: Issues in Practice, Policy, & Research, 17*(1), 83–101.

Bradford, J., & Ryan, C. (1988). *The National Lesbian Health Care Survey.* Washington, DC: National Lesbian and Gay Health Foundation.

Brotman, S., Ryan, B., & Cormier, R. (2002). *Gay and lesbian seniors.* National Advisory Council on Aging (Canada). Retrieved July 30, 2005 from http://www.naca-ccnta.ca/writings_gerontology/writ18/writ18_5_e.htm

Brotman, S., Ryan, B., & Cormier, R. (2003). The health and social service needs of gay and lesbian elders and their families in Canada. *Gerontologist, 43,* 192–202.

Cahill, S., South, K., & Spade, J. (2000). *Outing age: Public policy issues affecting gay, lesbian, bisexual, and transgender elders.* New York: The National Gay and Lesbian Task Force Policy Institute. Retrieved July 23, 2005 from www.thetaskforce.org/downloads/outingage.pdf

Chernin, J. N., & Johnson, M. R. (2002). *Affirmative psychotherapy and counseling for lesbians and gay men.* Thousand Oaks, CA: Sage.

Cook-Daniels, L. (2001). *Is your "T" written in disappearing ink? A checklist for Transgender inclusion.* Published by FORGE and Transgender Aging Network. Retrieved on July 30, 2005 from www.forge-forward.org/handouts/InclusionChecklist/pdf

Council on Scientific Affairs, American Medical Association. (1996). Health care needs of gay men and lesbians in the United States. *Journal of the American Medical Association, 275,* 1354–1359.

Dean, L., Meyer, I. H., Robinson, K., Sell, R. L., Sember, R., Silenzio, V. M. B., Bowen, D. J., Bradford, J., Rothblum, E., Scout, M. A., White, J., Dunn, P., Lawrence, A., Wolf, D., & Xavier, J. (2000). Lesbian, gay, bisexual, and transgender health: Findings and concerns. *Journal of the Gay and Lesbian Medical Association, 4,* 101–151.

Deevey, S. (1990). Older lesbian women: An invisible minority. *Journal of Gerontological Nursing, 16*(5), 35–37.

Elliott, P. (1996). Shattering illusions: Same-sex domestic violence. *Journal of Gay and Lesbian Social Services, 4*(1), 1–8.

Finnegan, D. G., & McNally, E. B. (2002). *Counseling lesbian, gay, bisexual, and transgender substance abusers.* Binghamton, NY: Haworth Press.

Gay and Lesbian Medical Association (GLMA). (2004). *Strategic plan.* Retrieved on July 22, 2005 from www.glma.org/images/GLMA_strat_plan_04.pdf

Gay and Lesbian Medical Association (GLMA). (2005a). *Community health centers serving the lesbian, gay, bisexual, and transgender community.* Retrieved June 12, 2005, from the worldwide web: http://www.glma.org/resources/Community_Health_Centers.shtml

Gay and Lesbian Medical Association (GLMA). (2005b). *Guidelines for creating a safe clinical environment for LGBTI patients.* Retrieved July 23, 2005 from http://www.glma.org/medical/clinical/lgbti_clinical_guidelines.pdf

Gay and Lesbian Medical Association and LGBT Health Experts (2001). *Healthy people 2010 companion document for lesbian, gay, bisexual, and transgender health.* San Francisco: Author. Gay City Health Project Wellness Center. (2005). Retrieved from the world wide web: http://www.gaycity.org/index1.html

GLBT Health Access Project. (2005). *Community standards of practice for provision of quality health care services for gay, lesbian, bisexual, and transgendered clients.* Retrieved July 27, 2005 from http://www.glbthealth.org/CommunityStandardsofPractice.htm

Haldeman, D. C. (1994). The practice and ethics of sexual orientation conversion therapy. *Journal of Consulting and Clinical Psychology, 62,* 221–227.

Harry Benjamin International Gender Dysphoria Association. (2001). *The standards of care for gender identity disorders,* (6th ed.). Düsseldorf: Symposium. Retrieved on July 25, 2005 from http://www.hbigda.org/soc.cfm

Herek, G. M. (1999, September). *Sexual prejudice: Survey research on heterosexual's attitudes toward lesbians and gay men.* Paper presented at National Institute of Health Workshop: New Approaches to Research on Sexual Orientation, Mental Heath and Substance Abuse, Rockville, MD.

Human Rights Campaign Fund. (2005). *What's happening in your state and your community.* Retrieved June 12, 2005 from the worldwide web: http://www.hrc.org/Template.cfm?Section=Your_Community&Template=/ContentManagement/ContentDisplay.cfm&ContentID=8471

Jacobs, E. (2003). A *housing boom for GLBT seniors.* Bay Windows Online, November 13, 2003. Retrieved July 19, 2005 from http://www.baywindows.com/media/paper328/news/2003/11/13/LocalNews/A.Housing.Boom.For.Glbt.Seniors-556210.shtml

Kaplan, B. J. (2002). Gay elders face uncomfortable realities in LTC. *Caring for the Ages, 3*(11). Retrieved from worldwide web: http://www.amda.com/caring/november2002/gayelders.htm

Klitzman, R. L., & Greenberg, J. D. (2002). Patterns of communication between gay and lesbian patients and their health care providers. *Journal of Homosexuality, 42*(4), 65–75.

L. A. Gay and Lesbian Center. (2000). *Advancing gay and lesbian health: A report from the gay and lesbian health roundtable.* Retrieved on July 20, 2005 from www.lgbthealth.net/downloads/research/LAGLCRoundTable2000.pdf

Lesbian and Gay Aging Issues Network (LGAIN). (2005). *About LGAIN.* Retrieved June 12, 2005 from the world wide web: http://www.asaging.org/networks/LGAIN/about.cfm

Leventhal B., & Lundy, S. (Eds.) (1999). *Same-sex domestic violence: Strategies for change.* Thousand Oaks, CA: Sage.

Marech, R. (2005, January 14). Retirement homes without the closets. *San Francisco Chronicle*. Retrieved February 1, 2005 from http://www.sfgate. com/cgi-bin/article.cge?8-c/a/2005/01/14/MNGE6AQEQN1.DTL

McGarry, K. A., Clarke, J. G., Cyr, M. G., & Landau, C. (2002). Evaluating a lesbian and gay health care curriculum. *Teaching and Learning in Medicine, 14*, 244–248.

Meyer, I. H. (2001). Why lesbian, gay, bisexual, and transgender health? *American Journal of Public Health, 91*, 856–859.

Michigan HIV News. (2002, summer). *Improving care for gays and lesbians.* Retrieved July 27, 2005 from www.mihivnews.com/features/scrubs.htm

Millman, M. (1993). *Access to health care in America.* Washington, DC: National Academy Press.

National Association of Lesbian, Gay, Bisexual, and Transgender Community Centers (NALGBTCC). (2005). *NALGBTCC Regional map.* Retrieved June 12, 2005, from the worldwide web: http://www.lgbtcenters.org/

National Coalition for LGBT Heath. (2004). *An overview of U.S. Trans health priorities.* Retrieved July 1, 2005 from www.nctequality.org/HealthPriorities.pdf

National Transgender Advocacy Coalition (NTAC). (2005). *Who we are/Activism.* Retrieved June 21, 2005 from the worldwide web: http://www.ntac.org/

New Leaf. (2005). New Leaf: Services for our community. Retrieved June 12, 2005, from the world wide web: http://www.newleafservices.org/index.htm

Newman, B.S. (1989). Including curriculum content on lesbian and gay issues. *Journal of Social Work Education, 25*(3), 202–209.

Peterkin, A., & Risdon, C. (2003). *Caring for lesbian and gay people: A clinical guide.* Toronto: University of Toronto.

Quam, J. K. (Ed.). (1997). *Social services for senior gay men and lesbians.* Binghamton, NY: Harrington Park Press.

Rainbow Gardens. (2005). *Rainbow Gardens: Stay at home assisted living for elderly lesbians, gay men, and friends & family of lesbians and gays.* Retrieved July 23, 2005 from www.rainbow-gardens.com

Randall, C. E. (1989). Lesbian phobia among BSN educators: A survey. *Journal of Nursing Education, 28*, 302–306.

Reid, J. C. (1995). Development in late life: Older lesbian and gay lives. In A. R. D'Augelli & C. J. Patterson (Eds.), *Lesbian, gay, and bisexual identities over the lifespan: Psychological perspectives* (pp. 215–242). New York: Oxford University Press.

Renzitti, C. M., & Miley, C. H. (Eds.) (1996). *Violence in gay and lesbian domestic partnerships.* New York: Harrington Park Press/Haworth Press.

Riddle, D. (1994). *The Riddle scale. In Alone no more: Developing a school support system for gay, lesbian, and bisexual youth.* St. Paul, MN: Minnesota State Department.

Roberts, S. J., Patsdaughter, C. A., Grindel, C. G., & Tarmina, M. S. (2004). Health related behaviors and cancer screening of lesbians: Results of the Boston Lesbian Health Project II. *Women & Health, 39*(4), 41–55.

Robinson, G., & Cohen, M. (1996). Gay, lesbian and bisexual health care issues and medical curricula. *Canadian Medical Association Journal, 155*, 709–711.

Rondahl, G., Innala, S., & Carlsson, M. (2004). Nurses' attitudes towards lesbians and gay men. *Journal of Advanced Nursing, 47,* 386.

Ross, M. W., & Rosser, B. R. (1996). Measurement and correlates of internalized homophobia: A factor analytic study. *Journal of Clinical Psychology, 52*(1), 15–21.

Rowen, C. J., & Malcolm, J. P. (2002). Correlates of internalized homophobia and homosexual identity formation in a sample of gay men. *Journal of Homosexuality, 43*(2), 77–92.

Sanchez, J. P., Meacher, P., & Beil, R. (2005). Cigarette smoking and lesbian and bisexual women in the Bronx. *Journal of Community Health, 30*(1), 23–47.

Schatz, B., & O'Hanlan, K. (1994). *Anti-gay discrimination in medicine: Results of a national survey of lesbian, gay and bisexual physicians.* San Francisco: American Association of Physicians for Human Rights.

Simkin, R. (1998). Not all patients are straight. *Journal of the American Medical Association, 159,* 370–375.

Skinner, W. F., & Otis, M. D. (1996). Drug and alcohol use among lesbian and gay people in a southern U.S. sample: Epidemiological, comparative, and methodological findings from the Trilogy Project. *Journal of Homosexuality, 30*(3), 59–92.

Solarz, A. L. (Ed.). (1999). *Lesbian health: Current assessment and directions for the future.* Washington, DC: National Academy Press, Institute of Medicine.

Substance Abuse Mental Health Services Administration (SAMHSA). (2005). *Survivor project.* Retrieved from the worldwide Web: http://www.survivor-project.org/

Szymanski, D. M., Chung, Y. B., & Balsam, K. F. (2001). Psychosocial correlates of internalized homophobia in lesbians. *Measurement & Evaluation in Counseling & Development, 34*(1), 27–39.

Tang, H., Greenwood, G. L., Cowling, D. W., Lloyd, J. C., Roeseler, A. G., & Bal, D. G. (2004). Cigarette smoking among lesbians, gays, and bisexuals: How serious a problem? (United States). *Cancer Causes and Control, 15,* 797–803.

Tesar, C. M., & Rovi, S. L. D. (1998). Survey of curriculum on homosexuality/bisexuality in departments of family medicine. *Educational Research and Methods, 30,* 283–287.

Transgender guide: Strategies for care providers. (2005). Retrieved June 12, 2005, from the worldwide Web: http://www.tgguide.com/

Transgender Law and Policy Institute. (2005). Retrieved June 12, 2005 from the worldwide web: http://www.transgenderlaw.org/

U.S. Department of Health and Human Services. (2005). *CSAP substance abuse resource guide: Lesbian, gay, bisexual, and transgender populations.* Retrieved from the worldwide web June 14, 2005.

Wainberg, M. L. (1999). The Hispanic, gay, lesbian, bisexual and HIV-infected experience in health care. *The Mount Sinai Journal of Medicine, 66,* 263–266.

Wallik, N. M., Cambre, K. M., & Townsend, M. H. (1992). How the topic of homosexuality is taught in US medical schools. *Academic Medicine, 67,* 601–603.

Wright, E., Shelton, C., Browning, M., Orduna, J. M. G., & Wong, F. Y. (2001). Cultural issues in working with LGBT individuals. In U.S. Department of Health and Human Services (USDHHS), SAMHSA, Center for Substance Abuse Treatments, *A provider's introduction to substance abuse treatment for lesbian, gay, bisexual, and transgender individuals.* Rockville, MD: USDHHS, SAMHSA, Center for Substance Abuse Treatments.

PART V

Older Adults with HIV/AIDS

Health Issues of Older Adults with HIV/AIDS

C. A. Emlet and K. M. Nokes

HIV/AIDS has traditionally been seen as a disease of younger persons. Thus, older adults with HIV/AIDS have been called a *hidden population* (Emlet, 1997) and the *invisible ten percent* (Genke, 2000), referring to the fact that approximately 10% of AIDS cases in the United States have been diagnosed in persons of age 50 and older. Older adults, often defined in HIV research as those aged 50 years and over, are increasingly recognized as being at-risk for HIV disease. Although health professionals are becoming increasingly aware of the impact that HIV/AIDS has on older adults, many stereotypes and ageist attitudes continue to exist, limiting the delivery of quality health care to this population. As with older adults in general, those infected with or affected by HIV disease are not a homogeneous group. A great deal of diversity exists within this emerging vulnerable population including gender, ethnicity, and sexual orientation. The purpose of this chapter is to present an overview of issues confronting older adults with HIV/AIDS, including a discussion of the various aspects of diversity. Health-related issues such as age-related changes, transmission risks, diagnostic issues, symptom management, and psychosocial factors will also be described. Strategies to meet these needs will be presented in the following chapter.

Although HIV disease has been most often viewed as affecting those in young adulthood and early middle age (Riley, 1989), individuals over the age of 50 years with AIDS have been consistently reported over the course of the pandemic (Ory & Mack, 1998). Throughout the tracking of AIDS cases by the Centers for Disease Control and Prevention (CDC, 2005), 10–12% of all diagnosed cases of AIDS in the United States have been in those aged 50 and over, translating to 114,951 AIDS cases as of December 2004 (CDC, 2005). This figure does not include older adults diagnosed with HIV (not yet AIDS) or those who received an AIDS diagnosis prior to age 50 and have "aged in" with the disease. According to Mack and Ory (2003), 18.9% of persons living with AIDS at the end of 2000 were of age 50 and over. Still, it is possible that numbers of older adults living with HIV/AIDS are even higher. According to Wooten-Bielski (1999), these figures may also underrepresent the actual number of AIDS cases among older persons, as HIV/AIDS goes undiagnosed in older people to a larger degree than in their younger counterparts. Because of the lack of accurate diagnosis, it is possible that many infected older adults die without having been properly diagnosed (Szirony, 1999). It is clear that there are now two distinct groups of older adults living with HIV/AIDS: those who are newly infected at the age of 50 or older, those who became infected at earlier ages and have survived into older age due to treatment advancements (Mack & Ory, 2003).

As seen in Figure 9.1, the largest proportion of AIDS cases is found in those aged 35–39 years. Although the number and proportion of AIDS cases decline in the older age groups, 154,513 cases had been diagnosed

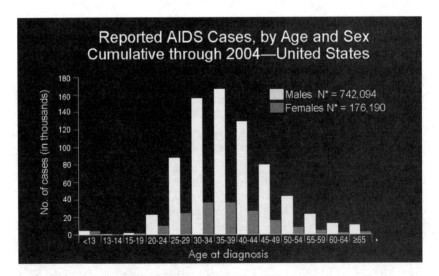

FIGURE 9.1   Persons diagnosed with AIDS through 2004.

Source: Center for Disease Control and Prevention, HIV/AIDS surveillance—general epidemiology. L178 slide series. Available at http:www.cdc.gov/hiv/graphics/surveill.htm

in individuals between 45 and 54 years of age by the end of 2004, with 60,082 cases diagnosed in persons aged 55 and over (CDC, 2005). The trend of fewer AIDS cases among older age groups is primarily associated with gender. Although cases of AIDS in older adults decline overall, this pattern changes among older women. More cases of AIDS have been reported to the CDC in women aged 65 and over than in the 60–64 years age group. Although infected blood products constituted a major source of HIV infection in the early years of the pandemic, particularly for older women, blood products in the United States have been carefully screened since 1985, making this mode of transmission negligible (Nichols et al., 2002). Recently, Zablotsky and Kennedy (2004) reviewed exposure trends and noted the increase in heterosexual exposure and injection drug use among older women. Older adults in general, and older adults living with HIV/AIDS specifically are far from a homogeneous population. The diversity seen in age at diagnosis may also reflect differences in history, values, willingness to disclose HIV status, available social support and help in seeking it.

GENDER

Throughout the epidemic, men have been disproportionately affected by HIV/AIDS. This pattern holds true for adults aged 50 and over. As shown in Figure 9.1, a considerably higher proportion of AIDS cases in all adult age groups are diagnosed in men. This pattern holds true for those aged 50 and over. Thus, older men represent a population in need of prevention and education efforts in addition to care and treatment. Because of the dominant impact on men, however, older women living with HIV/AIDS have historically been marginalized and overlooked. Little research has been conducted that examines older women relative to their risk for contracting HIV or their experiences of living with the disease (Zablotsky, 1998). Assumptions that older women are neither infected with, nor impacted by, HIV/AIDS continue to exist. Zablotsky and Kennedy (2003), however, documented that although women comprised only 8.9% of the AIDS cases in those aged 50 and over in 1988, by June of 2000 this figure had risen to 15%. We must recognize that women of all ages, especially older Black or Hispanic women, represent a specific vulnerable population with their own needs for prevention and education. It is critical that we understand the ideologies that place older women at risk, as well as these specific care and treatment needs.

With regard to prevention and education, older women are more likely than their younger counterparts to state that they know little or nothing about HIV (Zablotsky, 1998). In a recent study of 167 older

TABLE 9.1 Estimated AIDS Incidence in Women and Adolescent Girls by Exposure Category Through 2003

Proportion of AIDS Cases among Female Adults and Adolescents, by Transmission Category and Age at Diagnosis, 2003—United States					
	Age at diagnosis (in years)				
Transmission category	13-19	20-24	25-34	35-44	≥45
	%	%	%	%	%
Injection drug use	14	17	22	30	29
Heterosexual contact	63	82	76	68	68
Other/not identified*	23	1	2	2	3

Source: Centers for Disease Control and Prevention, HIV/AIDS surveillance—general epidemiology, L264 slide series. Available at http:www.cdc.gov/hiv/graphics/surveill.htm

African-American women, Willingham, Richter, Corwin, & Gore-Felton, (2004) found that approximately one third of the sample reported low perceived risk for HIV despite reporting self or partner high-risk behavior.

Older women, who are no longer concerned about pregnancy, may not see a need for condom use, and studies focusing on initiating condom use for disease protection have been conducted almost exclusively in women aged 45 and younger (Zablotsky & Kennedy, 2003). As seen in Table 9.1, 68% of all AIDS cases documented in women aged 45 years and older have heterosexual exposure as the means of contracting HIV disease.

Nichols et al. (2002) state that prevention efforts must not only include the basics of HIV/AIDS for older women, but should also discuss safe-sex practices such as protecting themselves and negotiating with sexual partners. These prevention efforts must also cover issues of power and control, the risks of drug and alcohol use, and the risk of injection drug use (Nichols et al., 2002). The ratio of sexually active older men to older women results in a small pool of available partners. Women may be particularly reluctant to negotiate safer sexual practices if they fear that these conversations would result in loss of the desired male partner.

Nurses, social workers, and other health care providers must recognize that older women, once infected, face differences in sociodemographic characteristics that can heighten their vulnerability. For example, in a study by Schable, Chu, and Diaz (1996), women over 50-years with

HIV/AIDS were more likely to be widowed, separated, or divorced; and to live alone and to have less than 12 years of schooling than their younger counterparts. Keigher, Stevens, and Plach (2004) conducted a qualitative study of older, HIV-infected women and found that the loss of vital roles and relationships due to HIV/AIDS to be a common experience of older women. The loss of the ability to work, as well as the loss of present and future sexual relationships, was identified by several of the women as a change in social roles and support after being diagnosed with HIV.

Older women have been found to have different support needs than their younger, HIV-infected counterparts. Emlet, Tangenberg, and Siverson (2002) reported on participants in a support group designed specifically for older women and found they could not relate to the issues addressed in (younger) women's HIV support groups. In those groups, topics often focused on pregnancy, vertical transmission, parenting, and childcare. As one woman in her mid 50s puts it, "It's about time that there's a group just for older women because we have different issues, like menopause, body changes, and relating to our adult children. I kind of feel left out sitting in a group hearing people talk about what their babies are doing" (p. 239).

Keigher, Stevens, and Plach (2004) remind us that survival rates for women with HIV have improved significantly so that we can now expect middle-aged women infected with HIV to live into old age. If the needs of older, HIV-infected and at-risk women are to be met, it must be recognized that older women continue to be sexually active. The historical elements of poverty, racism, sexism—and more recently HIV-stigma that will continue to impact their lives must be acknowledged. Tangenberg (2004) suggests the need for greater recognition of older women's sexuality by health and social service providers, increased HIV education for older adults, and further research on the physical, psychological, and social needs of older, HIV-positive women.

Gender differences have been identified in older samples living with HIV/AIDS. Conversations during group sessions revealed that sources of life stressors among older HIV-1-infected individuals varied widely with sex. Men frequently discussed the difficulties of adhering to complex medication regimens, toxic side-effects of treatment, changes in physical appearance due to normal aging, HIV-1 disease manifestations, and the difficulty of disclosing one's HIV status to others. In contrast, women more frequently spoke of the difficulty of informing their children of their illness, worries about the future well-being of their children, issues related to personal histories of psychoactive substance abuse, and the personal sense that HIV-1 infection had enhanced their spirituality. Hence, men appeared to be more body-focused, whereas women appeared to be more relationship-focused (Goodkin et al., 2003).

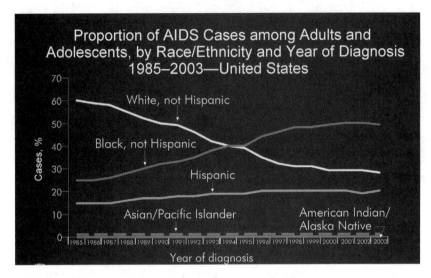

FIGURE 9.2   Proportion of AIDS cases by race/ethnicity and year of diagnosis.
Source: Centers for Disease Control and Prevention, HIV/AIDS surveillance—general epidemiology. L238 slide series. Available at: http:www.cdc.gov/hiv/graphics/surveill.htm

RACE/ETHNICITY

HIV/AIDS in the United States has heavily impacted people of color. In particular, African Americans and Hispanics have been disproportionately affected in recent years. As seen in Figure 9.2, the consistent rise in cases of AIDS among African Americans surpassed that in the nonHispanic White population in 1995. The proportion of newly reported cases among nonHispanic Whites has continually decreased while increasing in African Americans and Hispanics (CDC, 2000). Montoya and Whitsett (2003) have suggested that this disproportionality may result in negative labeling and blaming the victim.

The disproportionate number of cases of AIDS and HIV infection among people of color across ages appears to hold true for those aged 50 and over. According to CDC data (2002), the majority of AIDS cases (65%) in those diagnosed at age 50 or over were among people of color, primarily African Americans and nonWhite Hispanics. Older women of color are particularly impacted. Although 52.6% of AIDS cases among men in this age group are in people of color, the proportion among older women is 73.9%. In fact, among women aged 65 and over, more African American women have received an AIDS diagnosis than their White counterparts.

According to Brown and Sankar (1998), sociodemographic circumstances differ among elders of color, and these differences may influence how HIV/AIDS is experienced among older adults in ethnic minority communities. These differences may influence numerous issues, including awareness and knowledge of HIV, sexual practices and preventive behaviors, social support, access to health care, as well as service use (Brown & Sankar, 1998). For example, Montoya and Whitsett (2003) have suggested that older Hispanic women, for example, tend to be more reluctant to discuss sexuality and sexual disease prevention than their younger counterparts. Additionally, stigma associated with HIV among people of color may be a significant barrier to prevention, education, and testing (Nichols et al., 2002). Jimenez (2003) found in his study of 110 older men who have sex with men that the perception of being labeled gay and having HIV/AIDS was highly stigmatizing. The potential fear of stigma may result in nondisclosure of HIV status and sexual practices to other sexual partners.

Older adults from ethnic minority communities have been found to possess lower levels of knowledge about HIV/AIDS as compared to their White counterparts of the same age (LeBlanc, 1993). Once infected with HIV, elders of color face a variety of issues that may exacerbate support, care, and treatment. It is well documented that elders of color experience greater morbidity and mortality due to chronic health conditions such as diabetes, hypertension, and cardiovascular disease than Whites (Hooyman & Kiyak, 2004). These comorbid health conditions may serve to increase functional disability and complicate their treatment and prognosis. The increased incidence of comorbidity seen among older adults in general (Skeist & Keiser, 1997) may be more pronounced among African American and Hispanic elders.

It has been well documented that older adults in minority communities valued and received considerable informal social support from a variety of sources (Hooyman & Kiyak, 2004). Family and friends often provide both instrumental and emotional support. For many older persons, particularly African Americans, the church can be an important source of support in times of need (Hooyman & Kiyak, 2004). These assumptions, however, may not hold true with regard to older adults diagnosed with HIV/AIDS. For example, Mays and Cochran (1988) suggest that older African Americans with HIV/AIDS may face rejection from family members, friends, and religious congregations because of the socially stigmatizing behaviors typically associated with HIV disease. This supports recent findings from Emlet (2002), who noted that in a sample of 34 adults with HIV/AIDS over the age of 50 years, both Hispanic and African Americans received substantially less social support from friends, neighbors, and family than their White counterparts.

Although older adults from communities of color may face stigmatization and marginalization from informal social support networks, they also face barriers and challenges related to formal care and treatment. Hooyman and Kiyak (2004) suggest that cultural, economic, and structural barriers influence the use of and access to services by older adults of color. For example, the perceived stigma of using services, the fear of health care providers due to historical acts of racism, perception of experimentation as a result of the continuing changes in standards of care for HIV disease, real and perceived discrimination, the lack of knowledge of services, and geographical barriers may all serve to create barriers to care. Considering these barriers exist for the population of elders of color in general, the introduction of a stigmatizing condition such as HIV/AIDS may further limit and isolate them from formal service use.

SEXUAL ORIENTATION

Older adults, like their younger counterparts, vary in sexual orientation. Although sexual orientation is often used as a proxy for HIV risk, it has influences, particularly for older adults beyond its relevance to HIV risk. As HIV is a disease that is often sexually transmitted, older adults, service providers, and society must confront ageist views of older persons being either asexual or exclusively heterosexual. Older adults face different and specific challenges regarding HIV and AIDS as compared to their younger counterparts regardless of sexual orientation. Diversity in sexual orientation must also be seen in the context of history, cohort, and belief systems.

Older adults may have decreased sexual communication skills as compared to their younger counterparts. These differences may be the result of cohort effects that dictate what is considered "proper behavior" (University of California, San Francisco, 2000). They may be reluctant to disclose behaviors they view as being socially unacceptable and may lack negotiation skills that promote safe sex. Older women, for example, grew up prior to the sexual revolution of the 1960s and 1970s and were socialized to defer to male partners. As Genke (2000) points out, many of these women are now widowed or divorced and dating again after many years. HIV/AIDS did not exist during their previous dating experiences, however, thus diminishing their HIV awareness and prevention strategies. Many older adults who are in long-term monogamous relationships assume their partners to be completely faithful (University of California, San Francisco, 2000). This assumption may not always be accurate and could place both partners at risk.

Older gay and bisexual men also face unique challenges that are associated with age. Gay men aged 50 and over have lived half or more of their lives before the Stonewall Rebellion[1] of 1969 (Grossman, 1995).

---

[1]This street demonstration that occurred in New York in 1969 is often regarded as the start of the modern gay and lesbian rights movement.

Many of these men have felt a need to hide their sexual identities throughout their lives in order to protect themselves from stigma and discrimination (Szirony, 1999; Wooten-Bielski, 1999). Morrow (2001) reminds us that older sexual minorities came of age when gay-related hate and violence was pervasive, and when heterosexism and homophobia remained unchallenged (Grossman, D'Augelli, & O'Connell, 2001). According to Genke (2000), many gay men of this generation "took refuge in heterosexual marriages to shield themselves from the overwhelming fear and shame of familial disapproval and societal retribution" (p. 199). Findings from Kooperman (1993) suggest that older gay men often refuse to reach out to HIV/AIDS education and service organizations. A recent study by Jimenez (2003) found that over 50% of the men surveyed had limited or no exposure to family members regarding the types of their sexual relationships.

OLDER INJECTION-DRUG USERS

Although the overall rates of drug abuse among racial and ethnic minorities are similar, minority populations are disproportionately affected by the relationship between drug abuse and HIV/AIDS. For example, between 1985 and 1999 more than twice as many Blacks (94,700) as Whites (36,800) developed AIDS through injection drug abuse, even though there are only one-fourth as many Black injection-drug users. Roughly the same number of Hispanics (35,100) and Whites developed AIDS through injection-drug abuse, even though there are only one eighth as many Hispanic injection-drug users. Of the drug-related AIDS cases in women reported through June 2000, 56% were among African American women, 21% among Hispanic women, and 22% among White women (Leshner, 2001).

Kwiatkowski and Booth (2003) analyzed data from a National Institute of Drug Abuse investigation of drug use and HIV risk between 1992 and 1999 in which 1,508 participants were aged 50 and older. As compared to younger drug users ($N = 1,515$), older users were more likely to be Black, disabled, or retired; arrested at some point during their lifetime; injected intravenously but less frequently than younger users; and were equally likely to engage in high-risk sexual practices. In a study of veterans receiving HIV related care in three sites, 44% of the sample ($N = 881$) were aged 50 and older but in the New York City site, the mean age was 51 years and 54.3% reported their HIV exposure category as intravenous drug use (Smola et al., 2001). There are many opportunities to provide services to injection drug users for health and social service providers. They often have limited financial

218   OLDER ADULTS WITH HIV / AIDS

resources, unstable housing, fragmented relationships with social support networks, and illnesses resulting from injection drug use such as
bacterial endocarditis and hepatitic C. Preventing relapse is a lifelong
challenge for drug users in recovery and a harm-reduction approach
has shown to be an effective modality in working with persons who
abuse substances.

HEALTH-RELATED ISSUES

Age-Related Changes

Older adults, as both an HIV at-risk population and one that is seriously
affected by HIV infection in other ways, have largely been absent from
HIV/AIDS studies. Studying how older persons influence and are affected
by the epidemic however offers a valuable way to advance the study
of HIV biologically through consideration of its manifestation under
different age conditions (Levy, Holmes, & Smith, 2003). Physiologically,
older adults experience a natural senescence to their immune system,
particularly the part of the immune system that is also impacted by HIV.
The process of HIV infection, like the aging process, has been associated
with both a disproportionate loss of naive CD4 cells and decreased
T-lymphocyte proliferation (Goodkin et al., 2001). These changes may
be associated with more rapid disease progression. Age-related changes
affecting drug therapy and increased numbers of chronic illnesses associated with aging also contribute to decreased life expectancy of older
adults with AIDS.

   Older women may be at particular risk for HIV infection because of
physical age-related changes including atrophic vaginitis, possible shift
at menopause in the role of barrier contraceptives from use in blocking
fertility to preventing viral transmission, and change in marital status
as a result of widowhood or divorce, which propels some women into
dating and courtship at midlife or later without adequate knowledge.
Perimenopausal women frequently report hot flashes and sweats along
with fragmented sleep and may delay seeking input from a health care
provider because they attribute the symptoms to menopause and not to
a viral infection.

TRANSMISSION RISKS

The two major routes of HIV transmission are infected sexual fluids
or blood. Persons engaging in unprotected anal sex are at highest risk;

although vaginal sex is also a risky behavior, and there is some risk associated with oral sex. Blood is often exchanged by persons while injecting drugs, especially intravenously. Any person who engages in behaviors that are known to transmit HIV infection is at risk irrespective of their age.

The Centers for Disease Control and Prevention (CDC) classifies HIV transmission exposure categories as: male-to-male sexual contact, injection drug use, or heterosexual contact; however, a person may not know that they have engaged in risky behaviors with an HIV-positive person. According to CDC data, approximately 11% of adolescents and adults living with AIDS by the end of 2003 reported "other" as their exposure category. "Other" is defined as hemophilia, blood transfusion, perinatal, and risk not reported or not identified. During the HIV counseling and testing session, persons are asked about their sexual and drug use history, and most are able to identify a specific risk category. Mack and Ory's (2003) analysis of CDC data indicates a rise in those "exposure not identified" cases as age increases. They noted that of those aged 60 and over, 39.6% of men and 44% of women had HIV exposure falling into this category.

Generally, older adults are exposed to HIV through the same routes as younger people including: men having sex with men, injection-drug use, and heterosexual contact (CDC, 1998). There are, however, some important differences in HIV exposure for older persons. Notably, those over the age of 50 years are slightly less likely to be exposed to HIV through men having sex with men or injection drug use, but have an increased likelihood of exposure risk through heterosexual contact, blood products, or having an unknown or unidentified risk (CDC, 1998; Inungu, Mokotoff, & Kent, 2001). Specific to older women, normal age-related changes place postmenopausal women at greater risk as estrogen loss results in thinning of the vaginal mucosa, leaving them more susceptible to tears of the vaginal walls during sexual activity (Linsk, 2000; Szirony, 1999; Zelenetz & Epstein, 1998). The decreased knowledge of HIV transmission and perceptions of limited HIV risk among older persons may alter their ability to make informed decisions about risky sexual behavior (Nichols et al., 2002). This point is underscored by a study by El-Sadr and Gettler (1995), who examined 257 hospital patients, aged 60 and over, all of whom had no previous history of HIV disease. They found 13 of those older individuals to be infected with HIV, the majority of which were women.

There is little known about the sexual risk behaviors and drug use of older HIV-infected adults following their HIV/AIDS diagnosis. Through an extensive search of the literature, Savasta (2004) found a paucity of articles focusing on HIV-associated transmission risks in the late middle-aged and older population. A recent study of a sample of men aged 50 and older living in New York City ($N = 59$), 36% reported unprotected sex (vaginal, anal, or oral) in the 6 months preceding the interview, 22% reported crack, cocaine, or heroin use the previous year (Siegel, Schrimshaw, & Karus, 2004). Because most persons interact socially with persons in their own age group, HIV-related risk behaviors such as unprotected sex or sharing drug using equipment can clearly lead to exposure, especially in relatively high-prevalence areas such as New York City, San Francisco, and Miami. Interacting with younger populations where rates of HIV infection are high increases the risk of infection. An older person might be flattered that a younger person is interested in them sexually and be more reluctant to suggest use of a barrier method such as a male or female condom.

With the advent of drugs to treat erectile dysfunction, the gap in prevention efforts for older adults may be driving an increase in the number of cases in mid-life and older adults who embraced the implied message that AIDS is a problem for younger people. To quote Helen Hernandez (2004) who lives in the South Bronx in New York City when speaking about older women living in her predominantly Hispanic neighborhood: "A lot of them, they've never been out of the house, never been on the street, never been with anyone except their husband. But then Viagra came along and woke the dead. Their husbands starting having sex with younger women."

Regarding injection drug use, older drug users are more likely to be injectors but they inject less frequently than their younger peers, are less likely to use a previously used and unclean needle, share other drug paraphernalia, or smoke crack (Levy, Ory, & Crystal, 2003). Older drug users may have viral hepatitis B and/or C and attribute their fatigue to that viral liver infection and aging. They may perceive that their more careful drug use techniques have protected them against infection not realizing that sharing infected blood is the highest risk behavior and even one exposure many years ago could have resulted in infection. Older drug users who seek health care for other reasons related to ongoing intravenous drug use such as bacterial infections may assume that health care providers have tested their blood for HIV. In states such as New York, this assumption is inaccurate because blood can only be tested for HIV with the expressed consent of the person being tested. Testing is especially important because of the false assumption of low risk of HIV among older adults by the population in general including health care providers.

Diagnosis Issues and Testing

Deciding to take an HIV antibody test is a health promotion activity because treatment with highly active antiretroviral medications have clearly extended life-expectancy and HIV disease has evolved into a chronic condition for infected persons who take these drugs. Most consumers seek advice from health care providers when they have persistent and/or severe symptoms that are not alleviated by self-care strategies. Symptoms of HIV disease are generalized and can be attributed to a number of different pathological conditions including diabetes or dementia and developmental changes such as menopause. Based on different symptoms, health care providers choose to "rule out" different pathologies in order to make a diagnosis.

Because HIV is typically seen as an infection of younger people, HIV disease would probably not be one of the first problems assessed. Also, health care providers are often reluctant to ask about sexual or drug use history in midlife and older persons who they may not perceive as sexually active or drug users. Consumers might be embarrassed to suggest the need for an HIV test because of the stigma associated with the behaviors through which HIV is transmitted in addition to denying their possible risk. A comprehensive workup that results in no definitive diagnosis although symptoms persist may then prompt a suggestion that a relatively inexpensive HIV antibody blood test be taken. Consumers may get discouraged during this extensive workup or concerned about related costs, especially if health insurance is limited and so diagnosis of HIV disease is delayed.

This lack of awareness or denial of risk-related behaviors can lead to delays in diagnosis and treatment and increased mortality in mid-life and older persons with undiagnosed HIV/AIDS. Although advanced age has been associated with more rapid progression of disease and increased mortality (Perez & Moore, 2003), delay in diagnosis and treatment of infection for older individuals may be a significant confounding situation. Factors that may play a role in the delay include societal bias that HIV is a disease predominantly of the young, a variation in risk profile for infection in older individuals as compared with younger individuals, and misdiagnosis of other age-associated diseases due to decreased suspicion of HIV infection in this age group (Valcour & Sacktor, 2002).

SYMPTOM MANAGEMENT AND COMORBIDITIES

Successful management of HIV disease requires the recognition and treatment of significant symptoms. But total symptom counts were consistently lower in the older nonWhite population in a sample receiving

health care from the Veterans Administration and older subjects responding to the HIV Cost and Services Utilization Survey (HCSUS) (2000).
Older patients were more likely to report peripheral neuropathy, weight
loss, and hair loss but less likely to report headaches, depressed mood,
white oral patches, or diarrhea (Zingmond et al., 2003). Total symptom
count for 64 symptoms on the Revised Sign and Symptom Checklist for
Persons with HIV Disease (SSC-HIVrev) (Holzemer, Hudson, Kirksey,
Hamilton, & Bakken, 2001) were compared in an American sample of
HIV positive persons aged 50 and more ($N = 177$) and younger per-
sons ($N = 680$) and no difference in total symptom count was found
(Nokes et al., under review). These consistent findings are troublesome.
Although older persons have more comorbidities in addition to HIV/
AIDS, they do not report more symptoms. It is possible that older people
expect an increase in symptoms and disability to accompany aging, and
thus may underreport their symptoms.

Epidemiological studies suggest that older adults, once infected,
experience a variety of complicating factors with regard to treatment
and outcomes as compared to their younger counterparts. The weakened
immune system mentioned previously has been suggested as a factor associated with more rapid disease progression found among older persons.
Numerous studies have found shorter survival times among older persons
(Ferro & Salit, 1992; Inungu et al., 2001), in addition to higher rates of
mortality (CDC, 1998; Emlet & Farkas, 2002; Ferro & Salit, 1992). In
addition, older adults have higher rates of opportunistic infections that
frequently accompany AIDS (CDC, 1998). With the advent of HAART
(highly active antiretroviral treatment) medications that became widely
available after 1996 in the developed world, however, there have been
improvements in survival with HIV disease. These improvements can
be attributed to various factors, including earlier diagnosis, treatment
of opportunistic infections, and improved antiretroviral therapy. The
benefits of improved therapies only result if the person with HIV/AIDS
takes the medications without missing doses. This can be a particular
challenge for older HIV patients in that they are often diagnosed later in
their disease course than younger patients, and typically they take more
medications for concomitant therapy (Wutoh et al., 2003).

Another important epidemiological aspect of HIV among older
adults is the issue of comorbidity. The physical well-being of older persons may be impacted not only by HIV but also by age-related diseases
such as arthritis, nonHIV related respiratory or cardiac disease, or other
disease processes. Numerous studies have found that persons aged 55 and
over have significantly higher rates of concurrent nonHIV-related chronic
health conditions than their younger counterparts (Skeist, & Keiser, 1997,
Nokes et al., 2000, Shah, McGowan, Smith, Blum, & Klein, 2002).

These multiple comorbidities mean that older persons living with HIV/AIDS are medically diverse and can range from experiencing few symptoms to having a complex interplay of serious HIV-related symptoms coupled with symptoms arising from age-related diseases. As a provider of HIV services, the first author was surprised to learn from some older clients that they were more concerned about age-related chronic conditions, such as cardiac disease or diabetes, than about the management of their HIV disease. They are also at higher risk of medical harm especially from adverse drug reactions (Justice et al., 2001).

COGNITIVE DYSFUNCTION

A pattern of marked increase in cognitive dysfunction has been found among older HIV-infected persons. Older HIV-infected individuals tended to have slower information processing speeds, decreased abstraction abilities, and impaired learning (Wilkie et al., 2003). Preliminary analysis of the first 35 individuals enrolled in a study conducted by Valcour and Sacktor (2002) revealed a marked increase in neurocognitive dysfunction in the older group (aged 50 and older) compared with the younger group (less than 40). Eleven percent of younger individuals (2/18) compared with 41% of older individuals (7/17), had mild to moderate dementia. Low educational attainment, head trauma, developmental factors, and genetic factors can also contribute to a decreased brain reserve. These cognitive changes can impact on self-care abilities related to coordinating multiple medications, keeping appointments, and increased social isolation. Providers, recognizing the potential of greater cognitive changes in older persons with HIV/AIDS, need to tailor their interventions to include multiple strategies to convey information and also to provide the time needed to ensure that clients understand what is expected of them.

MEDICATION ISSUES

There are now at least 20 medications approved by the Food and Drug Administration to treat HIV disease. There are additional protocols to treat or prevent opportunistic infections associated with AIDS. Midlife and older adults are also taking medications to treat their other comorbidities. One study (Shah et al., 2002) found that patients aged 55 or older ($N = 198$) were using an average of 2.7 medications in addition to antiretroviral drugs to treat their HIV infection. All of these medications have side and toxic effects, and the possibilities of drug/drug interactions are significant. But self-reported adherence rates are the same or superior in older compared with younger HIV-seropositive individuals despite a larger number of reported adverse reactions in older HIV-seropositive individuals (Valcour & Sacktor, 2002). Body changes were significantly greater ($p = 0.000$) for older compared to younger persons taking HIV medications, and yet there were no differences in their feelings or confidence about HIV drugs (Nokes et al., in review).

Because older persons report liver problems as a common co-morbidity and most drugs are detoxified by the liver, there is greater potential for serious liver-related problems which needs to be monitored carefully. The risks of taking antiretroviral medications are outweighed by the benefits because there was no significant difference in survival for older persons on highly active antiretroviral therapy but mortality was higher in untreated older compared to younger persons with HIV (Perez & Moore, 2003).

Recent research regarding the use and efficacy of antiretroviral medications (including HAART) among older adults is encouraging. Older adults are prescribed antiretroviral therapy at equal proportions to their younger counterparts (Emlet & Berghuis, 2002; Wellons et al., 2002), and these therapies are equally as effective in lowering the HIV viral load (Wellons et al., 2002). In fact, Wellons et al. found older adults to be more compliant with HIV medication regimes than their younger counterparts. One complicating factor, however, is the increased likelihood of contraindications or drug–drug interactions between medications prescribed for HIV/AIDS and other medical conditions. Drugs like simvastatin (Zocor), used to lower cholesterol and triglycerides, interacts with many of the drugs used to treat HIV disease (Ernst, 2004). Self-reported adherence rates were the same or superior in older compared with younger HIV-seropositive individuals, although a larger number of adverse reactions were reported by older HIV-seropositive individuals (Valcour & Sacktor, 2002).

PSYCHOSOCIAL ISSUES

Older adults with HIV/AIDS experience many of the same psychosocial issues as their younger counterparts, such as feeling stigmatized, marginalized, and afraid (Linsk, 2000). They may fear disclosing their diagnosis, and confront strained relationships with family and friends (Zelenetz & Epstein, 1998). They can experience lack of support from the community, dwindling financial resources, and diminished quality of life (Szirony, 1999). At the same time, older adults may also experience the intersection of ageism and HIV phobia, as well as a combination of issues and problems faced by both older adults and persons living with HIV/AIDS. These issues can be categorized as intrapersonal, interpersonal, and related to the broader service delivery system.

Although many older adults living with HIV/AIDS have adjusted well to their illness, Heckman et al. (2002) found a "sizable minority of HIV-infected older adults" with psychological symptomatology (p. 126). In a study of 113 individuals aged 45 or older with HIV or AIDS, Kalichman et al. (2000) found 27% reported having thought of suicide in the past week. Parallel findings come from a recent study by Heckman, Kochman, and Sikkema (2002) who found that approximately one-quarter of adults aged 50 and more with HIV/AIDS reported elevated levels of depression.

Researchers have found an association between psychiatric symptomology and issues of disclosure and social support. Both studies mentioned above found an association between the symptoms being studied and lower levels of social support. As several studies have found that older persons are more likely to live alone than their younger counterparts (Crystal & Sambamoorthi, 1998; Emlet & Berghuis, 2002; Emlet & Farkas, 2002), it is important to recognize that decreased social support can be a complicating and serious issue. Recently, Nokes et al. (2000) found older adults with HIV disease less likely than younger adults to disclose their HIV status. Although not disclosing HIV status may act as a protective mechanism against stigma, it can also serve to exacerbate social isolation–a topic particularly relevant to this population.

Older adults living with HIV disease must also face prejudice and discrimination of an ageist society as whole. As Fowler (1999) describes, "in a society that does not respect or value the aging population, older HIV infected people may confront social and professional bias regarding allocation of health care services and resources available to the AIDS community" (p. 4). Older adults can be caught between aging and HIV services, wherein their HIV issues may not be addressed by aging programs, although AIDS support services are typically geared to a younger population (Genke, 2000). Heckman et al. (2002) found decreased social support to be associated with higher barriers to health care and social services. Older adults living with HIV may be the unwitting victims of multiple programs working at cross-purposes and lack the knowledge of where to turn for help.

Social support has been found to affect a variety of health-related issues including medication adherence (Cox, 2002), feelings of distress (Chesney, Chambers, Taylor, & Johnson, 2003), and the ability to manage stress and access needed personal care assistance (Crystal et al., 2003). Age, however, has been found to impact the social networks of adults with HIV/AIDS in various ways. Numerous studies have found older adults living with HIV/AIDS to be more likely to live alone than their younger counterparts (Emlet & Berghuis, 2002; Emlet & Farkas, 2002; Crystal et al., 2003). This may contribute to social isolation and limit personal care assistance when needed.

Crystal et al. (2003) documented that in addition to the potential for smaller social networks, older adults may experience differences in the quality of their relationships. In a study of 2,864 adults living with HIV disease, those over 50-years reported more conflicts with family, friends, and others than their younger counterparts. The quantity and quality of social networks may be important for managing various aspects of HIV disease. For example, in a recent study of 88 individuals living with HIV/AIDS, social support, in particular the availability of a relative or friend as a confidant, was associated with decreased levels of HIV stigma (Emlet, 2005). Chesney et al. (2003) recently found that the association between social support and distress was stronger for older (versus younger) individuals, and that higher levels of social support were associated with higher levels of positive affect. These findings suggest that older adults living with HIV/AIDS may be more vulnerable to decreased levels of social support and the subsequent impact of those reductions.

CAREGIVING AND AFFECTED OLDER ADULTS

Older adults infected with the HIV virus are slowly becoming recognized as a population of elders needing care, resources, and attention. Still, a growing number of older adults are what Poindexter (2001) refers to as *HIV-affected*. HIV-affected "refers to those family members who have responsibilities of caregiving for an adult or child who has HIV disease" (p. 525). Mullan (1998) suggests that age is particularly relevant to caregiving and HIV, as: (a) younger infected individuals and their caregivers are aging; (b) older people contract AIDS; and (c) older people become informal caregivers to those with HIV/AIDS. Estimates suggest as many as one third of persons living with AIDS are dependent on older relatives (often parents) for financial, emotional, and physical support (Allers, 1990).

Older, HIV-affected caregivers face numerous challenges and rewards for accepting their caregiving role. The caregivers' own health-related and aging issues, unexpected role change, as well as stigma and disclosure, are all examples of issues that can present as problems and barriers for older caregivers. Many caregivers for persons living with HIV/AIDS are not only older, but also women of color. In these instances, the compounding effects of vulnerability and marginalization from racism, sexism, and ageism must be recognized. Additionally, however, recent research serves to remind us that taking on these caregiving roles can be a personally rewarding and even a transformative experience (Poindexter, 2001).

Older HIV-affected caregivers must contend with their own aging and concomitant health problems. Older caregiving grandparents often report poorer health than their noncaregiving counterparts (Joslin & Harrison, 2002) and have a higher incidence of depression (Fuller-Thomson & Minkler, 2000). In their study of 20 caregivers living in New Jersey, Joslin and Harrison (2002) reported that over half of the respondents described their health as *fair* or *poor*. These figures contrast with those nationally where 72% of adults aged 65 and over rate their health as *good* or *excellent* (Federal Interagency Forum on Aging-Related Statistics, 2000). HIV caregivers also report numerous somatic symptoms including chronic fatigue, physical exhaustion, and backaches. The Joslin study found that over half of the caregivers in their sample also rated their emotional health as *fair* or *poor*. As these data suggest, HIV-affected caregivers are individuals vulnerable to physical and emotional distress.

Accepting the role as caregiver for a loved one with HIV/AIDS may initiate changes in expected or anticipated life roles. Some parent caregivers may need to confront lifestyle and behavioral aspects of their adult child's life that were heretofore ignored. For example, parents may simultaneously learn of a child's drug use or homosexuality, while at the same time learning of their HIV or AIDS diagnosis (Levine-Perkell, 1996). Accepting the role of caregiver may require one to reassess career direction, retirement, social relationships, and the issue of "out of time" role change (Mullan, 1998). The acceptance of such change is not limited to spouses or parents of an individual with HIV/AIDS but to grandparents as well.

As Joslin (2000) points out, catastrophic illness and death have always served as a reason for grandparents to accept parenting roles. She estimates that as many as 20,000 grandparents in the US are raising approximately 41,000 children orphaned by AIDS. These grandchildren may or may not themselves be HIV-infected. Grandparents in this role often experience compromised health and well-being. Grandparent caregivers in Joslin's study reported an average of three chronic illnesses including cardiac disease, arthritis, hypertension, and diabetes. In fact, according to Joslin (2000), participants in this study from New Jersey reported poorer self-reported health than grandparents from California raising grandchildren in the wake of the crack cocaine epidemic reported in another study.

Like those infected with HIV, affected caregivers confront issues of stigma and the potential benefits and detriments of disclosure. Fear of stigma and further marginalization may cause HIV-affected caregivers to limit their disclosure of HIV issues or not disclose at all. As Poindexter and Linsk (1999) suggest, disclosure of HIV must precede the experience of being stigmatized, yet it is the fear of being stigmatized that precedes disclosure. In their qualitative study of 19 older African-American caregivers, Poindexter and Linsk found that ascribing the illness of the care receiver to another cause, i.e., cancer, was a common method of avoiding or minimizing stigma. In fact, none of the four caregivers in this study who were grandparents disclosed the HIV status to their infected minor grandchildren "in an effort to protect the children from feeling stigmatized" (p. 53). The fear of potential stigma may also result in the elimination of potential sources of care and support for the caregiver. Poindexter and Linsk found 11 of the participants in their study who attended church had not disclosed the issue of HIV to anyone in the church—including the pastor. As these researchers put it, "it is a tragedy that these caregivers and their HIV-positive loved ones often live in terror of disclosure and, thus, do not gain access to informal and formal support because of this fear" (pp. 57–58).

Despite the fact that many caregivers of persons with HIV or their survivors face obstacles of stigma, disclosure, and physical as well as mental health problems, caregiving is not without its rewards. In a qualitative study of seven HIV-affected older caregivers, Poindexter (2001) noted that these women gained a variety of personal and societal benefits from their experience. She notes particularly the development of a strong reciprocal relationship with the HIV-positive care recipient. It was this relationship that sustained the caregivers and helped them get through their challenges. Another positive result in her study was the commitment to social justice by the caregivers. They developed "impassioned belief in the right of adults and children with HIV to participate fully in society and not be neglected" (p. 530). Some caregivers have called this experience transformative.

Much of the literature and research on HIV caregivers early in the epidemic focused on gay men and their infected partners; however, caregivers have become much more diverse in the past three decades. It is now recognized that HIV-affected caregivers vary in relationship to the care recipient, and represent diversity in gender, ethnicity, and age. Types of coping strategies, informal support networks, and willingness to seek formal services may depend upon history, knowledge, and trust (or lack of) in the health and social service system.

SUMMARY

It can be seen from this brief review that older persons are demographically different and experience physiological, psychological, and historical differences as compared to their younger counterparts. Older adults living with HIV/AIDS vary in age, gender, ethnicity, sexual orientation, and exposure to HIV. Ageist and sexist stereotypes will need to be confronted by all as the twenty-first century progresses, and there is a continued increase in the number of older persons becoming infected and living with HIV/AIDS. Additionally, the confounding intersection of racism, ageism, sexism, homophobia, and HIV-stigma will continue to create tremendous barriers for these older adults. The combination of HIV and old age also brings special problems related to the disease itself and its treatment. Health and social service providers must recognize this growing population of vulnerable elders as individuals with special needs requiring a sensitive and knowledgeable approach to care.

Health and social service providers must also recognize the diverse population that comprises HIV-affected caregivers. Because many of these caregivers are older women of color, they are likely to have faced discrimination and prejudice throughout their lives and often have limited financial resources. For both older persons infected with and affected by HIV, better communication and coordination between health and social service systems will need to be forged. More research into the health care needs of this population is necessary and will help to inform future directions in care. Professionals providing services designed for persons living with HIV will need to better understand the needs of their older consumers, whereas the aging network will need to recognize the differences and special needs of an emerging and diverse population of vulnerable older adults.

REFERENCES

Allers, C. T. (1990). AIDS and the older adult. *Gerontologist, 30*, 405–407.

Brown, D. R., & Sankar, A. (1998). HIV/AIDS and aging minority populations. *Research on Aging, 20*, 865–884.

Centers for Disease Control and Prevention. (1998). AIDS among persons aged ≥50 years—United States, 1991–1996. *Morbidity and Mortality Weekly Report, 47*(2), 21–27.

Centers for Disease Control and Prevention. (2005). *HIV/AIDS surveillance,* Vol. 16. Atlanta, GA: Author.

Centers for Disease Control and Prevention. (2004). *HIV/AIDS surveillance report* (year end edition), *15*, 1–46.

Centers for Disease Control and Prevention. (2002). *HIV/AIDS surveillance report* (year end edition) 13, 1–46.

Chesney, M. A., Chambers, D. B., Taylor, J. M., & Johnson, L. M. (2003). Social support, distress and well-being in older men living with HIV infection. *Journal of Acquired Immune Deficiency Syndromes, 33*(Suppl. 2), S185–S193.

Cox, L. (2002). Social support, medication compliance and HIV/AIDS. *Social Work in Health Care, 35*, 425–460.

Crystal, S., Akincigil, A., Sambamoorthi, U., Wenger, N., Fleishman, J., Zingmond, D., et al. (2003). The diverse older HIV-positive population: A national profile of economic circumstances, social support, and quality of life. *Journal of Acquired Immune Deficiency Syndromes 33*(Suppl. 2), S76–S83.

Crystal, S., & Sambamoorthi, U. (1998). Health care needs and service delivery for older persons with HIV/AIDS: Issues and research challenges. *Research on Aging, 20*, 739–759.

El-Sadr, W., & Gettler, J. (1995). Unrecognized human immunodeficiency virus infection in the elderly. *Archives of Internal Medicine, 155*, 184–186.

Emlet, C. A. (1997). HIV/AIDS in the elderly: A hidden population. *Home Care Provider, 2*, 69–75.

Emlet, C. A. (2002, November). *Older adults living with HIV/AIDS: An emerging vulnerable population.* Paper presented as part of the symposium Emergent Issues in Contexts of Care for Vulnerable Populations of Elders. The 55th Annual Scientific Meeting of the Gerontological Society of America. Boston, MA.

Emlet, C. A., & Berghuis, J. P. (2002). Service priorities, use and needs: Views of older and younger consumers living with HIV/AIDS. *Journal of Mental Health and Aging, 8*, 307–318.

Emlet, C. A., & Farkas, K. J. (2002). Correlates of service utilization among midlife and older adults with HIV/AIDS: The role of age in the equation. *Journal of Aging and Health, 14*, 315–335.

Emlet, C. A., Tangenberg, K., & Siverson, C. (2002). A feminist approach to practice in working with mid-life and older women with HIV/AIDS. *Affilia: Journal of Women and Social Work, 17*, 229–251.

Emlet, C. A. (2005). Measuring stigma in older and younger adults with HIV/AIDS: An analysis of an HIV stigma scale and initial exploration of subscales. *Research on Social Work Practice, 15*, 291–300.

Ernst, J. (2004). It's always something. . . . Medical complications of aging with HIV. *ACRIA Update, 13*(3), 8–10, 12.

Federal Interagency Forum on Aging Related Statistics. (2000). *Older Americans 2000: Key indicators of well-being.* Washington, DC: U.S. Government Printing Office.

Ferro, S., & Salit, I. E. (1992). HIV infection in patients over 55 years of age. *Journal of Acquired Immune Deficiency Syndrome, 5*, 348–355.

Fowler, J. P. (1999). *HIV in People Over 50. Focus: A Guide to AIDS Research and Counseling, 14*(9), 1–4.

Fuller-Thomson, E., & Minkler, M. (2000). The mental and physical health of grandmothers who are raising their grandchildren. *Journal of Mental Health and Aging, 6*, 311–323.

Genke, J. (2000). HIV/AIDS and older adults: The invisible ten percent. *Care Management Journals, 2*(3), 196–205.

Goodkin, K., Wilkie, F., Concha, M., Hinkin, C., Symes, S., Baldewicz, T., et al. (2001). Aging and neuro-AIDS conditions and the changing spectrum of HIV-1 associated morbidity and mortality. *Journal of Clinical Epidemiology, 54*, S35–S43.

Grossman, A. H. (1995). At risk, infected, and invisible: Older gay men and HIV/ AIDS. *Journal of the Association of Nurses in AIDS Care, 6*(6), 13–19.

Grossman, A. H., D'Augelli, A. R., & O'Connell, T. S. (2001). Being lesbian, gay, bisexual and 60 or older in North America. *Journal of Gay and Lesbian Social Services, 13*(4), 23–40.

Heckman, T. G., Heckman, B. D., Kochman, A., Sikkema, K. J., Suhr, J., & Goodkin, K. (2002). Psychological symptoms among persons 50 years of age and older living with HIV disease. *Aging and Mental Health, 6*(2), 121–128.

Heckman, T. G., Kochman, A., & Sikkema, K. J. (2002). Depressive symptoms in older adults living with HIV disease: Application of the chronic illness quality of life model. *Journal of Mental Health and Aging, 8*, 267–279.

Hernandez, H. (2004, Auguat 17). Aging with HIV: Four profiles. *New York Times*. F6.

Holzemer, W. L., Hudson, A., Kirksey, K., Hamilton, M. J., & Bakken, S. (2001). The Revised Sign and Symptom Check-List for HIV (SSC-HIV rev). *Journal of the Association of Nurses in AIDS Care, 12*(5), 60–70.

Hooyman, N. R., & Kiyak, H. A. (2004). *Social gerontology: A multidisciplinary perspective* (7th ed.). Boston: Allyn and Bacon.

Inungu, J. N., Mokotoff, E. D., & Kent, J. B. (2001). Characteristics of HIV infection in patients fifty year or older in Michigan. *AIDS Patient Care and STDs, 15*, 567–573.

Jimenez, A. D. (2003). Triple Jeopardy: Targeting older men of color who have sex with men. *Journal of Acquired Immune Deficiency Syndromes, 33* (Suppl. 2), S222–S225.

Joslin, D. (2000). Grandparents raising children orphaned and affected by HIV/ AIDS. In C. Cox (Ed.), *To grandmother's house we go and stay: Perspectives on custodial grandparents* (pp. 167–183). New York: Springer Publishing.

Joslin, D., & Harrison, R. (2002). Physical health and emotional well-being. In D. Joslin (Ed.), *Invisible caregivers: Older adults raising children in the wake of HIV/AIDS* (pp. 90–112). New York: Columbia University Press.

Justice, A., Landefeld, C. S., Asch, S., Gifford, A., Whalen, C., & Covinsky, K. (2001). Justification for a new cohort study of people aging with and without HIV infection. *Journal of Clinical Epidemiology, 54*, S3–S8.

Kalichman, S. C., Heckman, T., Kochman, A., Sikkema, K., & Bergholte, J. (2000). Depression and thoughts of suicide among middle-aged and older persons living with HIV-AIDS. *Psychiatric Services, 51*, 903–907.

Keigher, S. M., Stevens, P. E., & Plach, S. K. (2004). Midlife women and HIV: Health, social, and economic factors shaping their future. *Journal of HIV/ AIDS and Social Services, 3*(1), 43–58.

Kooperman, L. (1993, March). *AIDS and the elderly*. Paper presented at the 39th Annual Meeting of the American Society on Aging, Chicago.

Kwiatkowski, C., & Booth, R. (2003). HIV risk behaviors among older American drug users. *Journal of Acquired Immune Deficiency Syndromes, 33*(Suppl. 2), S131–S137.

LeBlanc, A. J. (1993). Examining HIV-related knowledge among adults in the US. *Journal of Health and Social Behavior, 34*, 23–36.

Leshner, A. (2001). Meeting the Challenge of Reducing Health Disparities. *NIDA NOTES 16*(1) March, 1.

Levy, J., Ory, M., & Crystal, S. (2003). HIV/AIDS interventions for midlife and older adults: Current status and challenges. *Journal of Acquired Immune Deficiency Syndromes, 33*(Suppl. 2), S59–S67.

Linsk, N. L. (2000). HIV among older adults: Age-specific issues in prevention and treatment. *AIDS Reader, 10*, 430–440.

Mack, K. A., & Ory, M. G. (2003). AIDS and older Americans at the end of the twentieth century. *Journal of Acquired Immune Deficiency Syndrome, 33*(Suppl. 2), S68–S75.

Mays, V. M., & Cochran, S. D. (1988). Issues in the perception of AIDS risk and risk reduction activities by Black and Hispanic women. *American Psychology, 43*, 949–957.

Montoya, I. D., & Whitsett, D. D. (2003). New frontiers and challenges in HIV research among older minority populations. *Journal of Acquired Immune Deficiency Syndrome, 33*(Suppl.2), S218–S221.

Morrow, D. F. (2001). Older gays and lesbians: Surviving a generation of hate and violence. *Journal of Gay and Lesbian Social Services, 13*(1/2), 151–169.

Mullan, J. T. (1998). Aging and informal caregiving to people with HIV/AIDS. *Research on Aging, 20*, 712–738.

Nichols, J. E., Speer, D. C., Watson, B. J., Watson, M. R., Vergon, T. L., Valee, C. M., et al. (2002*). Aging with HIV: Psychological, Social and Health Issues*. San Diego: Academic Press.

Nokes, K., Hamilton, M. J., Bunch, E., Corless, I. B., Kemppainen, J., Nicholas, P., Reynolds, N., Coleman, C., Bunch, E., Holzemer, W., Wantland, D., Tsai, Y., Rivero-Mendez, M., & Canaval, G. (2006). *Identifying age-related differences in chronically ill persons with HIV/AIDS*. Unpublished manuscript.

Nokes, K. M., Holzemer, W. L., Corless, I. B., Bakken, S., Brown, M. A., Powell-Cope, G. M., et. al. (2000). Health-related quality of life in persons younger and older than 50 who are living with HIV/AIDS. *Research on Aging, 22*, 290–310.

Ory, M. G., & Mack, K. A. (1998). Middle-aged and older people with AIDS. *Research on Aging, 20*, 653–664.

Perez, J., & Moore, R. (2003). Greater effect of highly active antiretroviral therapy on survival in people aged 50 and older years compared to younger people in an urban observational cohort. *Clinical Infectious Diseases, 36*, 212.

Poindexter, C. C. (2001). "I'm still blessed": The assets and needs of HIV-affected caregivers over 50. *Families in Society, 82*, 525–536.

Poindexter, C. C., & Linsk, N. L. (1999). HIV-related stigma in a sample of HIV-affected older female African American caregivers. *Social Work, 44*, 46–61.

Riley, M. W. (1989). AIDS and older people: The overlooked segment of the population. In M. W. Riley, M. G. Ory, & D. Zablotsky (Eds.), *AIDS in an aging society: What we need to know* (pp. 3–26). New York: Springer Publishing.

Savasta, A. M. (2004). HIV: Associated transmission risks in older adults–An integrative review of the literature. *Journal of the Association of Nurses in AIDS Care, 15*(1), 50–59.

Schable, B., Chu, S., & Diaz, T. (1996). Characteristics of women 50 years of age and older with heterosexually acquired AIDS. *American Journal of Public Health, 86*, 1616–1618.

Shah, S., McGowan, J., Smith, C., Blum, S., & Klein, R. (2002). Comorbid conditions, treatment, and health maintenance in older persons with HIV infection in NYC. *Clinical Infectious Diseases, 35*, 1238–1243.

Siegel, K., Schrimshaw, E., & Karus, D. (2004). Racial disparities in sexual risk behaviors and drug use among older Gay/Bisexual and Heterosexual men living with HIV/AIDS. *Journal of the National Medical Association, 96*, 215–223.

Skeist, D. J., & Keiser, P. (1997). Human immunodeficiency virus infection in patients older than 50 years. *Archives of Family Medicine, 6*, 289–294.

Smola, S., Justice, A., Wagner, J., Rabeneck, L., Weissman, S., & Rodriguez-Barrada, M. (2001). Veterans aging cohort three-site study (VACS 3): Overview and description. *Journal of Clinical Epidemiology, 54*, S61–S76.

Szirony, T. A. (1999). Infection with HIV in the elderly population. *Journal of Gerontological Nursing, 25*(10), 25–31.

Tangenberg, K. M. (2004). Mental health dimensions of HIV/AIDS in women over 50. In C. A. Emlet (Ed.), *HIV/AIDS and older adults: Challenges for individuals, families and communities* (pp. 73–91). New York: Springer Publishing.

University of California–San Francisco. (2000). HIV and older adults. *HIV Counselor Perspectives, 9*(5), 1–7.

Valcour, V., & Sacktor, N. (2002). HIV-associated dementia and aging. *Journal of Mental Health and Aging, 8*(4), 295–306.

Wellons, M. F., Sanders, L., Edwards, L. J., Bartlett, J. A., Heald, A. E., & Schmader, K. E. (2002). HIV infection: Treatment outcomes in older and younger adults. *Journal of the American Geriatrics Society, 50*, 603–607.

Wilkie, F., Goodkin, K., Khamis, I., vanZuilen, M., Lee, D., Lecusay, R., et al. (2003). Cognitive functioning in younger and older HIV-1 infected adults. *Journal of Acquired Immune Deficiency Syndromes, 33*(Suppl. 2), S93–S105.

Willingham, A., Richter, D., Corwin, S., & Gore-Felton, C. (2004). Perceptions of vulnerability to HIV among older African American women: The role of intimate partners. *Journal of HIV/AIDS and Social Services, 3*(1), 25–42.

Wooten-Bielski, K. (1999). HIV & AIDS in older adults. *Geriatric Nursing, 20*, 268–272.

234 OLDER ADULTS WITH HIV/AIDS

Wutoh, A., Elekwachi, O., Clarke-Tasker, V., Daftary, M., Powell, N., & Campusano, G. (2003). Assessment and predictors of antiretroviral adherence in older HIV-infected patients. *Journal of Acquired Immune Deficiency Syndromes, 33*(Suppl. 2), S106–S114.

Zablotsky, D. L. (1998). Overlooked, ignored and forgotten: Older women at risk for HIV infection and AIDS. *Research on Aging, 20,* 760–775.

Zablotsky, D. L., & Kennedy, M. (2003). Risk factors and HIV transmission to midlife and older women: Knowledge, options, and the initiation of safer sexual practices. *Journal of Acquired Immune Deficiency Syndrome, 33*(Suppl. 2), S122–S130.

Zablotsky, D., & Kennedy, M. (2004). Assessing the progress and promise of research on midlife and older adults and HIV/AIDS. In C. A. Emlet (Ed.), *HIV/AIDS and older adults: Challenges for individuals, groups and communities* (pp. 1–20). New York: Springer Publishing.

Zelenetz, P. D., & Epstein, M. E. (1998). HIV in the elderly. *AIDS Patient Care and STD's, 12,* 255–262.

Zingmond, D., Kilbourne, A., Justice, A., Wenger, N., Rodriguez-Barradas, M., Rabeneck, L., et al. (2003). Differences in symptom expression in older HIV+ patients: The Veterans Aging Cohort 3 site study and HIV Cost and Service Utilization Study Experience. *Journal of Acquired Immune Deficiency Syndromes, 33*(Supp. 2), S84–S92.

CHAPTER TEN

Health Care Strategies for Older Adults with HIV/AIDS

K. M. Nokes and C. A. Emlet

HIV/AIDS is a highly stigmatized, life threatening, and disabling condition that presents difficult challenges for older adults with the disease. Midlife and older persons are a heterogeneous group, and HIV-related interventions must be tailored to meet their unique needs. The previous chapter discussed increased risk and vulnerability to HIV infection among older women, people of color, gay men, and injection-drug users. Health-related issues for older adults were also discussed including age-related changes that increase risk, delays in diagnosing and treating, more rapid disease progression, accompanying comorbidities, cognitive dysfunction, and increased problems with medications.

Older adults with HIV/AIDS are often more marginalized because of the added stigma of age. They are generally more reluctant to disclose their HIV status than younger adults and may experience more depression and social isolation. These difficult problems of older adults with HIV/AIDS present unique challenges for health professionals who are often specialists in either geriatrics or HIV/AIDS care, but not both.

In contrast to infections that occur through exposure to inanimate objects, insects, or animals, HIV is transmitted from one person to another; therefore, infections occur in a social context. A diagnosis of HIV infection is interpreted through cultural mores, gender roles, stigma, and marginalization along with ageism, racism, and homophobia. Health professionals are not immune to biases embedded in the dominant culture. Practitioners and educators need to be aware of their own biases and ageist beliefs related to sexuality, aging, and sexual orientation. Anderson (1998) suggests the importance of ascertaining the knowledge base of clients about HIV without assumption. "To assume that the older gay man is well informed because of his ties to the gay and lesbian community would be a mistake" (p. 445). He points out that the biggest barrier to success in working with this population may be health professionals' unwillingness to overcome ageism. It is the responsibility of social workers, states Anderson, and all health professionals to create an environment that will encourage older persons to "share in the work of surviving HIV/AIDS" (p. 448).

The course of HIV disease is characterized by uncertainty because, despite being in the third decade of the HIV epidemic, changes in treatment protocols continue to evolve rapidly. With the advent of each new category of drugs to treat HIV disease and strategies to prevent development of AIDS, living with HIV/AIDS has evolved into more of a chronic illness in contrast to the acute, life-threatening experiences of persons sick during the early years of the epidemic. This chapter addresses strategies targeting both the individual level and the larger system level. Health care strategies for caring for the needs of older adults with HIV/AIDS, as well as strategies for prevention and education, are discussed. Five different sectors offering care to this population are also described with a call for an increase in interdisciplinary, coordinated care across sectors.

IDENTIFYING THE SCOPE OF THE PROBLEM

The course of HIV infection evolves over years and a diagnosis of AIDS reflects severe immune damage. Although AIDS cases have been reported to the CDC for years, the implementation of HIV reporting has differed from state to state. To better monitor the patterns of HIV diagnosis, most states have now implemented HIV surveillance (Janssen, 2004). Daniels, Curtis, Klevens, and Lee (2004) reported that rates of new HIV diagnosis among older adults declined or were stable and lower than the rates for younger adults but used data from cases reported during the period 1994 through 2000 from states in which name-based reporting was implemented before 1994. States such as New York, Florida, or Texas that reported 64% of the HIV cases in 2002 (Janssen, 2004, p. 8) initiated confidential name-based HIV reporting after 1994 and were not included in the analysis of Daniels et al. (2004). It is unclear why these CDC authors did not use more complete data to analyze age-related trends in HIV diagnosis.

PRIMARY PREVENTION AND EDUCATION

Societal attitudes including those of health care providers have hindered primary prevention and educational efforts for prevention of HIV among older adults. The following myths continue to be pervasive:

- Older people are no longer interested in sex.
- If they do have sex, it is within a long-term monogamous relationship.
- Older people do not use injectable drugs.
- Those who were injection drug-users have died before reaching old age.
- Older people are all heterosexual.

Older adults themselves seem to share the misconception that they are not at risk. A national study (Stall & Catania, 1994) found that older adults over the age of 50 years who engaged in high-risk sexual behaviors were only one sixth as likely as young adults to use condoms and only one fifth as likely to be tested for HIV. It is imperative to develop educational initiatives for both the public and health care professionals to dispel these myths.

Currently there are few HIV prevention and education programs aimed specifically at older adults as this age group has been largely ignored in prevention messages (Bay, 2004). Some efforts are being made to meet this need, however. One such program is the Senior HIV Intervention Project (SHIP) (Agate, Mullins, Prudent, & Liberti, 2003) developed by the Broward County Health Department in Florida. This was a senior initiative program, which involved peer educators who did outreach in senior centers. They identified fundamental elements of these programs as: (a) to be sensitive to the beliefs and values of your audience, with special attention paid to the cultural and social circumstances of older adults; (b) to package the educational program in labels and titles that will be acceptable to the intended older audience; (c) to locate HIV/AIDS programming for older adults within the context of other adult programming; (d) to tailor programming to match the physical needs and limitations of an older population; and (e) to tailor programs to recognize the special characteristics and needs of transient/seasonal residents.

Another HIV prevention program, the Senior HIV Prevention and Education (SHAPE) program, was discontinued as of December 2002 (University of South Florida, n.d.). Prevention and education messages may not be presented in ways that are culturally sensitive or may not be presented in a fashion that older adults accept as relevant to themselves. Montoya and Whitsett (2003) recently suggested that educational messages delivered in English may be confusing or even useless when targeting older individuals whose native language is one other than English. A videotape, entitled *HIV/AIDS and Older Americans*, produced by the National Minority AIDS Council (2001), is a good example of age-sensitive messages regarding prevention and education from a multicultural perspective.

Health and social service providers, serving a predominantly older Hispanic population in New York City, adapted many of these elements by using a soap opera approach that has been well received and has a dedicated following eager to learn about the ongoing relationship of Isis and Valentino (Engle, 2001). This ongoing story, which has extended over 3 years, chronicles the adventures and challenges of a mature Hispanic couple who met on a cruise, decided to have a relationship including sex with a condom, which was particularly fortunate because it turns out that Valentino did not know that he was HIV-infected. The vignette is one ongoing component of 1-hour health lecture series about topics of particular interest to seniors.

Video releases discussing HIV and AIDS among older adults are also making important contributions to the prevention efforts. The American Association of Retired Persons (AARP, 1997) has produced a video, *It Can Happen to Me*, available for free loan or purchase from the AARP. In 2004, the national public television gay and lesbian news magazine *In the Life* produced a segment on aging with AIDS. This story included interviews with racially and ethnically diverse older adults and addressed diagnostic, clinical, social, and financial issues for persons with HIV who had not expected to live into midlife (Outword Online, 2005). Although this broadcast was focused more on the challenges of aging with HIV rather than on prevention, it increases awareness that older adults are not immune to HIV/AIDS. These video releases have contributed to "successful media and social marketing campaigns [to] raise awareness of HIV/AIDS in older people and reinforce the need for educational programs, while promoting respect and validation for the elderly as a group" (National Association of HIV Over Fifty [NAHOF] [2005]). Media and marketing campaigns are identified as necessary actions by the NAHOF, an organization of professionals and consumers working together to promote the availability of a full range of educational, prevention, service, and health care programs for persons over 50 years of age affected by HIV.

TESTING AND DIAGNOSIS

A diagnosis of HIV is often overlooked in the older persons as early symptoms of HIV such as weight loss, fatigue, or memory problems may mimic more common age-related conditions. The older person may not share these symptoms with their health care provider because they attribute them to "old age." When providers are made aware of the symptoms, their biases and acceptance of the myths may prevent their thinking of HIV as a possible diagnosis until extensive testing rules out other possible alternatives (Baldwin, 2005). Even when opportunistic infections are diagnosed, the possibility of HIV infection may still not be considered (Wooten-Bielski, 1999).

Early identification of impending health crises may be avoided if persons know how to interpret symptoms and take action. It is not clear why older HIV-infected persons do not report more symptoms. It may be due to expectations that advancing age brings increasing disability, and it may be due to reluctance to engage or bother their health care providers. In anticipation of the possible underreporting of symptoms, health care providers need to be more vigilant in assessing symptoms in older populations living with HIV/AIDS.

A careful health history should be done with all older adult clients, including assessment of sexual and substance abuse histories. Clinicians are often uncomfortable asking questions about sexual practices; however, indications are that older people are willing to talk about their sexual history in relation to their own health (Stall & Cantania, 1994). Questions about sexual and substance use history must be included in a thorough diagnostic workup. Older people themselves may also suspect HIV infection and can request that their health care provider test their blood. Early diagnosis is key in order to begin antiretroviral therapy as soon as possible if HIV has significantly depressed the immune system.

In some high-incidence states such as New York, there are legislated parameters required for HIV testing and special consent forms that must be used. Although these regulations were designed to ensure informed consent and recognize the stigma associated with an HIV diagnosis, they also increase the burden for health care providers who suspect HIV infection because the counseling and testing requirements can take much longer than the 7–12 minutes allocated for the patient/provider visit.

HEALTH CARE INTERVENTIONS

As discussed in the previous chapter, older people are more likely to be diagnosed later in the disease, and have more rapid progression of HIV infection and shorter survival times. They also often have comorbidities that add further complications and difficulty in assessment and disease management. Discussions of specific clinical treatment of symptoms and medication management are beyond the scope of this chapter. General approaches to identified problem areas, however, will be discussed.

It is difficult to determine which symptoms stem from HIV, the aging process, lifestyle issues such as lack of exercise, or from comorbidities. This requires early assessment and testing to identify the disease. Increased awareness of HIV as potential diagnosis is necessary among health care providers caring for older adults.

Because care of HIV/AIDS in older adults is much more complex, an interdisciplinary team approach is imperative. Interdisciplinary teams of specialists in HIV/AIDS working with professionals from several disciplines who are specialized in gerontology/geriatrics can provide coordinated care that addresses complex psychosocial and medical treatment issues.

Some special concerns of older adults with HIV/AIDS result from comorbidities, which may influence highly active antiretroviral therapy (HAART) choices. In general, older people are treated with the same HAART as younger people. Some conditions such as insulin resistance and medications may interact with certain antiviral drugs requiring modification of the HAART regimen. With all older adults, as number of medications increase, numbers of adverse drug events, including drug–drug interactions, also increase. For older adults with HIV/AIDS with other comorbidities, the number of medications may be high, placing them at high risk for adverse drug events. In addition, as the complexity of the medical regimen increases, adherence rates may decrease. For the older person who is depressed, motivation to continue a complicated, expensive drug regimen may be low. The interdisciplinary team is best able to help the older person deal with these issues to facilitate the best quality of life possible.

Because of age changes in the immune system, older adults have increased difficulty with opportunistic infections. Latent tuberculosis or other dormant infections can be reactivated when the person's immune system is depressed by HIV infection. Health care providers must be vigilant in their assessment and treatment of infections, and special measures must be taken to prevent the spread of infections.

Cognitive decline often accompanies HIV/AIDS and/or may also be due to diseases of aging such as Alzheimer's disease. These cognitive changes can impact on self-care abilities related to coordinating multiple medications, keeping appointments, and increased social isolation. Providers, recognizing the potential of greater cognitive changes in older persons with HIV/AIDS, need to tailor their interventions to include multiple strategies to convey information and also to provide the time needed to ensure that clients understand what is expected of them.

Psychosocial needs including social support are key to quality of life. To address the need for social support, SAGE (Senior Action in a Gay Environment) partnered with the New York Association on HIV over 50, Inc. and offered two 10-week telephone-based support groups to increase knowledge about health-related self-care strategies and social support specifically targeting older gay men (Nokes, Chew, & Altman, 2003). Although these telephone-based groups have been discontinued due to funding cuts, SAGE-NY continues to offer in-person support groups on a weekly basis for their older clients with HIV/AIDS.

Although health care providers may often look to formal networks for assistance with chronic diseases such as HIV, it is also important to consider the adequacy of the informal support system for older adults living with HIV/AIDS. Health care providers working with older adults with HIV/AIDS should pay particular attention to social networks, the quality and quantity of those networks, and carefully determine the strengths and deficits of those support systems.

SYSTEMS OF CARE

Emlet and Poindexter (2004) recently suggested that systems of care, influenced by public policy, have historically centered on particular needs or populations. Such foci have tended to separate issues that may be connected, such as aging and HIV disease. Although pieces of legislation may need to be viewed separately (by necessity), it is imperative that attention is directed to how care and services at the local level can be improved through coordination and collaboration. For example, older adults living with HIV disease could obtain assistance from case management services through multiple mechanisms.

There are at least five sectors that could provide services to older adults; however, these appear to operate independently. They do not typically communicate or attempt to coordinate services, and thus cannot see the whole picture (Topolski, Gotham, Klinkenberg, O'Neill, & Brooks, 2002). The burden of integration of services then falls on the midlife and older person living with HIV/AIDS. These five sectors are: (a) AIDS Service Organizations; (b) Health/Medical sector; (c) Behavioral Health Treatment Sector; (d) Public Health Sector; and (e) Aging Services Sector.

AIDS Service Organizations

In the early 1980s, gay men, responding to a severe lack of services for their friends and colleagues dying from AIDS, created a system of social service agencies devoted to the needs of persons with AIDS. This network has evolved over the 20 years plus of the epidemic to address broader populations of persons with HIV/AIDS and provide comprehensive services uniquely tailored to the needs of their target population. Until recently, AIDS service organizations have not responded to the needs of midlife and older persons with HIV/AIDS perhaps because of ageist bias or because of the perception that older persons should have made plans to care for themselves. Advocacy groups like the New York Association on HIV over 50, Inc. (Nokes, 2004) and the National Association on HIV over 50, Inc. (Linsk, Fowler, & Klein, 2003) emerged to meet this unique need, but they have been severely underfunded.

The Ryan White Comprehensive AIDS Resources Emergency [CARE] Act (PL101-381) of 1990 was the first federal service delivery mechanism to aid persons with HIV. The CARE Act addresses the unmet health needs of persons living with HIV disease by funding primary health care and social support services. Services for persons of all ages living with HIV may be provided through numerous mechanisms, including public health and social services, university medical centers and clinics, and AIDS Service Organizations (ASOs). ASOs are community-based agencies that developed to ensure the delivery of health-related and social services to HIV-affected individuals and families (Burrage & Porche, 2003). ASOs and other providers of services may not specifically target midlife and older adults through the Ryan White CARE Act; however, CARE Act programs can easily be used to serve older persons with HIV, as well as offer support to older persons who are taking care of HIV-infected adult or child family members. An example of Title I of the Ryan White CARE Act is the provision of emergency assistance to Eligible Metropolitan Areas (EMAs) that are most severely affected by the HIV/AIDS epidemic. Title II provides grants to all 50 states, the District of Columbia and U.S. territories. Unlike Title I, grants may include non-profit as well as public entities. Through both titles, individuals with HIV disease may receive a variety of services, including ambulatory and home-based health care, early intervention services including HIV testing and counseling, and a wide variety of supportive social services. An important component of the Ryan White CARE Act is the AIDS Drug Assistance Program (ADAP). ADAP provides medications for the treatment of HIV disease (U.S. Health Resources and Services Administration [USDHHS, HRSA], 2002).

The graying of the HIV epidemic is reflected in services provided through the Ryan White CARE Act. According to a recently released study, 29% of the people served through Title I and 26% of the people served through Title II were aged 45 or older in 2000, compared to 20% in 1998 (HRSA, 2002–2003). Although few AIDS services throughout the country have developed special programs for older adults, some data suggest that older adults may choose to receive assistance through ASOs rather than through other mechanisms. Emlet (2004) surveyed 44 older adults living with HIV/AIDS ranging in age from 50 to 72 years. These individuals were aware of significantly more services provided through the HIV network as compared to the aging network and used significantly more services from the same system of care.

Most American government funding is categorical in nature and programs emerge based not only on need but also on availability of funding to support the program. Although the number of persons diagnosed with AIDS after 50 years of age has been steady at 11% since the beginning of the epidemic, the midlife and older age group, unlike younger age groups such as the unborn or adolescents, has not been identified as a developmental category with special needs. The other four sectors identified previously (Health/Medical, Behavioral Health Treatment, Public Health, and Aging) also look to the AIDS Service Organizations to advocate for the needs of populations living with HIV/AIDS. These organizations have a long history of activism and are respected for their skill in communicating about the needs of persons with HIV/AIDS. The silence of the AIDS community unfortunately lends false credibility to claims that midlife and older persons do not have special needs that should be addressed in either prevention or treatment programs.

Health/Medical Sector

The health/medical sector is fraught with many barriers. Inadequate insurance or a total lack of health insurance is a major reason why persons with many symptoms fear learning their HIV diagnosis. Although Medicaid is the major insurer for most people with HIV/AIDS, qualifying for this federal/state government benefit often requires proving limited financial resources. Assuming that the person has health insurance, many health care providers specialize in either HIV/AIDS or geriatrics, and the aging person might be receiving primary health care from two providers in different settings. As mentioned in chapter 9, persons aged 50 and older, compared to younger people with HIV/AIDS have more comorbidities, such as liver disease, diabetes, and cardiovascular problems. As one ages, there is an increase in the number of age-associated medical illnesses, the number of medications taken, and the risk for poorer outcomes to medical conditions (Valcour & Sacktor, 2002).

Older adults who have been diagnosed with HIV/AIDS may also benefit from services developed through the Medicaid home and community-based waiver program. The Omnibus Reconciliation Act of 1981 added section 1915 (c) to the Social Security Act which authorized the waiver of certain Medicaid limitations to allow states to cover home- and community-based services to individuals as an alternative to institutional care (U. S. General Accounting Office, 2003). The same Act was amended in 1985 to allow the creation of waiver program specific to persons living with AIDS (Buchanan & Chakravorty, 1997). These home- and community-based waiver programs provide a wide range of services to targeted subgroups of individuals. Focusing originally on frail older adults and those with developmental disabilities, the targeted populations have been expanded to include individuals with AIDS, working age individuals with physical disabilities, and children with a variety of conditions. Waiver programs are developed on a state-by-state basis and may provide nonmedical services such as case management, homemaker services, personal care services and adult day-care as well as medical care such as nursing services in the home (Miller, Ramsland, & Harrington, 1999). An older adult with HIV could, depending on age, disability status, and diagnosis, be eligible for services through a variety of waiver program categories. Waiver programs may target frail elderly specifically, combine frail older adults with disabled adults over 18 years of age, as well as specifically targeting those disabled from AIDS.

Behavioral Health Treatment Sector

The older person with an addiction history will probably also interface with the Behavioral Health Treatment Sector. Within the United States, rates of HIV infection tend to be highest in economically disadvantaged high-crime areas where illicit drug use and sex work are common sources of income. Many low-income older adults live in publicly subsidized housing in poor urban neighborhoods where rates of HIV infection are high, thus increasing the odds of exposure to the virus when practicing unsafe sex or sharing unclean needles (Levy, Ory, & Crystal, 2003). Using the HIV Cost and Services Utilization Survey (HCSUS) data from 1996 through 1998, Crystal et al. (2003) found that more than half of the older injection-drug users were Black (56%), reported the least emotional support of any subgroup, were significantly lower than those of their younger counterparts (by more than 10 points on the scale from 0–100) on physical functioning scores, and scored the worst of all subgroups on role functioning, with less than half of the optimal score. Because of their illegal drug use, many older persons with HIV/AIDS also report a history of incarceration and need to interface on a regular basis with the criminal justice system. Short stays in prison resulting from parole violation interrupts medication treatment plans and promotes viral resistance, because most clients will not be able to access their medications while in detention. There is little coordination between the criminal justice system and any other sector interfacing with older persons with HIV/AIDS. Older persons with HIV/AIDS may not feel physically able to keep the many appointments required by their parole officer, methadone program, and health care provider.

Public Health Sector

The public health sector has largely ignored midlife and older adults in their prevention messages. This invisibility has prompted some older people to perceive that AIDS is not their issue. The Centers for Disease Control and Prevention (Daniels et al., 2004) reported that rates of new HIV diagnosis among older adults declined or were stable and lower than the rates for younger adults, and concluded that increases in the rates of HIV diagnoses were not likely to be the cause of the increase in the proportion of AIDS diagnoses for persons aged 45 and older, but rather the graying of persons infected at an earlier age. As mentioned earlier, the CDC report used HIV infection rate data from states reporting HIV infection prior to 1994. In contrast, as of June 1, 2000, New York State began to require reporting new diagnoses of HIV (not AIDS). Using New York City data for 2002, 11.9% of the new HIV cases were in persons aged 50–59 and 4.3% of the new HIV cases were reported in persons aged 60 and older (New York City, 2004). Because New York City supplies surveillance data to the Centers for Disease Control and Prevention, it is not clear why the CDC concluded that an AIDS diagnosis in the over-50 age group were not new HIV infections but rather infections from an earlier age. This confusing message reinforces the public's perception that midlife and older persons, irrespective of their sexual and drug use behaviors, are somehow "immune" from HIV infection.

AGING SERVICES SECTOR

Another viable system of support for older adults infected with or affected by HIV disease is commonly known as the "aging network." These are programs funded through the Older Americans Act of 1965 as amended. The Older Americans' Act (OAA) of 1965 was one of several major federal initiatives of President Lyndon B. Johnson's Great Society programs designed to benefit older persons (Estes, 1979). The Act created the Administration on Aging and authorized grants to States for community planning and services programs, as well as for research, demonstration, and training projects in the field of aging. The OAA calls for specific attention to those elders who are in the greatest social and economic need; anyone who is aged 60 older, or the legal spouse of someone over 60 years can access OAA services. Today the OAA has firmly established the aging network, which includes 57 state units on aging, approximately 650 Area Agencies on Aging and 220 tribal organizations representing 300 native tribes (Takamura, 2001).

Titles III, V, VI, and VII provide a wide array of services that may be relevant to older adults who are living with HIV disease, as well as to HIV-affected caregivers. Title III authorizes funds to states and Area Agencies on Aging for a variety of in-home and supportive services (AoA, 2001). Part C focuses on the provision of nutrition services, nutrition education and counseling, whereas Part D provides disease prevention and health promotion services to older adults (AoA, n.d.). The Administration on Aging provides a listing of each State Unit on Aging and Area Agency on Aging through their Web site at: http://www.aoa.gov/eldfam/How_To_Find/Agencies/Agencies.asp

It is difficult to think of the elderly as persons over the age of 50 years, and aging services are more familiar with the issues of persons aged 60 or 65 and older. The American population continues to age, and many more persons reach the age of 100 years. As one ages, the number of chronic illnesses increase along with the need for assistive services. Although the aging sector would not deny services to a 62-year-old person with HIV/AIDS, their target population is all older people in general. Funding for aging programs such as Meals on Wheels has been decreasing since the 1970s, and the aging network finds itself torn by conflicting priorities and great need.

Although an older adult with HIV/AIDS could receive services from one or more of these service delivery systems, there is an overall lack of cross-system knowledge among health professionals and poor communication between systems. Joslin and Nazon (1996) suggest that older HIV-positive persons often present themselves to service providers with needs that can only be partially met within one service system. It is incumbent upon health care providers to develop an understanding across systems of care if the needs of this emerging vulnerable population are to be met. Not-for-profit organizations serving midlife and older persons, such as the AARP (AARP, 2004), have not adequately addressed HIV/AIDS, although they do provide information on other chronic illnesses such as diabetes and heart disease.

Components of an Integrated System of Care

Topolski et al. (2002) identified the components of an integrated system as: communication, cross-training, cross-disciplinary consultation, co-ordinated treatment planning, colocation of services, integrated service teams, and integrated funding sources. Achievement of these components will require a major paradigm shift in programs funded to serve persons with HIV/AIDS. To start, each program should poll their midlife and older clients and ask three questions: (a) are the services meeting your unique needs; (b) what unique services do you, as a person of 50+ believe should be offered by the agency; and (c) have you experienced age discrimination while receiving services from this agency (Nokes, 2001).

SUMMARY

In summary, health and social service providers must act as advocates and expert clinicians to assist midlife and older persons with HIV/AIDS to successfully age. Through skilled and caring interventions, depression can be decreased, morale improved, meaning found in a life often marginalized and stigmatized but nonetheless of value, and social supports maintained and strengthened. As with many vulnerable populations, system fragmentation exists and methods to improve coordination will need to occur. In May of 2005, the Senate Select Committee on Aging convened an historical hearing on this topic entitled "HIV Over Fifty: Exploring The New Threat." As our elected officials begin to recognize the unique needs and circumstances of this emerging vulnerable population, we can look toward increased visibility, recognition, and perhaps even funding to meet the need of a population that will continue to grow in the coming years.

REFERENCES

Administration on Aging [AOA]. (2001). *Selected highlights: Side by side comparison of OAA as amended in 1992 with OAA as amended in 2000.* Retrieved May 24, 2004 from the World Wide Web: http://www.aoa.gov/Oaa/2000/side-by-side-fin.html

Administration on Aging. (n.d.). *A layman's guide to the Older Americans Act.* Retrieved May 24, 2004: http://www.aoa.gov/about/legbudg/oaa/laymans_guide/laymans_guide.asp#TitleIII

Agate, L., Mullins, J., Prudent, E., & Liberti, T. (2003). Strategies for reaching retirement communities and aging social networks: HIV/AIDS prevention activities among seniors in South Florida. *Journal of Acquired Immune Deficiency Syndromes, 33*(Suppl. 2) S238–S242.

American Association of Retired Persons (AARP) (1997). *It Can Happen to Me* video kit. Washington, DC: Author.

American Association of Retired Persons (AARP) (2004). *AARP: Making the most of life after 50.* Retrieved September 28, 2004 from http://www.aarp.org/ leadership/Articles/a2003-01-12-aarphistory.html

Anderson, G. (1998). Providing services to elderly people with HIV. In D. M. Aronstein & B. J. Thompson (Eds.), *HIV and social work: A practitioner's guide* (pp. 443–450). New York: Harrington Park Press.

Baldwin, P. (2005). *Disease and democracy: The industrialized world faces AIDS.* Berkeley, CA: University of California Press.

Bay, E. (2004, July). *Teaching old dogs new tricks: HIV prevention for senior citizens.* Abstract #D12930. 15th International Conference on AIDS. Burrage, J., & Porche, D. (2003). AIDS service organization partnerships: A method to assess outcomes of community service organizations for vulnerable populations. *Journal of Multicultural Nursing and Health, 9*(1), 7–12.

Buchanan, R. J., & Chakravorty, B. J. (1997). Medicaid home and community-based waiver programs: Providing services to people with AIDS. *Health Care Financing Review, 18*(4), 83–103.

Centers for Disease Control and Prevention. (200x). Table 21. *Number of adolescents and adults living with AIDS, by age as of December 31, 2002, sex, and exposure category – United States, 2000 .* Accessed August 26, 2004. http://www.cdc.gov/hiv/stats/hasrsupp91/table21.htm

Crystal, S., Akincigil, A., Sambamoorthi, U., Wenger, N., Fleishman, J., Zingmond, D., et al. (2003). The diverse older HIV-positive population: A national profile of economic circumstances, social support, and quality of life. *Journal of Acquired Immune Deficiency Syndromes, 33*(Suppl. 2), S76–S83.

Daniels, D., Curtis, A., Klevens, R., & Lee, L. (2004, July). *Status report on HIV diagnosis rates in older adults in the United States Rates decline or remain stable.* Abstract #D6513. 15th International Conference on AIDS.

Emlet, C. A. (2004). Knowledge and use of AIDS and aging services by older, HIV infected adults. *Journal of HIV/AIDS and Social Services, 3*(1), 9–24.

Emlet, C. A., & Poindexter, C. C. (2004). The unserved, unseen and unheard: Integrating program for HIV-infected and affected elders. *Health and Social Work, 29*(2), 86–96.

Engle, L. (2001). HIV and older adults: A novela approach. *Body Positive, 14*(9). http://www.thebody.com/bp/sept01/older.html

Estes, C. L. (1979). *The aging enterprise.* San Francisco: Jossey-Bass.

Janssen, R. (2004). *HIV/AIDS surveillance report 2002: 14.* Also available at http://www.cdc.gov/hiv/stats/hasrlink.htm

Joslin, D., & Nazon, M. C. (1996), HIV/AIDS and aging networks. In K. Nokes (Ed.), *HIV/AIDS and the older adult* (pp. 129–141) Bristol, PA: Taylor & Francis,

Levy, J., Ory, M., & Crystal, S. (2003). HIV/AIDS interventions for midlife and older adults: Current status and challenges. *Journal of Acquired Immune Deficiency Syndromes, 33*(Suppl. 2), S59–S67.

Linsk, N., Fowler, J., & Klein, S. (2003). HIV/AIDS prevention and care services and services for the aging: Bridging the gap between service systems to assist older people. *Journal of Acquired Immune Deficiency Syndromes, 33*(Suppl. 2), S243–S250.

Miller, N. A., Ramsland, S., & Harrington, C. (1999). Trends and issues in the Medicaid 1915 (c) waiver. *Health Care Financing Review, 20*, 139–160.

Montoya, I. D., & Whitsett, D. D. (2003). New frontiers and challenges in HIV research among older minority populations. *Journal of Acquired Immune Deficiency Syndromes, 33*(Suppl. 2), S218–S221.

National Association of HIV Over Fifty. Educational Tips Sheet: Necessary actions. Retrieved May 10, 2005 at http://www.hivoverfifty.org

National Minority AIDS Council (Producer). (2001). *HIV/AIDS and older Americans* [Video recording]. Available from the National Minority AIDS Council, 1931 13th Street, N.W. Washington, DC 20009).

New York City. (2004). HIV/AIDS surveillance statistics 2002. New York: New York City Department of Health and Mental Hygiene. 2004. Posted August 25, 2004. Retrieved August 30, 2004 from http://www.nyc.gov.html/doh/html/ah/hivtables2002.html

Nokes, K. (2001). *Needs assessment: Primary/secondary prevention targeting HIV infected persons 50+.* Unpublished report. Available from The Prevention Planning Unit, 225 Broadway, 23rd floor, Box A-2, New York, New York.

Nokes, K. (2004). Sustaining a coalition: A case study of the New York Association on HIV over Fifty. 181–190. In C. Emlet (Ed), *HIV/AIDS and older adults: Challenges for individuals, families and communities.* New York: Springer Publishing.

Nokes, K., Chew, L., & Altman, C. (2003). Using a telephone support group for HIV-positive persons aged 50+ to increase social support and health-related knowledge. *AIDS Patient Care and STDs, 17*, 345–351.

Outword–Online (2005). *PBS news magazine looks at aging with AIDS.* Retrieved April 15, 2005 from www.asaging/networks/LGAIN/outword_online/2005/mar.cfm.

Stall R., & Catania, J. (1994). AIDS risk behaviors among late middle-aged and elderly Americans. The National AIDS Behavioral Surveys. *Archives of Internal Medicine, 154*(1), 57–63.

Takamura, J. C. (2001). Older Americans Act. In M. D. Mezey (Ed.). *The encyclopedia of elder care: The comprehensive resource on geriatric and social care* (pp. 468–471). New York: Springer Publishing.

Topolski, J., Gotham, H., Klinkenberg, W. D., O'Neill, D., & Brooks, A. (2002). Older adults, substance use, and HIV/AIDS: Preparing for a future crisis. *Journal of Mental Health and Aging, 8*, 349–363.

University of South Florida. (n.d.). *Department of Aging and Mental Health, SHAPE project* Update. Retrieved April 17, 2003 from the world wide Web: http://amhserver.fmhi.usf.edu/shape/index.html

U. S. General Accounting Office. (2003). *Federal oversight of growing Medicaid home and community-based waivers should be strengthened.* Publication No. GAO-03-576. Washington, DC: Author.

U.S. Department of Health and Human Services, Health Resources and Services Administration, HIV/AIDS Bureau. (2002). *Ryan White CARE Act Programs*: Available at: http://hab.hrsa.gov/programs.htm

U. S. Health Resources and Services Administration. (2002–2003). *The AIDS epidemic and the Ryan White CARE Act: Past progress and future challenges 2002–2003* . Available at: http://hab.hrsa.gov/tools/progressreport/

Valcour, V., & Sacktor, N. (2002). HIV-associated dementia and aging. *Journal of Mental Health and Aging, 8*, 295–306.

Wooten-Bielski, K. (1999). HIV & AIDS in older adults. *Geriatric Nursing, 20*, 268–272.

Epilogue

Having reviewed the issues, needs, and strategies for frail older adults; older prisoners; older homeless people; older people who are lesbian, gay, bisexual, and transgender; and those with HIV/AIDS; this is a call to action. McKinlay (1979), in his classic article on the frustrations of medical practice, uses Zola's story of standing by a swiftly flowing river and hearing the cries of a drowning man. He quickly pulls him out of the river, applies artificial respiration, and just as he begins to breathe, he hears the cry of another person. He pulls this person out of the river, resuscitates him, and then hears another cry. And so it goes, on and on—jumping into the river, pulling people out, resuscitating, breathing, followed by another cry for help. The sequence continues without end. He is so busy rescuing them that he has no time to go upstream to see who the hell is pushing them in.

Health providers often focus downstream on the rescue efforts. Health education and prevention efforts occur more at midstream, but still at the individual level. McKinlay (1979) argues that health providers must move toward broader upstream strategies aimed at the political and economic forces pushing the people in the river. He makes a case for going upstream to search for the "manufacturers of illness" and intervening at the sociopolitical level. Manufacturers of illness are those organizations and groups who benefit from and have a stake in the continuance of the illness or condition; for example, the tobacco industry as a manufacturer of illnesses associated with smoking. Using a critical perspective, one can gain insight into the manufacturers of illness by asking "Who benefits?" from the marginalization of the vulnerable populations described in this book.

"Upstream thinking" requires us to look at the larger system causes or the manufacturers of illness for each of the populations discussed in this book. For frail older adults, consider the change in American culture following World War II emphasizing the development products and technology for entertainment and to make life easier, thus systematically reducing the amount of physical activity in daily life. The cultural effects of a sedentary lifestyle, along with societal expectation that the condition of frailty, accompanies old age contribute to the incidence of frailty among our elders.

The United States incarcerates more people than any other industrialized country, with the privatized prison industrial complex reaping increased profits as the number of prisoners grows. The homeless population, including homeless older adults, in the United States is growing as the lack of affordable housing increases. A societal bias against LGBT people and people with HIV/AIDS is evident in many areas, including health care. By asking the question "who benefits?" we can gain insight into these difficult problems.

To improve the quality of life and health for these five vulnerable populations of older adults, downstream, midstream, and upstream interventions are needed. Downstream, quality care at the individual level based on knowledge of the client's unique needs is necessary. This type of care is described in each of the strategy chapters in this book. A midstream approach focuses on interventions aimed at prevention such as efforts to increase exercise to forestall frailty.

There is a paucity of research on each of the vulnerable groups of elders described here, a reflection of the interest of researchers and funding resources. Recent attention on research aimed at discovering the causes of frailty and interventions to reduce frailty show promise. *Healthy People 2010* (U.S. Department of Health and Human Services, 2000), by making eliminating health disparities one of their two major goals, has set the stage for more research with incarcerated older adults, older homeless people, LGBT elders, and older people with HIV/AIDS. It is our hope that funding resources will follow.

Educational efforts must include both continuing education with practicing health professionals and curricular change in schools for students in the health professions. In addition to improving knowledge about the population at risk, education should include an examination of attitudes toward the population group. Few health professionals are attracted to caring for these groups of elders. Few new graduates of professional programs express their delight in starting a new job in a nursing home caring for frail elders, or excitement at caring for homeless older adults in the emergency rooms. In addition to bias against these populations, the complexity of their needs makes delivery of care to them at the individual level extremely challenging and often frustrating. Just as with care of older adults in general, it requires a change in focus from a curative model of care to a caring model. Health care providers must be taught to assess the strengths of individual clients, to set small goals with clients and measure progress in small steps, and to be detectives in seeking the multiple factors underlying the constellation of problems, both in the individual and in society. Once a shift in perspective from curative to caring has taken place, the rewards are great; as seemingly small interventions may have great effects, and there is much potential for improving the quality of life of elders.

A caring model requires advocacy and empowerment for vulnerable older adults. Because all of these groups of vulnerable older adults lack social power and are at risk for discrimination and bias, advocates are often necessary for them in the health care system and beyond. Caution must be taken, however, to join empowerment with advocacy in such a way as to avoid being patronizing or promoting dependence on the advocate. A collaborative partnership between the advocate and the individual or group being advocated for may be the most effective way to move toward equal access to equal resources.

Lastly, truly upstream-interventions include political action aimed at the manufacturers of illness. To do this effectively, a consideration of the sociopolitical and economic advantages is inherent in maintaining the vulnerability of these population groups. Actions here include legislative interventions, lobbying, and public education to raise awareness of issues. Many health professionals are not taught to think in economic terms. This is a disservice to our students as improvements in health care must be cost effective. Without at least a general understanding of economic principles and how they work within systems, health professionals are at a disadvantage in working upstream. Regardless of our moral responsibility to provide quality health care, changes will not be made without financial resources to do so. Political action must be based on a sound knowledge base about the issues and go further than protesting inequalities and calls for change. Effective political action offers practical strategies for change based on knowledge of the issues, of the resources available, and of the agendas of people in power. Potentially successful strategies minimize the barriers, examine attitudes, avoid blaming the victim, analyze the economic and political factors, and maximize the benefits of change for as many groups of those involved as possible.

Years ago I taught an undergraduate clinical group in community health nursing. One of my experiences was particularly distressing and I found myself, the next day, in tears getting onto the elevator in our College of Nursing building. A colleague saw me and asked what had happened. I related the story of one of my student's clients who was a young mother with a beautiful new baby. The night before our visit, the mother's boyfriend had shaken the baby and killed her. I was at a loss as to what to do, feeling a responsibility not only to my student and the young mother, but also to address the larger issue of child abuse. There are so many injustices and issues in the world that are in desperate need of attention. My colleague wisely told me that we are each only one person and have our own areas of expertise and interest. Mine was with older adults. Although that advice was not meant to discourage me from working in the area of child abuse, it did help me realize that one person cannot intervene on all fronts. We need to choose our areas of activism and our battles based on our expertise and what is in our hearts. As health professionals, we have a great deal of credibility and power and are in excellent positions to be change agents. The situation is not hopeless. We need to discover the possibilities for change and to take action. These groups of vulnerable older adults deserve to have improved health and quality health care.

P. Burbank

REFERENCES

McKinlay, J. B. (1979). A case for refocusing upstream: The political economy of illness. In E. G. Jaco (Ed.), *Patients, physicians, and illness* (3rd. ed.). New York: Free Press.

U.S. Department of Health and Human Services (2000). Healthy people 2010: Understanding and improving health (2nd ed.). Washington, DC: U.S. Government Printing Office.

Index

Page numbers followed by f or t indicate figures and tables, respectively.

Food pantries. *See* Food service
   programs
Food service programs
   for homeless, 102, 112, 115,
     124, 125, 126, 131, 137
   Meals on Wheels as, 36, 43, 246
   nutrition in, 126
   for women, 126
Foucault, M., 141
Fowler, J.P., 225
Frailty
   abuse/neglect due to, 19, 20
   acceptance of, xv–xvi
   acute care for, 8
   adaptation for, 5, 6
   ADLs/IDLs and, 17, 18, 25
   aging and, 5
   alcohol use and, 8
   Alzheimer's and, 14
   attributes of, 6–7
   biology of, 6
   care systems for, 42
   caregivers for, 9
   CGA for, 26–27
   chronic conditions for, xiv, 6, 7,
     8f, 11, 18, 19
   comorbid diseases and, 25
   cognitive ability and, 14
   confusion and, 9
   cycle of, 6–7, 8, 20
   definition of, 3, 4–6
   delirium and, 8, 15, 16–17, 20
   dementia and, 8, 20
   depression and, 20
   disability and, 8
   disease and, 5, 14, 113
   empowerment from, 253
   exercise regiment for, xv–xvi,
     26, 39–40, 41t, 46
   falls and, 3, 10–11, 20, 33
   free radicals and, 6
   functional impairment and, 8
   health care and, 3
   homeostasis and, 5
   hormones and, 6, 42
   hydration for, 40
   immobility and, 9
   immunity and, 6
   immunizations for, 32
   incontinence and, 8, 9
   long-term care for, 8, 18, 25
   malnutrition and, 9, 40
   marginalization and, xiv
   morbidity for, 8, 20
   mortality for, 3, 8
   pharmacotherapy effects for, 12
   polypharmacy and, 8–9, 11, 20
   predictors of, 7–8
   prevention of, 4, 25
   public policy on, 251–52
   reduction of, 4
   research into, xv–xvi,
     xvi–xvii, 252
   reversal of, 19, 25
   risk factors for, 6, 46
   sarcopenia for, 7, 40, 42
   in senior population, 3
   social isolation and, 8
   support services for, 8, 10
   syndrome of, 4–5, 6, 32
   tobacco use and, 8
   treatment plan for, 27, 39
   trigger events for, 7–8, 11
   vulnerability of, 3
Frailty and Injuries: Cooperative
    Study of Intervention
    Techniques (FICSIT), 34
Frailty Index (FI), 33
Free radicals, 6
Freely, M., 61
Fried, L.P., 5, 6, 7f, 8f, 25
Friend, R.A., 154
Functional decline, 9, 43

Gagnon, J.H., 151
Gay and Lesbian Medical Association
   (GLMA), 181, 181t, 200
*Gay and Lesbian Mental
   Health: A Sourcebook for
   Practitioners* (Alexander), 190

University of Texas Medical
  Branch at Galveston, 91–92
Urinary incontinence. *See*
  Incontinence, urinary
U.S. correctional system. *See also*
  Health care, prison
  administrative subculture in,
    63, 78t
  advance directives for, 88
  aging offender in, 57, 65–66, 85
  batch living in, 62
  compassionate release from,
    90, 94
  correctional officer in, 63
  counseling within, 81
  criminal risk factors and, 61
  demographics of, 58–60, 70
  early release from, 89–90, 94
  environment of, 58
  formal policy v. con code, 62
  HIV/AIDS in, 67, 67t, 68, 80,
    82, 91, 92, 245
  hospice in, 87–89
  infectious diseases within,
    81–82
  inmate delirium in, 81
  inmate dementia in, 70, 81, 87
  inmate depression within, 69,
    81, 85
  inmate subculture in, 62–63
  lawsuits in, 64
  long-term care within, 86–87
  medical cost containment in, 77,
    85, 91
  Medical Parole Law for, 90
  nutrition within, 88
  older adults in, xiv, xvi
  organization of, 63
  parole from, 90
  predation in, 63, 65
  preventive health care in, 83–84
  release from, 65, 76, 84
  specialty units within, 84–86, 94
  stress within, 57, 69, 85
  substance abuse in, 68
  substance abuse treatment
    in, 81
  systems of, 58
  telemedicine within, 91
  transinstitutionalization to, 68
  vocational training in, 84
U.S. Department of Health and
  Human Services (USDHHS),
  128, 188
U.S. Department of Justice, 85
U.S. Housing and Urban
  Development (HUD), 136
USDHHS. *See* U.S. Department of
  Health and Human Services

Valcour, V., 223
Valee, C.M., 212
Validation therapy, 38
Vergon, T.L., 212
Veterans Administration, 222
Veterans Affairs Medical
  Center, 91
Viagra, 220
Victimization. *See also* Violence
  in health care system, 162
  of homeless, 108, 110, 112,
    114, 125, 140
  of transgender, 162
Villareal, D.T., 41t
Violence
  homeless as victims of, 108,
    110, 112, 114, 125, 140
  by prisoners, 63, 69
  towards LGBT, 158–59, 188
  towards transgender, 158–59
*Violence in Gay & Lesbian
  Domestic Partnerships*
  (Renzetti & Miley), 188
Volunteers of America. *See*
  GRACE project
Vulnerability
  cognitive impairment for, 13–15
  definition of, xiii–xiv